Handbook for Public Health
Social Work

Robert H. Keefe, PhD, ACSW, is an associate professor of social work at the University at Buffalo, State University of New York, where he teaches courses in social work practice and human behavior and conducts research on macro-level factors that lead to negative health outcomes. Dr. Keefe's research has been funded by the National Institutes of Health, the Metanexus Institute, the Health Resources and Services Administration, the Centers for Disease Control and Prevention, and the Administrations on Aging and Developmental Disabilities. His published research articles have focused on the topics of health disparities in birth outcomes, HIV/AIDS, childhood lead poisoning, teen pregnancy, and managed care. He has held elected offices in the American Public Health Association, and his awards and honors include being awarded the Insley/Evans Public Health Social Worker of the Year by the American Public Health Association and being named to Who's Who in Medicine and Healthcare and Who's Who Among Executives and Professionals in Healthcare. He has also received teaching awards at both the University at Buffalo and Syracuse University. Among his other scholarly activities he is a member of the editorial board of several journals including the *Journal of Adolescent Health, Journal of Healthcare for the Poor and Underserved, American Journal of Managed Care,* and *Medical Science Monitor.* Dr. Keefe's community service includes serving as a member of the board of directors for various not-for-profit health care agencies.

Elaine T. Jurkowski, PhD, MSW, is a professor and graduate program director at Southern Illinois University at Carbondale's School of Social Work, where she teaches courses in health and aging policy, research, and program evaluation; she also holds a joint appointment with the Department of Health Education. Dr. Jurkowski's early career experience working as a social worker in a community public health interdisciplinary setting in Manitoba, Canada, exposed her to mental health, disability, vocational rehabilitation, and aging programs. These early experiences, coupled with her training in community health sciences and epidemiology, have shaped Dr. Jurkowski's research and practice interests. Dr. Jurkowski conducts research on factors that influence access to care in rural communities, and intervention strategies that lead to positive health and public health outcomes. She has also served as a Great Cities Research Scholar through the University of Illinois at Chicago and as a Social Work Leadership Fellow for the New York Academy of Medicine. Dr. Jurkowski's research has been funded by the National Institutes of Health, The Hartford Foundation, the U.S. Department of Health and Human Services, the Administration on Aging, and the Illinois Department on Aging. Her published research articles have focused on the topics of health disparities, access to mental health and health care services, aging, and disability issues. She has held elected offices in the American Public Health Association, National Association of Social Workers, the Gerontological Society of America, and the Illinois Rural Health Association. Her public health social work experiences have included consultation within public health settings in Niger, Hong Kong, India, China, Russia, and Egypt, and employment as a public health social worker in Canada. Dr. Jurkowski's community service includes serving as a member of the board of directors for various not-for-profit health care agencies within the southern Illinois area.

Handbook for Public Health Social Work

Edited by
Public Health Social Work Section of the
American Public Health Association

Robert H. Keefe, PhD, ACSW
Elaine T. Jurkowski, PhD, MSW
Managing Editors

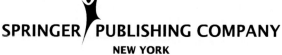

SPRINGER PUBLISHING COMPANY
NEW YORK

Springer Publishing Company, LLC
11 West 42nd Street
New York, NY 10036
www.springerpub.com

Acquisitions Editor: Allan Graubard
Composition: Techset

ISBN: 978-0-8261-0742-8
E-book ISBN: 978-0-8261-0743-5

12 13 14 15/ 5 4 3 2 1

The author and the publisher of this Work have made every effort to use sources believed to be reliable to provide information that is accurate and compatible with the standards generally accepted at the time of publication. The author and publisher shall not be liable for any special, consequential, or exemplary damages resulting, in whole or in part, from the readers' use of, or reliance on, the information contained in this book. The publisher has no responsibility for the persistence or accuracy of URLs for external or third-party Internet websites referred to in this publication and does not guarantee that any content on such websites is, or will remain, accurate or appropriate.

Library of Congress Cataloging-in-Publication Data

CIP data is available at the Library of Congress.

Special discounts on bulk quantities of our books are available to corporations, professional associations, pharmaceutical companies, health care organizations, and other qualifying groups.

If you are interested in a custom book, including chapters from more than one of our titles, we can provide that service as well.

For details, please contact:
Special Sales Department, Springer Publishing Company, LLC
11 West 42nd Street, 15th Floor, New York, NY 10036-8002
Phone: 877-687-7476 or 212-431-4370; Fax: 212-941-7842
Email: sales@springerpub.com

Printed in the United States of America by Gasch Printing.

7609553

This book is dedicated to public health social work practitioners and students who continue to effect change and improve the lives of individuals, families, groups, and communities throughout the world.

Contents

Contributors

Chris Anne Rodgers Arthur, Ph, MPH, MCHES   Associate Professor, Director of Faculty Development and Medical Education, Department of Family Medicine, The University of Mississippi Medical Center, Jackson, Mississippi

Julie Cederbaum, PhD, MSW, MPH   Assistant Professor, School of Social Work, University of Southern California, Los Angeles, California

Elaine Congress, DSW, LCSW   Professor and Associate Dean, Fordham University Graduate School of Social Service, New York, New York

Bari Cornet, MSW, MPH,   Field Consultant and Lecturer Emeritus, School of Social Welfare, University of California at Berkeley, Berkeley, California

Patricia A. Ely, MSW candidate   School of Social Work, Southern Illinois University at Carbondale, Carbondale, Illinois

Theora A. Evans, PhD, MPH, MSW   Past Chair, Social Work Section, Memphis, Tennessee

William J. Hall, MSW   Doctoral Student, School of Social Work, University of North Carolina at Chapel Hill, Chapel Hill, North Carolina

Julia F. Hastings, PhD, MSW   Assistant Professor, School of Public Health, School of Social Welfare, University at Albany, State University of New York, Albany, New York

Mary Helen Hogue, MSW, LCSW   Department of Health Education & Recreation, Southern Illinois University at Carbondale, Carbondale, Illinois

Elaine T. Jurkowski, PhD, MSW   Professor and Graduate Program Director, School of Social Work, Southern Illinois University at Carbondale, Carbondale, Illinois

Karun Karki, MSW, MA   Doctoral Student, Louisiana State University, Baton Rouge, Baton Rouge, Louisiana

Robert H. Keefe, PhD, ACSW   Associate Professor, School of Social Work, University at Buffalo, State University of New York, Buffalo, New York

Michele A. Kelley, ScD, MA, ACSW   Associate Professor, School of Public Health, Division of Community Health Sciences, University of Illinois at Chicago, Chicago Illinois

Gary Lounsberry, PhD, LCSW   Professor, Social and Behavioral Sciences, Alfred State College, State University of New York, Alfred, New York

Whitney E. Mendel, MSW   Doctoral Student, School of Social Work, University at Buffalo, State University of New York, Buffalo, New York

Mizanur Miah, PhD, MPH, MSW   Professor and Director, School of Social Work, Southern Illinois University at Carbondale, Carbondale, Illinois

Abigail M. Ross, MSW, MPH   Doctoral Student, Boston University School of Social Work, Boston, Massachusetts

Kathleen Rounds, PhD, MPH, MSW   Professor, School of Social Work, University of North Carolina at Chapel Hill, Chapel Hill, North Carolina

Betty J. Ruth, MSW, MPH   Clinical Associate Professor, Director, MSW/MPH Program, Boston University School of Social Work, Boston, Massachusetts

Patricia Welch Saleeby, PhD, MSW   Assistant Professor, School of Social Work, University of Missouri–St. Louis, St. Louis, Missouri

Edward Saunders, PhD, MSW, MPH   Associate Professor and Director, School of Social Work, The University of Iowa, Iowa City, Iowa

Jeanne Saunders, PhD, LISW   Associate Professor and MSW Program Director, School of Social Work, The University of Iowa, Iowa City, Iowa

Tammie L. Scamell, MSW, LMSW, CADC   Clinical Therapist, Bootheel Counseling Services, Sikeston, Missouri

Derek R. Smith, MSW, MPH   Program Director, Tobacco Prevention Program, San Mateo County Health System, San Mateo, California

Joseph Telfair, DrPH, MSW, MPH   Professor, Public Health Research and Practice, Director, UNCG Center for Social, Community, and Health Research and Evaluation, University of North Carolina at Greensboro, Greensboro, North Carolina

Foreword

SOCIAL WORK AND PUBLIC HEALTH: TWO SIDES OF THE SAME COIN

I am fortunate to have degrees in both social work and public health. As a result, I have always been comfortable with the overlap of paradigms, the transference of skill sets, the lack of clarity of definitions, and the transdisciplinary aspects of practice. I have never been concerned about role blurring but instead see the clear advantages of role blending.

I am a stronger advocate, a better rounded professional, and a more qualified health care practitioner because of my social work and public health linkage. Whether looking at the person-in-environment or the person-in-population; whether working in prevention or intervention; whether focusing on the micro, mezzo, or macro levels; whether using the methods of epidemiology or ecology, the combined knowledge and skills from public health and social work provide a unique framework and lens that are crucial to health care and social welfare today and in the future. In fact, public health social work will have a major role in the delivery of the health care of the future (Van Pelt, 2009).

Perhaps public health and social work can best be described as two sides of the same coin. Although there are certain differences—for example, more of an emphasis on prevention for public health and on intervention for social work—the connections far outweigh the divisions between the two disciplines. Both professions seek to promote individual and public health; both want to reduce social, psychological, and environmental risk factors; and both want to promote self-sufficiency and self-determination.

Linked Roots

The similarities between social work and public health are partially a result of linked historical roots beginning in the late 1800s and early 1900s, as social reformers worked to bring about positive social change. Many of the names of the historic activists found in the chronology of events of each profession are the same: Lillian Wald, Jane Addams, Jeanette Rankin, Julia Lathrop, Grace Abbott, Harry Hopkins, Frances Perkins, Ida Cannon, Virginia Insley, Elizabeth Watkins, and Ruth Knee (National Association of Social Workers Foundation, 2012; Stuart, 2008), to name just a few.

The original organizations and government programs that underpin both professions—including settlement houses, health clinics, social insurance, and maternal and child health programs—were essential to, and heralded by, pioneers of social work and public health.

The founding of the Children's Bureau in 1912, by Julia Lathrop, a social worker, is well known to most public health social workers (Sable, Schild, & Hipp, 2012). However, the efforts of social workers Frances Perkins and Harry Hopkins may be less well-known examples of the impact of social work on early public health efforts.

The Children's Bureau came into existence after a decade of advocacy and activism. It grew out of the settlement house movement and was assisted by the labor movement as well as by social work educators in schools of social work that were established at the end of the 19th century. The goal was to protect the well-being of children.

During its first 50 years, four of the five leaders (Julia Lathrop [1912–1921], Grace Abbott [1921-1934], Katherine Lenroot [1934-1952], and Katherine Oettinger [1957-1968]) were social workers. The main areas of focus in the early days included child labor, maternal and child health, and infant mortality, all of which are still clearly linked to public health (Copeland & Henry, 2008). During the Depression in the 1930s, the Children's Bureau also helped to frame the social welfare program, Aid to Families With Dependent Children (U.S. Department of Health, Education, and Welfare, 1962).

In a similar fashion, much of the social safety net we rely upon today, including Social Security, was fashioned by Perkins and Hopkins. Perkins was the first woman (and social worker) to be appointed to a presidential cabinet position. She served as Secretary of Labor from 1933 until 1945, throughout Franklin Delano Roosevelt's entire presidency. Perkins had worked with Jane Addams at Hull House before moving to New York City, where she became a crusader for improved factory safety—a serious public health issue of the time. Before accepting her cabinet position, Perkins had gotten Roosevelt to agree to support her major unemployment relief program and workers' rights protections, such as minimum wage, maximum hours of work, and ending child labor (Cohen, 2009). She also served as chairwoman of the President's Committee on Economic Security, which ultimately crafted the Social Security Act of 1935 (Downey, 2009).

Hopkins was from Iowa, and he moved to New York City after college where he, too, worked in a settlement house on New York's Lower East Side. Hopkins understood the linkage of environment and social issues to health and well-being. Roosevelt chose Hopkins to head the first state emergency relief agency in New York during the early days of the Depression. Hopkins persuaded Roosevelt to create a $500 million federal relief program, which he then administered (Cohen, 2009).

Regardless of historical figures or era of activism, or the social problems each profession has had to face, the focus of both public health and social work has been unwavering. The common goals—the elimination of health disparities and the promotion of social, economic, and environmental justice (Sable et al., 2012) remain firmly entrenched and continue to guide the practice and actions of both fields.

Public health has greatly affected Americans' health care. Public health's focus on fairness and common rights for all citizens is consistent with American values of equal rights for all. Despite the positive impact of public health, social and health disparities remain in all aspects of the U.S. health care service delivery system. *Health disparities*, defined as "persistent differences in health conditions and illness rates that cut across many illness categories and demographic groups" (Keefe, 2010, p. 238), have led to poor health outcomes, unequal access to care, and premature death for many population groups. Consequently, health disparities has been a hotly contested issue for many years and will continue to be one through the foreseeable future.

As early as 1959, René Dubos in his book, *The Mirage of Health*, noted:

> It is generally assumed that . . . the cause of all diseases can and will be found in due time—by bringing the big guns of science to bear on the problems. In reality, however, search for *the* cause may be a hopeless pursuit because most disease states are an indirect outcome of a constellation of circumstances rather than the direct result of single determinant factors. (pp. 86–87)

In 1988, Sloane, in a supplementary statement to an Institute of Medicine (1988) study, *The Future of Public Health*, noted, "There is overwhelming evidence from this report, and from a myriad of studies, that the financial problems confronting the poor must be solved before we can have a significant impact on the other health issues confronting the American people" (p. 160).

Smedley, Stith, and Nelson (2008) also emphasized that disparities exist in different contexts and are rooted in the discriminatory and inequitable distribution of health care resources.

Disparities remain an area of concern for our government. Every 10 years, the U.S. Department of Health and Human Services drafts a comprehensive set of health objectives that form the priorities for our nation's health. The most current objectives were released in December 2010 in *Healthy People 2020*, which embraces public health social work values. The *Healthy People 2020* document underscores the need to continue focusing on disparities in health care among various racial/ethnic, socioeconomic, gender, age, disability, sexual orientation, and geographic groups (U.S. Department of Health and Human Services, 2010).

Common Values

Of particular significance with regard to social–health disparities is the similarity of the value structure of both fields. The Code of Ethics of the National Association of Social Workers lists six ethical principles that delineate social work's core values of service, social justice, dignity and worth of the person, importance of human relationships, integrity, and competency (National Association of Social Workers, 2008). The code further requires social workers to challenge social injustice and to work for social justice for all people, but especially those who are marginalized and who are targets of discriminatory practices.

Public health also takes a "social justice" approach. The Public Health Code of Ethics lists 12 Principles of the Ethical Practice of Public Health. Principle 4, in particular, links directly to social work practice: "Public health should advocate for, or work for the empowerment of, disenfranchised community members, ensuring that the basic resources and conditions necessary for health are accessible to all people in the community" (Thomas, Sage, Dillenberg, & Guillory, 2002, p. 1058).

Given these values, social work and public health have an interlocking social justice mandate to improve and to ameliorate social health problems (Ruth et al., 2008). The two professions routinely intersect at points of social action and advocacy. The points of intersection, when taken together, map the breadth and depth of public health social work.

Social Justice Philosophy

Social justice from the social work perspective is defined as "an ideal condition in which members of a society have the same rights, protections, opportunities, obligations, and social benefits.... A key social work value, social justice, entails advocacy to confront discrimination, oppression, and institutional inequities" (Barker, 2003, p. 405).

In 1998, while celebrating 150 years of public health, Krieger and Birn noted that during the formative years of public health in the mid-1840s, social justice was seen as the foundation of both the movement and the profession. They noted the importance of looking back:

> Because knowing the paths our field has traversed and identifying which dreams of the early public health visionaries have been fulfilled, and which have not can help us understand our current situation, put contemporary conflicts in perspective. . .and inform options for future endeavors (p. 1603).

Beauchamp (1976) contended that "public health should be a way of doing justice, a way of asserting the value and priority of all human life" (p. 8). He further defined justice as meaning that "each person in society ought to receive his due and that the burdens and benefits of society should be fairly and equitably distributed" (p. 8).

These common values form the foundation for common agendas. Both public health and social work have an obligation to work for social justice to eliminate health disparities. Advocacy at all levels is needed and, working together, public health and social work can amplify their efforts. It would be useful for the two professional associations to establish a combined action agenda. The beginning framework for such an agenda is set out below.

SUGGESTED ACTION AGENDA

- Forge a common policy agenda and collaborate for its greatest impact.
- Expand professional understanding and commitment to a collective *human rights* perspective.
- Locate and understand domestic social justice issues within the global context (Finn & Jacobson, 2008).
- Integrate social and economic justice concepts into research and academic curricula (Vincent, 2012).
- Engage in transdisciplinary research, especially comparative effectiveness research (Social Work Policy Institute, 2010).
- Encourage evidence-based practice and practice-based research (Epstein, 2011).
- Coauthor publications and expand publication in journals outside of the fields of social work and public health (Institute for the Advancement of Social Work Research, 2003; Social Work Policy Institute, 2010).
- Work together to advance *Healthy People 2020* goals to eliminate health disparities.
- Translate the value of social justice into public health social work practice (Finn & Jacobson, 2008).
- Strengthen the ability of public health and social work to influence the political and corporate landscape at the federal, state, and local levels (National Association of Social Workers, 2005).
- Build coalitions and partnerships to effect better policies and to advance needed legislative change at state and federal levels.
- Provide written and spoken testimony from an integrated public health social work perspective.
- Review ethical standards and professional competencies and cross-list in both fields as appropriate.

- Continue the national dialogue on the importance and future of public health social work (Ruth & Sisco, 2008).

This handbook helps to map the direction forward for public health social work. It not only marks existing obstacles and challenges but also highlights strategies for moving beyond the current constraints. The chapter authors, all public health social work experts, provide a comprehensive look at the field. Their writings include past successes, life span analyses, practice settings, and what the future might hold for the field of public health social work and the health issues we may face as a nation.

As we move forward with health care reform and the implementation of the Patient Protection and Affordable Care Act, with its emphasis on outcomes, effectiveness, and efficiency, the need for public health social work has rarely been stronger. Recent political changes will affect the future delivery of health care, leading to more emphasis on prevention and wellness and on integrated and transdisciplinary care. The ability of public health social workers to bridge prevention and intervention; to practice at both the individual and community levels; and to link research, practice, and policy will become increasingly valued. In fact, public health social work may well be the future of health care.

Elizabeth J. Clark, PhD, MSW, MPH
Chief Executive Officer
National Association of Social Workers

REFERENCES

Barker, R. L. (2003). *The social work dictionary.* Washington, DC: National Association of Social Workers.

Beauchamp, D. E. (1976). Public health as social justice. *Blue Cross and Blue Shield Inquiry, 13,* 1-14.

Cohen, A. (2009). *Nothing to fear: FDR's inner circle and the hundred days that created modern America.* New York: Penguin Group.

Copeland, V. C., & Henry, B. N. (2008). Maternal and child health. In T. Mizrahi & L. E. Davis (Eds.), *Encyclopedia of social work* (20th ed., Vol. 3, pp. 192-195). Washington, DC: National Association of Social Workers.

Downey, K. (2009). *The woman behind the new deal: The life of Frances Perkins.* New York: Random House.

Dubos, R. (1959). *Mirage of health: Utopias, progress, and biological change.* New York: Harper.

Epstein, I. (2011). Reconciling evidence-based practice, evidence-informed practice, and practice-based research: The role of clinical data-mining. *Social Work, 56,* 284-286.

Finn, J. L., & Jacobson, M. (2008). Social justice. In T. Mizrahi & L. E. Davis (Eds.), *Encyclopedia of social work* (20th ed., Vol. 4, pp. 44-52). Washington, DC: National Association of Social Workers.

Institute for the Advancement of Social Work Research. (2003). *Social work contributions to public health: Bridging research & practice in preventing violence— Lessons from child maltreatment & domestic violence*. Retrieved from http://www.socialworkpolicy.org/publications/iaswr-publications/social-work-contributions-to-public-health-bridging-research-practice-in-preventing-violence-%e2%80%93-lessons-from-child-maltreatment-domestic-violence.html

Institute of Medicine. (1988). *The future of public health*. Washington, DC: National Academies Press.

Keefe, R. H. (2010). Health disparities: A primer for public health social workers. *Social Work in Public Health, 25,* 237–257.

Krieger, N., & Birn, A. E. (1998). A vision of social justice as the foundation of public health: Commemorating 150 years of the spirit of 1848. *American Journal of Public Health, 88,* 1603–1606.

National Association of Social Workers. (2005). *Social Work Congress—Final report*. Washington, DC: Author.

National Association of Social Workers. (2008). *Code of ethics of the National Association of Social Workers*. Washington, DC: Author.

National Association of Social Workers Foundation. (2012). *Social work pioneers biographies*. Retrieved from http://naswfoundation.org/pioneers/default.asp

Ruth, B. J., & Sisco, S. (2008). Public health. In T. Mizrahi & L. E. Davis (Eds.), *Encyclopedia of social work* (20th ed., Vol. 3, pp. 476–483). Washington, DC: National Association of Social Workers.

Ruth, B. J., Sisco, S., Wyatt, J., Bethke, C., Bachman, S., & Piper, T. (2008). Public health and social work: Training dual professionals for the contemporary workplace. *Public Health Reports, 123*(Suppl. 2), 71–77.

Sable, M. R., Schild, D. R., & Hipp, J. A. (2012). Public health and social work. In S. Gehlert & T. Brown (Eds.), *Handbook of health social work* (pp. 64–99). Hoboken, NJ: Wiley.

Sloane, H. I. (1988). Supplementary statements. In *The Future of Public Health* (pp. 160–161). Washington, DC: National Academies Press.

Smedley, B. D., Stith, A. Y., & Nelson, A. R. (2008). *Unequal treatment: Confronting racial and ethnic disparities in health care*. Washington, DC: National Academies Press.

Social Work Policy Institute. (2010). Comparative effectiveness research and social work: Strengthening the connection. Retrieved from http://www.socialworkpolicy.org/wp-content/uploads/2010/03/SWPI-CER-Full-RPT-FINAL.pdf

Stuart, P. H. (2008). Social work profession: History. In T. Mizrahi & L. E. Davis (Eds.), *Encyclopedia of social work* (20th ed., Vol. 3, pp. 156–164). Washington, DC: National Association of Social Workers.

Thomas, J. C., Sage, M., Dillenberg, J., & Guillory, V. J. (2002). A code of ethics of public health. *American Journal of Public Health, 92,* 1057–1059.

U.S. Department of Health and Human Services (2010). *Healthy People 2020* (Publication No. B0132). Washington, DC: U.S. Government Printing Office.

U.S. Department of Health, Education, and Welfare (1962). *Five decades of action for children: A history of the children's bureau*. Washington, DC: Author.

Van Pelt, J. (2009). Social work and public health. *Social Work Today, 9*(1), 28.

Vincent, N. J. (2012). Exploring the integration of social justice into social work research curricula. *Journal of Social Work Education, 48,* 205–222.

Preface

For well over 100 years, public health social workers have been at the forefront of promoting the health and well-being of, and eliminating negative health outcomes for, individuals, families, groups, and communities. Throughout the past century, the field of public health social work has grown to include primary, secondary, and tertiary prevention efforts in various contexts around the United States and abroad. Public health social workers practice in any number of settings, helping an individual address issues of diabetes management, a family access health care services for a sick child, or a community center obtain funds for an obesity-management clinic. Whereas public health social work students 25 years ago were largely from the United States, students from various nations now come to this country to pursue social work degrees and learn the necessary skills to practice effectively as public health social workers in their home countries.

Throughout the years, public health social workers have advocated on behalf of people everywhere whose voices are not heard by legislative bodies. We have worked to eliminate infant mortality, improve the quality of care in nursing homes, and promote legislation that will allow people with limited financial means to receive competent and culturally appropriate health care. We continue today by addressing these and additional pressing challenges, including the ever-increasing numbers of returning veterans who are unable to access treatment for post-traumatic stress disorder; poor families who are unable to find service providers willing to accept Medicaid; frail elderly individuals who are homebound and unable to access community-based services; and people living with chronic health conditions whose insurance companies refuse to reimburse services for long-term care.

As the field of public health social work moves forward, we face many ongoing challenges. Various legislative efforts, developed ostensibly to facilitate better health care for all Americans, have languished as politicians looking to further their own careers vote to slash funding for health services, including reproductive health care for young mothers, clean-needle exchange programs for intravenous drug users, and behavioral health care services for people living with severe and persistent mental illnesses. The uncertain economic forecasts leave many voters unwilling to use tax dollars to pay for much-needed services in spite of the services' proven effectiveness. Shifts toward political conservatism lead many citizens living with stigmatizing conditions such as HIV to avoid reaching out for services due to the shame and stigma associated with receiving care.

As we move well into the second decade of the 21st century, we are faced with ever-widening disparities in health outcomes in all branches of health care. *Healthy People 2020* addresses many of these issues and charges us, as public health social workers, with developing solutions that will eliminate these disparities and enhance the well-being of all Americans. To accomplish this charge, public health social workers must be skilled in working at all levels of intervention including the micro, mezzo, and macro levels.

The idea for this book came about a few years ago, during a business meeting of the Public Health Social Work Section at the annual American Public Health Association conference. Many of the section's members have been in practice for over 30 years in various health care settings. Our concern over the condition of many health care services, the upward predicted job growth for social workers nationwide, and the ever-challenging and ever-changing health care needs of our fellow citizens served as the motivating forces for the section members to propose this book. The profits from the sales of the book will go directly to the Public Health Social Work Section, which will use the profits to support mentoring students and new professionals into the public health social work profession, provide funding for students to attend the annual conference of the American Public Health Association, and promote the public health social work profession around the country and abroad.

I am proud to be associated with this project and with all of you, who, as aspiring public health social workers, strive to enhance the well-being of citizens wherever they may live and remove barriers to care so that we can all live fulfilling and healthy lives.

Robert H. Keefe
Chairperson, Public Health Social Work Section
Pittsford, NY

Acknowledgments

As any well-practiced public health social worker knows, large-scale efforts require the assistance of many people. Our efforts to bring this book to completion would have been in vain without the ongoing support and tempered guidance of the staff of Springer Publishing Company. Our thanks to Jennifer Perillo for helping us broaden our ideas for the handbook and for setting the project in motion; Sheri W. Sussman, Executive Editor, for providing ongoing support and guidance to help us bring this project to conclusion; and Kathryn Corasaniti, Associate Editor, for offering quick feedback on each chapter and thereby assuring the book would be completed in a timely and thorough manner.

We also wish to thank the members of the Public Health Social Work (formerly Social Work) Section of the American Public Health Association who stepped forward to share their ideas and experience gained from many years of practice by coauthoring several chapters, in particular Bari Cornett, who developed the format for each chapter.

We extend thanks to Sarah DeWolfe and Thuy Duong, students at the School of Social Work, Southern Illinois University at Carbondale, who spent many hours proofreading manuscripts and checking references and tables for accuracy.

Lastly, we would like to acknowledge the many public health social work students and practitioners who continue to inspire us with their never-ending quest for excellence in providing services to individuals, families, groups, and communities around the United States and abroad. Without their passion to learn and to share the wealth of their experiences in the field, this book would be severely limited in its contribution to the important field of public health social work.

Robert H. Keefe and Elaine T. Jurkowski

PART I

Introduction

*P*ublic health social workers are employed in many different areas throughout the world. Their roles are as diverse as the places in which they work. To be effective, public health social workers must learn multiple skills, be adept at multitasking, have excellent oral and written communication skills, and be competent working with individuals from various professional disciplines.

The first chapter of this book introduces the student to the fields of public health and social work, including the purpose, mission, and history of each discipline, and how professionals in each discipline began to work together in response to the ever-changing and increasingly complex health and social needs communities face. The authors discuss the emergence of social work as a pivotal entity within the American Public Health Association and the important role social workers have played within this large organization. Additional areas of focus include the core functions of public health (assessment, policy development, and assurance), key objectives of *Healthy People 2020*, (US DHHS) public health social work standards and competencies, and the education and professional experience necessary to be a competent public health social worker. The chapter concludes by providing the reader key dates in public health social work history.

Chapter 2 addresses the complex issue of public health ethics. The values of both the public health and social work professions are detailed along with each profession's standards and competencies. Case scenarios and websites are provided to enhance student learning regarding how to address various issues, to assure as public health social workers that we are rendering services that are culturally competent, ethically sound, and pertinent to clients' needs.

While reading these chapters, write down some of the important health issues residents in your community face, how these issues have changed over time, and the services that have been put into place to address them. As you develop your thoughts, think about the role of the public health social worker, what should he/she do to be of service, and how would he/she reach out in a way that is culturally sensitive and ethically astute. When you finish, discuss your answers with other classmates and your instructor and think about recommendations you could make to improve the public health service system in your communities.

CHAPTER 1

Introduction to Public Health Social Work

Robert H. Keefe and Theora A. Evans

HISTORICAL PERSPECTIVES ON PUBLIC HEALTH AND SOCIAL WORK

*T*he origins of public health and social work are rooted in antiquity. However, most people are familiar only with the American adaption of these disciplines, which were procured from England during the 19th century when John Snow, a renowned physician of that time, helped to stop the great cholera outbreak of 1848 in London. Snow collected statistics from various neighborhoods to prove that cholera was caused by "poisoned" drinking water, which devastated certain neighborhoods. Although few people today know of Dr. Snow, many people are familiar with his methods to contain the spread of disease: mapping the location of a disease outbreak, tracing the names of individuals who may have contracted an illness, and developing sanitary methods to dispose of waste. Consequently, many Americans today think of "public health" for its role in disease control and surveillance, campaigns for yearly flu vaccines, and public service warnings to boil water during times of flood and other natural or bio-terrorist emergencies.

The social work profession also began to grow during the 19th century when Dorothea Dix, a well-known activist, lobbied state legislatures and the U.S. Congress to create the first American mental asylums. Later, pioneers such as Jane Addams and Lillian Wald helped to bring forth political activist strategies that would lead to women's suffrage and services that promoted the health needs of new-born children and communities. Because of the well-known efforts put forth by Dix, Addams, Wald, and other activists many Americans today think of "social work" for its roles in government lobbying, case and cause advocacy, and neighborhood change.

Over the past many decades public health and social work professionals have grown to rely increasingly on each other's skills (Ruth, Wyatt, Chiasson, Geron, & Bachman, 2006). Public health professionals have become more aware of the psychosocial determinants of health (Awofeso, 2004; Krieger & Birn, 1998; Northridge, 2004) and social workers have become more aware of the importance of epidemiology (Ruth et al., 2006). Today, professionals in each discipline practice in all countries and with all populations. They hold elected office, administer large-scale organizations, and conduct research in various settings around the globe. Public health social workers fill many different roles including educators, case managers, and program evaluators (Sable, Schild, & Hipp, 2012). The purpose of this book is to fuse the principles and practices that underlie the public health and social work professions in their relationship to our nation's health and to help the reader learn of various roles public health social workers play in various settings.

To begin discussion of the interrelationship of public health and social work, a definition of each must be put forward. Charles Edward Amory Winslow, a professor of public health at Yale University in 1920, defined public health practice as,

> The science and art of preventing disease, prolonging life, and promoting physical health and efficiency through organized community efforts for the sanitation of the environment, the control of community infections, ... the organization of medical and nursing services for the early diagnosis and preventive treatment of disease, and the development of the social machinery which will ensure to every individual ... a standard of living adequate for the maintenance of health. (Winslow, 1920, p. 30)

Over time, numerous definitions of social work have been offered. For our purposes we will use the following definition:

> Social Work is the professional activity of helping individuals, groups or communities enhance or restore their capacity for social functioning and creating societal conditions favorable to this goal. (Standards for social service manpower, 1973, pp. 3–4)

Public health social work expands this definition to include:

> ... an epidemiological approach to identifying social problems affecting the health status and social functioning of all population groups with an emphasis on intervention at the primary prevention level. (Practice Standards Committee, 2005, p. 4)

These definitions make clear that although the public health and social work professions vary in their practice methods, their intended goals are similar: to improve the health, welfare, and social well-being of society-at-large. Both professions share an ecologic perspective for problem-solving, and a systemic approach toward intervention that calls upon various sources to bring about change to complex social problems (Volland, Berkman, Stein, & Vaughn, 1999). Likewise, each profession shares a core value of "social justice" and an essential role of "service provision" targeted at enhancing the lives of the disadvantaged (Krieger, 2003; Krieger, & Birn, 1998; Stover & Bassett, 2003). Both professions use social action and advocacy in numerous domains including community health (Wallerstein, Yen, & Syme, 2011); maternal, child, and adolescent health (Jaffee & Perloff, 2003); substance abuse (Skiba, Monroe, & Wodarski, 2004); immigrant health (Chang-Muy & Congress, 2008); HIV/AIDS (Smith & Bride, 2004); primary prevention (Vourlekis, Ell, & Padgett, 2001); bioterrorism (Mackelprang, Mackelprang, & Thirkill, 2005); and the uniformed services (Wheeler & Bragin, 2007).

THE EMERGENCE OF PUBLIC HEALTH IN AMERICA

Since antiquity, countries around the world have been concerned about upholding the health of their citizens. In 1798 the U.S. Congress required the provision of health care and compulsory insurance to merchant seaman via the Marine Hospital Service. In 1902, the program was expanded and reorganized as the United States Public Health Service (USPHS). The goal of the USPHS was to limit the spread of disease. Seamen were afforded benefits through the Marine Hospital Service because of their risk for contracting diseases while serving in the import/export industry, which put them in contact with people from far-off lands. Upon return from international travel on tall sailing ships, seamen were clinically evaluated for any diseases they may have contracted.

One of the principal tasks of the USPHS has been the diagnosis, mandatory reporting, and quarantining of individuals who are carriers of infectious diseases. Consequently, some people perceived public health as serving a sanitation function. That narrow focus was broadened by the work of Louis Pasteur and Robert Koch who in 1870 put forth "germ theory" as the cause of disease. Germ theory gained much momentum in the United States as more and more individuals moved to large, urban areas where frequent exposure to strangers living in nearby and often cramped housing gave rise to the spread of various communicable illnesses for which there were no known cures.

Germ theory helped people understand that the etiology of disease (i.e., germs) leads to the spread of illness, and the subsequent morbidity and mortality of citizens. In turn, public health moved toward the field of medicine to carry out its mission. This move was facilitated by scientific progress of the 19th century that included the dawn of bacteriology and the invention of the stethoscope in the mid-1800s, the introduction of antisepsis in England in 1876 (through the practice of hand washing with carbolic acid introduced by Dr. [Sir] Joseph Lister), and the discovery of ether in Boston in 1867 (Starr, 1982).

Public health services were later expanded to include direct-service interventions to stop the spread of illnesses. The ability to diagnose and provide primary intervention versus curative care put public health at odds with the American Medical Association (AMA), which was more interested in the treatment of illnesses once they developed than arresting the spread of disease outbreaks. Additionally, public health conflicted with the values of individuals who believed that providing services such as vaccinations, maternal and infant care, tuberculosis (TB) and venereal disease (VD) (or in today's nomenclature, sexually transmitted infections [STI]) prevention, and establishing clinics (known as dispensaries) for the poor was in opposition to groups who supported Social Darwinism and eugenics. Social Darwinists believed that only the healthiest members of society survived, thus ridding society of individuals who were unable to contribute to it. This way of thinking changed with more forward-thinking men and women who believed social reform was needed so that all people could receive necessary care and take part in society.

SOCIAL REFORMERS AND THE ADVENT OF SOCIAL WORK

The Social Reform Movement, begun in the 1890s, was brought about by individuals who were typically from well-educated and privileged backgrounds, who opposed Social Darwinism and laissez-faire ideology. Philosophically, the reformers had moved from a "blaming the victim" mindset of the 19th century to the realization that systemic evolution was necessary for the impoverished to subsist in America.

The women of the progressive movement took on leadership roles and were often among the first generation of women to have acquired a college education. They were typically from well-educated and privileged backgrounds, with fathers who were well-regarded attorneys, legislators, or businessmen. Many of their fathers supported equality for women and the right for women to vote. The reformers shared avid supporters during their formative years from settlement house reformers, labor union leaders, Children's Bureau (CB) staff, and the Women's Bureau's affiliate—

the Women's Joint Congressional Committee (Chambers, 1963). In large part due to their efforts, the field of social work grew and "scientific" methods were applied to charity work.

The reformers understood that good health was a key to longevity and one way to assure that people had good health was to impose strict laws (such as child labor laws) to ensure that children remained in school and were not forced to do dangerous jobs that often led to serious illnesses and injuries. In turn, the child labor movement became the means by which social reformation was to occur. The reformers teamed with union activists to support compulsory education for children and to press industrialists for better wages, unemployment compensation, safety codes/devices, and shorter work hours. They tied child labor to poverty, ill health, and limited opportunities for upward mobility. Social justice became fashionable and the "sleeping dog" (i.e., the indigent), was awakened and mobilized. Their efforts helped lead to the ratification of the 19th Amendment to the Constitution in 1921, whereby women were given the right to vote. Having achieved legislative success at the local, state, and national levels, the reformers moved to formulate federal programs that would impact poverty, child welfare, disabled persons, and the elderly. As a result, social work and public health were launched and national social policy (i.e., the Social Security Act [SSA]) was mandated.

Public health social work took active roles during the Great Depression of the 1930s by advocating for the passing of the SSA including the formulation of Maternal and Child Health Services (Title V), and the implementation of the New Deal programs. Public health social workers also pushed for passing The Great Society programs of the mid-to-late 1960s, which focused on social justice and empowerment (no doubt encouraged the Mental Health section's governing councilor, Ruth I. Knee [a social worker], and others to encourage the re-emergence of a Social Work section within APHA).

During the 1970s and 1980s, public health social work focused much of its efforts on community-based care. Fiscal cuts in health care led to shorter hospital stays, increased nursing home admissions and greater use of home health care and outpatient services. Thanks to vaccines, many communicable diseases were curable, or at least treatable. Long-term, chronic diseases, however, became ubiquitous. Consequently, although Americans were living longer, they were doing so with greater pain, more frequent visits to health care providers, and less adequate insurance coverage. Today, legislative changes including The Affordable Care Act place a spotlight on public health and community organizing. Forever present are the societal issues that continue to pit individual rights against the national agenda to maintain our society. Our ethics and values and our global responsibilities are competing forces requiring a wider lens to address our challenges.

THE FOUNDING OF THE AMERICAN PUBLIC HEALTH ASSOCIATION
AND THE SOCIAL WORK SECTION

The American Public Health Association (APHA) was founded in 1872 by Dr. Stephen Smith. Its members were primarily physicians who worked as state and local health officials (Starr, 1982). APHA's early agenda focused on the development of a centralized and systematic demographic database as well as preventive and primary interventions for children.

During the first annual APHA meeting in 1875, Dr. Elisha Harris stressed the need for an effective system of birth registration and primary prevention methods that would insure the health of Americans. His goal was to ensure cities and states had proper techniques for sanitation and a mode for vaccinating infants against smallpox. At this time, the smallpox vaccine was not in widespread use in the United States and generally was provided as a charity service (About the Cover, 1985; Schmidt & Wallace, 1982). For his efforts, Elisha Harris was remembered as a pioneer in American public health.

Social Work's roots within APHA date back to 1910, under the auspices of the Sociological section, one of five sections initially organized within the association. The leadership of the Sociological section was credited with introducing the concept of "social context" to the diagnosis of population-based assessment. They argued that the environments in which people live serve to enhance or undermine health. Julia Lathrop, the first chief of the Children's Bureau, referred to her work (eradicating infant mortality, initiating a national birth registry, and launching a program of child health conferences) as a "public health" line of attack whereby social workers could help to eliminate child health problems and promote the health and wellbeing of children. Lathrop touted her agenda and accomplishments as representative of a "sociological" perspective of public health practice (Parker & Carpenter, 1981).

Homer Folks, the first chair of the Sociological section, is credited with supporting Lathrop's intent to address the preventable phenomenon of infant mortality. In 1903, Folks studied the context of tuberculosis and realized that living in crowded housing conditions gave rise to the spread of the disease. Consequently, if individuals were removed from their home environments they were less likely to spread tuberculosis. Having pioneered the importance of integrating social and economic indices and an eco-systemic approach to assessing communicable disease to impact public health issues, the section moved on to introduce Mental Hygiene (1916) as an area in need of attention (Rosen, 1971).

Despite its work within APHA, the Sociological section disbanded in 1922 and many social workers migrated to the newly organized Maternal and Child Health section (1921) and subsequently to the Mental Hygiene section. Numerous reasons have emerged to explain the demise of the Sociological section, but the most prudent rationale was the social work profession's decision to shift its attention away from social reform and prevention to casework and treatment.

PUBLIC HEALTH VERSUS MEDICAL SOCIAL WORK PRACTICE

As we have seen so far in this chapter, public health and social work share many of the same goals and objectives. However, public health social work and medical social work practice differ in two very essential ways: (1) public heath social work practice stresses health promotion and primary prevention, and (2) targets groups rather than solely individuals in need of services (Watkins, 1985). Public health social workers recognize the need to provide culturally relevant services at all levels of intervention (micro, mezzo, and macro) (Sable et al., 2012) and acknowledge that there are few interventions that have been tested on each level and are generalizable across cultural groups (Chin Walters, Cook, & Huang, 2007).

Public health social workers also bring additional skills to their practice including social epidemiology, which examines the effect of social variables on health and behavioral variables that effect a community (Oakes & Kaufman, 2006) (such as the effects of socioeconomic status on health status (Lynch & Kaplan, 2000)) and Geographic Information Systems (GIS), a software package used to map spatial correlations of particular interest to public health workers including access to healthy food options for pregnant women living in neighborhoods that lack fully stocked food markets (Lane et al., 2008). Another skill is community assessment, used to identify strengths and weaknesses in a community. Community members meet to implement projects that may help eradicate community health problems (Kelley, Benson, Estrella, & Lugardo, 2009). Community members in turn may collaborate with public health researchers to evaluate the impact.

CORE FUNCTIONS OF PUBLIC HEALTH AND ESSENTIAL SERVICES

Public health social work practice emphasizes the identification, reduction, or elimination of social stressors associated with poor health (including poverty, discrimination, limited access to care, and fragmented service delivery), and determines the social supports that promote well-being and provide protection against poor health outcomes. Identifying populations at risk of poor health outcomes and providing primary prevention services to arrest the possibility of contracting an illness are rooted in epidemiology. Social epidemiology assumes that diseases, disparities in access to care, outcomes of care, as well as poverty are not randomly distributed throughout society. Therefore, subgroups within a population differ in their frequency of exposure to social problems that lead to poor health. Understanding the social context of an at-risk population is essential for public health social workers to render the most appropriate intervention (Krieger, 2001). Therefore, knowledge of the uneven distribution of risk factors as well as awareness of the economic and cultural indicators can be utilized to formulate programs for health promotion, illness control, and prevention (Mausner & Kramer, 1985, p. 1).

The funding for public health programs and services comes from federal, state, and local dollars. Data including the rates of diagnoses, morbidity, and mortality, and demographic information are aggregated at state and local levels from both public and private health care providers and reported to federal agencies including the Centers for Disease Control and Prevention (CDC) for analysis. These data are in turn shared with the World Health Organization (WHO), which monitors the spread of various diseases around the world.

THE CORE FUNCTIONS OF PUBLIC HEALTH PRACTICE

The three core functions of public health practice and their essential services that address public health problems are assessment (surveillance of disease/injury), policy development (to address problems discussed through assessment), and assurance (implementation of policy that in turn leads to service delivery for all citizens regardless of their ability to pay), which dictate how public health social workers render services. The professional public health community works to identify not only the bio-medical (e.g., virus) and psychological aspects of disease (e.g., trauma), but the social determinants (e.g., poverty) as well. By addressing the determinants, public health social workers are better able to render care at the primary, secondary, and tertiary levels. Public health social workers are employed within every level of service from surveillance, research, policy development and planning, to the delivery of care.

MEDICAL SOCIAL WORK

In contrast to the role that public health social workers play, the role of social work practitioners in medical practice is more restricted. In general, medical social workers are hospital-centered, acute-care focused, and their community interaction is usually limited to making referrals for patients post discharge for ongoing medical care (Silverman, 2008). Once highly regarded and considered a staffing necessity, today's medical social worker role has largely been usurped by the field of nursing. Many hospitals no longer employ social workers and those that do, often relegate them to discharge planning, minimizing their supportive counseling role, while increasing interdisciplinary collaboration with the goal of limiting lengths of hospital stays (Lechman & Duder, 2009). Often, hospital settings do not provide medical social workers with clear promotional tracks to administration, and supervision is often provided by non-social work professionals.

This model is not universal. For example, medical social workers employed by Veteran Administration (VA) hospitals are well compensated, integral members of interdisciplinary teams. They frequently have numerous opportunities for upward mobility, research activity, and public health service. The VA model for social work practice was the ultimate goal for medical social work envisioned by Ida M. Cannon. This pioneer of medical social work acknowledged the need for individualized patient care within medical settings, but also saw a place for social workers in public health programs (Bartlett, 1975).

It seems that although pioneering social work leaders promoted clinical practice, the need for prevention and population-based interventions supported by a social epidemiological perspective was also an ongoing goal. Mary Richmond engaged in social action to address social injustice and Jane Addams employed casework methods as a fact-finding vehicle that recognized a sudden tendency of social work practitioners to limit social work to casework. Richmond declared,

> I have spent twenty-five years of my life in attempt to get social casework accepted as a valid process in social work. Now I shall spend the rest of my life trying to demonstrate to social caseworkers that there is more to social work than casework. (Bruno, 1948, pp. 186–187)

Unfortunately, Richmond was unable to complete her task, leaving future generations of social workers to ponder the validity of cause versus function.

HEALTHY PEOPLE 2020

The initial goals and indices of *Healthy People* were the brainchild of Julius B. Richmond who served as Surgeon General during the Carter administration (1977–1981). *Healthy People* has been published every decade since 1990. (The website www.HealthyPeople.gov provides information for the current and prior editions of *Healthy People*.) Richmond has been lauded for his attempts to address the public health needs of all Americans.

(Julius) Richmond remains best known for his leadership in devising and implementing quantitative goals for public health, first published in 1979 as *Healthy People: The Surgeon General's Report on Health Promotion and Disease Prevention. Healthy People* moved PHS beyond its limited capabilities to lessen disparities in health services provision, to spur change by getting information out to journalists, health departments, and others about gains already made in reduced mortality from noninfectious causes. (http://www.surgeongeneral.gov/about/previous/biorichmond.htm, 2007)

The goals of *Healthy People 2020* are to (1) attain high quality, longer lives free of preventable disease, disability, injury, and premature death; (2) achieve health equity, eliminate disparities, and improve the health of all groups; (3) create social and physical environments that promote good health for all; and (4) promote healthy development and healthy behaviors across every stage of the life cycle (*Healthy People 2020*). A glaring reality is the inclusion of indices that are clearly within the practice domains of the social work profession. Note, this chapter does not include content on all of the newly added indices, but we do incorporate many of them, as well as many of those identified earlier that are of ongoing importance. The *Healthy People 2020* goals differ from previous goals in the addition of the following indices: Adolescent Health; Blood Disorders and Blood Safety; Dementias (including Alzheimer's Disease); Early and Middle Childhood; Genomics; Global Health; Health-Related Quality of Life and Well-Being; Healthcare-Associated Infections; Lesbian, Gay, Bisexual and Transgender Health; Older Adults; Sleep Health; and Social Determinants of Health.

PUBLIC HEALTH SOCIAL WORKER STANDARDS AND COMPETENCIES

By definition, professionals have standards and competencies that are used to assess and measure their practice performance. Prior to 2004, public health social work practitioners had not developed their own standards and competencies. A growing national movement of transparency, evidence-based practice, and outcomes measurement, compelled public health social workers to assess the required knowledge and skill sets needed for effective practice.

The task of formulating standards and competences was led by Kathleen Rounds and Dot Bon, who were the co-directors of the *Beyond Year 2010: Public Health Social Work Practice Project* in 1998. The *Public Health Standards and Competences* (Practice Standards Development Committee, 2005) was a collaborative effort of numerous public health social work practitioners, educators, members of the Association of State and Territorial Public Health Social Workers, community advocates, representatives of national organizations and foundations, policymakers, and consumers. (For a complete list of Standards Development Committee members see www. oce.sph.unc.edu/cetac/phswcompetencies_may05.pdf.) Consultation was provided by Paul Halverson (CDC). Many of those providing input were also members and leaders of the APHA's Social Work section including Loretta Fuddy, Deborah Stokes, and Delois Dilworth-Berry. Funds to publish the resulting brochure were secured by Deborah Stokes from the Health Community Access Program and The Maternal and Child Health Block Grant of the Ohio Department of Health.

Fourteen standards and accompanying performance indicators were identified. The standards define and highlight practice skills across public health functions and essential services. The document defines and provides the application of a social epidemiologic approach to empowerment and resiliency-focused practice models across ecological systems. The competencies' section includes measurement content in the following broad areas: theoretical knowledge base of practice, methodological and analytical processes, leadership and communication, policy and advocacy, and values and ethics. Ongoing evaluation of public health social work standards and competencies is essential for the profession to move forward and continue addressing the many pressing needs of health care across the country.

BECOMING A PUBLIC HEALTH SOCIAL WORKER

Becoming a public health social worker requires a passion for service, hard work, and a belief that good health should be afforded to all individuals. As you embark on a career in public health social work, employers will expect that you have a sound knowledge base in practice at the micro-, mezzo-, and macro-levels of intervention. Many employers will expect that you will have taken courses not only in social work, but in health as well. You can meet this expectation by enrolling in MSW courses that focus on health care and also by completing a field placement at a public health agency. There are now many dual MSW/MPH degree programs in the United States that help prepare students to enter the field of public health social work (Ruth et al., 2006, 2008). Although many MSW programs do not offer a dual MSW/MPH degree, many offer concentrations in health, gerontology, mental health, and child welfare that are also helpful to prepare you for a career as a public heath social worker.

Continuing education programs offer additional opportunities to develop and enhance one's skills. These programs typically charge a fee and can run as long as one day to several weeks. Some offer certificate programs in various areas that will enhance career opportunities. Professional organizations such as APHA and the Association of State and Territorial Public Health Social Work (ASTPHSW) provide excellent opportunities to develop professional skills and to network with other public health social workers around the country.

Finally, professional journals including the *American Journal of Public Health, Health & Social Work, The Journal of Social Work and Health, Social Work in Health Care,* and *Social Work in Mental Health* are excellent sources of up-to-date research studies that will help you to fine-tune your skills as an effective public health social worker.

THE PURPOSE AND STRUCTURE OF THIS BOOK

For this book, well-respected public health social work practitioners and scholars collaborated to produce a volume that we hope will educate the reader about today's practice realities in the field of public health social work. Social work educators will likely find the book useful for either undergraduate or graduate-level social work classes in social work practice, human behavior and the social environment, and social work/welfare policy courses. The chapters are structured in such a way as to provide background on the core functions of public health including assessment, assurance, and policy development; link to relevant *Healthy People 2020* objectives; educate the readers on disparities in health care among racial and ethnic groups; discuss relevant public health social work standards and competencies; provide exercises and case scenarios for class discussions; and provide useful websites for additional reading.

The book is divided into six sections: The first section provides an overview of public health social work, the second section focuses on public health social work across the lifespan, the third section focuses on chief medical topics public health social workers face, the fourth section is devoted to public health social work in selected settings, the fifth section takes a look at public health social work administration and policy, and the sixth section considers the future of public health and public health social work practice.

Unlike many social work health texts that focus on the social worker as a member of an interdisciplinary/transdisciplinary team, this book focuses on the role of the public health social worker as an independent professional who, while working collaboratively with other professionals, has a skillset and a set of resources to call upon. As with any good professional, the public health social worker's skills are always in development and require continuous updating. Health care in the United States requires the public health social worker to be continuously working on developing skills and practice methods to be an effective practitioner. This chapter provides web-based resources to be of help to students interested in pursuing rewarding and fulfilling careers as public health social workers. We hope this book is useful to each of you as you move forward in your careers in the field of public health social work.

APPENDIX 1.A

ABRIDGED PUBLIC HEALTH AND SOCIAL WORK MILESTONES

- 1872 APHA founded
- 1874 Society for the Prevention of Cruelty to Children founded
- 1875 APHA 1st Annual Meeting—Dr. Elisha Harris pushes for a birth registration system in the United States, and a mechanism for vaccinating infants against smallpox
- 1887 First American settlement house (NY Neighborhood Guild) established
- 1889 Hull House established in Chicago
- 1892 Milk stations open in New York City
- 1893 Jane Addams provides medical care to the indigent—dispensary in Hull House
- 1894 School-based medical services initiated in Boston
- 1895 Reports linking contaminated milk to disease in children leads to pasteurization
- 1896 The National Association of Colored Women (NACW) was co-founded by Mary Church Terrell and Josephine St. Pierre Ruffin. Among the agenda items for NACW members was advocacy for community development
- 1897 Compulsory vaccinations in New York City schools
- 1902 United States Public Health Service founded, replaces the Marine Hospital Service
- 1902 Committee on the Prevention of TB headed by Edward T. Devine, editor of *Charities and The Commons* and Executive Director of NY Charities Organization Society
- 1902 Meeting of 32 settlement house representatives (subsequently known as the National Child Labor Committee) to discuss child labor in NYC. The meeting was hosted by Lillian Wald (www.nwhm.org/education-resources/biography/biographies/lillian-wald/) and Florence Kelley (florencekelley.northwestern.edu)
- 1903 First comprehensive analyses of TB cases in the United States. The study was conducted and data were collected by social workers. The results led to social action and policy formulation on sanitation initiated by Hull House residents and Charity Organization Society members
- 1906 National Health Insurance Program proposed by Progressive Party members, including Jane Addams, contained a public health agenda

- 1908   NYC Health Department establishes program to eradicate contagious disease in children
- 1908   Lugenia   Burns   Hope   (www.georgiaencyclopedia.org/nge/Article. jsp?id=h-3513) opens the Neighborhood Union in Atlanta, Georgia. Mrs. Hope is further credited with pioneering satellite maternal and child health clinics, neighborhood schools, and adult education for Blacks
- 1909   First White House Conference on the Care of Dependent Children
- 1910   The Sociological Section of APHA is organized, "to bring social workers and health officer into closer touch . . ." (John M. Glenn, Russell Sage Foundation) (Glen, 1913)
- 1911   Mother's Pension in Illinois
- 1912   Children's Bureau headed by Julia Lathrop a former Hull resident (social worker) national birth registration initiated
- 1912   Theodore Roosevelt and the Progressive party endorse social insurance as part of their platform to include health insurance
- 1912   Jane Addams endorses Theodore Roosevelt's presidential nomination because of his agenda to sanction a National Health Service and social insurance programs, if elected
- 1918   Compulsory education mandated nationwide
- 1920   Jessie O. Thomas, Lugenia Burns Hope, and E. Franklin Frazier are credited with establishing the first school of social work for Blacks in the United States at Atlanta University
- 1921-1929   Sheppard–Towner Act (previously introduced by Jeanette Rankin, a social worker and 1st woman in Congress)
- 1921-1934   Grace Abbott represented United States on the League of Nations' Advisory Committee re: the Traffic in Women and Children
- 1930   Social Workers preempt coup to remove Title V programs from Children's Bureau
- 1931   Jane Addams awarded Nobel Peace Prize
- 1932-1935   New Deal programs shaped by Harry Hopkins, a social worker
- 1935   Under Franklin Delano Roosevelt's leadership, the Social Security Act passed by Congress and includes grants for Maternal and Child Health
- 1938   Fair Labor Standards Act—abolishes child labor nationally and ends racial discrimination in hiring practices of federal agencies, defense-related industries were specifically targeted with this mandate; Lenroot (www.columbia.edu/cu/lweb/archival/collections/ldpd_4079022/) and Abbott (www.americaslibrary.gov/jb/gilded/jb_gilded_abbott_1.html) were among the architects who crafted and secured this legislation
- 1941   Lenroot convened a conference that led the way to day care for working mothers
- 1944   Social Security Board calls for compulsory national health insurance as part of the Social Security system
- 1946   President Harry Truman signs National Mental Health Act
- 1949   President Harry Truman signs the Housing Act

- 1953   Federal Security Agency made a cabinet level agency and renamed as the Department of Health Education and Welfare (DHEW)
- 1954   President Dwight Eisenhower signs Vocational Rehabilitation Act
- 1963   President John Kennedy signs into law the Community Mental Health Centers Act
- 1964   Great Society Programs/War on Poverty inspired by Whitney Young's (a social worker) proposal for a domestic Marshall Plan
- 1964   President Lyndon Johnson signs the Economic Opportunity Act
- 1965   President Lyndon Johnson signs into law the Medicare and Medicaid programs
- 1965   President Lyndon Johnson signs Head Start Program
- 1969   The Public Health Service (PHS) takes over the administration of Title V with the organization of the Department of Health Education and Welfare, child welfare and health were and remain separated. An earlier coup to over-take Title V from the Children's Bureau was pre-empted by social workers in 1930
- 1955–1969   Virginia Insley is named Chief, Medical Social Work section, U.S. Children's Bureau
- 1969–1973   Chief, Medical Social section, Maternal and Child Health Services, USPHS
- 1973–1980   Chief, Medical Social Work section, Bureau of Community Health Services, USPHS
- 1970   The Social Work section established as a free-standing section of APHA
- 1972   President Richard Nixon signs the Social Security Amendment extending Medicare coverage to those under 65 who have long-term disabilities or end-stage renal disease
- 1972   WIC program established as part of the Child Nutrition Act on 1966
- 1974   President Richard Nixon signs Child Abuse Prevention and Treatment Act
- 1980   President James Carter signs Adoption Assistance and Child Welfare Act
- 1980–2000   Juanita Evans appointed Chief of the Office of Adolescent Health, U.S. Dept. of Health and Human Services, HRSA, Maternal and Child Health Bureau
- 1986   President Ronald Regan signs into law the Omnibus Budget Reconciliation Act, allowing workers and their families who lose health benefits to continue receiving benefits for a certain period of time
- 1997   The State Children's Health Insurance Program extends health coverage to children from low-income families that do not qualify for Medicaid
- 1995   Health Resources and Services Administration (HRSA) provides funding to establish the Center for School Mental Health Assistance, Maternal and Child Health Bureau
- 1996   AFDC program ends
- 1997   TANF program begins
- 2003   President George W. Bush signs the Medicare Prescription Drug Improvement and Modernization Act (i.e., Medicare Part D)

- 2009 President Barack Obama extends the State Children's Health Insurance Program through 2013
- 2010 President Barack Obama signs into law the Affordable Care Act

REFERENCES

About the Cover. (1985, July). *American Journal of Public Health, 75*, 7.

Awofeso, N. (2004). What's new about the "New Public Health"? *American Journal of Public Health, 94*, 705–709.

Bartlett, H. M. (1975). Ida M. Cannon: Pioneer in medical social work. *Social Service Review, 49*(2), 208–229.

Bruno, F. J. (1948). *Trends in social work: As reflected in the Proceedings of the National Conference of Social Work, 1874–1946*. New York: Columbia University Press, pp. 186, 187.

Chambers, C. A. (1963). *Seedtime of reform: American social service and social action 1918–1933*. Minneapolis, MN: University of Minnesota Press.

Chang-Muy, F, & Congress, E. (2008) Social work with immigrants and refugees: Legal issues, clinical skills, and advocacy. New York: Springer Publishing Company.

Chin, M. H., Walters, A. E., Cook, S. C., & Huang, E. S. (2007). Interventions to reduce racial and ethnic disparities in health care. *Medical Care Research Review, 64*(5 Suppl), 7S–28S.

Glenn, J. M. (1913). Sociological section. Report of the section committee. *American Journal of Public Health, 3*, 645–647.

Jaffee, K. D., & Perloff, J. D. (2003). An ecological analysis of racial difference in low birthweight: Implications for maternal and child health in social work. *Health and Social Work, 28*, 9–22.

Kelley, M. A., Benson, M., Estrella, M., & Lugardo, J. (2009). Jóvenes sin fronteras: Latino youth take action for social justice & well-being (GCP-09-01 (Working Paper Series ed.). Chicago, IL: University of Illinois at Chicago Great Cities Institute. Retrieved from http://www.uic.edu/cuppa/gci/

Krieger, N., & Birn, A. (1998). A vision of social justice as the foundation of public health: Commemorating 150 years of the spirit of 1848. *American Journal of Public Health, 88*, 1603–1606.

Krieger, N. (2001). A glossary for social epidemiology. *Journal of Epidemiology & Community Health, 55*(10), 693–700.

Krieger, N. (2003). Latin American social medicine: The quest for social justice and public health. *American Journal of Public Health, 93*, 1989–1991.

Lane, S. D., Keefe, R. H., Rubinstein, R. A., Levandowski, B. A., Webster, N. J., Cibula, D. A., Boahene, A. K., Dele-Michael, O., Carter, D., Jones, T., Wojtowycz, M. A., & Brill, J. (2008). Structural violence, urban retail food markets, and low birth weight. *Health & Place, 14*(3), 415–423.

Lechman, C., & Duder, S. (2009). Hospital length of stay: Social work services as an important factor. *Social Work in Health Care, 48*(5), 495–504.

Lynch, J., & Kaplan, G. (2000). Socioeconomic position. In L. F. Berkman, & I. Kawachi (Eds.), *Social epidemiology* (pp. 12–25). New York: Oxford University Press.

Mausner, J. S., & Kramer, S. (1985). *Epidemiology: An introductory text* (2nd ed., p. 1). Philadelphia: Saunders.

Mackleprang, R. W., Mackelprang, R. D., & Thirkills, A. D. (2005). Bioterrorism and smallpox: Policies, practices and implications for social work. *Social Work, 50,* 119–127.

Northridge, M. E. (2004). Building coalitions for tobacco control and prevention in the 21st century. *American Journal of Public Health, 94,* 178–180.

Oakes, J. M., & Kaufman, J. S. (2006). Introduction: Advancing methods in social epidemiology. In J. M. Oakes, & J. S. Kaufman (Eds.), *Methods in social epidemiology* (pp. 3–20). San Francisco: Jossey-Bass.

Parker, J. K., & Carpenter, E. M. (1981). Julia Lathrop and the children's bureau: The emergence of an institution. *Social Service Review, 55*(1), 60–77.

Practice Standards Development Committee, Beyond Year 2010: Public health social work practice project at the UNC School of Social Work. (2005). *Public health social work standards and competencies.* Columbus, OH: Ohio Department of Health. Retrieved March 5, 2012, from http://oce.sph.unc.edu/cetac/phswcompeten cies_May05.pdf

Rosen, G. (1971). Public health: Then and now. The sociological section of the American Public Health Association, 1910–1922. *American Journal of Public Health, 61*(12), 2515–2517.

Ruth, B. J., Sisco, S., Wyatt, J., Bethke, C., Bachman, S. S., & Piper, T. M. (2008). Public health and social work: Training dual professionals for the contemporary workforce. *Public Health Reports, 123*(Suppl 2), 71–77.

Ruth, B. J., Wyatt, J., Chiasson, E., Geron, S. M., & Bachman, S. (2006). Social work and public health: Comparing graduates from a dual-degree program. *Journal of Social Work Education, 42*(2), 429–439.

Schmidt, W. M., & Wallace, H. M. (1982). The development of health services for mothers and children in the United States. In Helen M. Wallace, Edwin M. Gold, & Allan C. Oglesby (Eds.), *Maternal and child health practices* (pp. 3–37) (2nd ed.). New York: John Wiley & Sons.

Silverman, E. (2008). From ideological to competency-based: The rebranding and maintaining of medical social work's identity. *Social Work, 53*(1), 89–91.

Skiba, D., Monroe, J., & Wodarski, J. S. (2004). Adolescent substance use: Reviewing the effectiveness of prevention strategies. *Social Work, 49,* 343–353.

Smith, B. D., & Bride, B. E. (2004). Positive impact: A community-based mental health center for people affected by HIV. *Health and Social Work, 29,* 145–148.

Standards for Social Service Manpower. (1973). Washington, DC: National Association of Social Workers.

Starr, P. (1982). *The social transformation of American medicine: The rise of a sovereign profession and the making of a vast industry.* New York: Basic Books.

Stover, G. N., & Bassett, M. T. (2003). Practice is the purpose of public health. *American Journal of Public Health, 93,* 1799–1801.

U.S. Department of Health and Human Services. Office of Disease Prevention and Health Promotion. Healthy People 2020. Washington, DC. Available at http://healthypeople. gov/2020/default.aspx. Accessed September 14, 2012.

Volland, P., Berkman, B., Stein, G., & Vaughn, A. (1999). *Social work education for practice in health care: Final report.* New York: New York Academy of Science.

Vourlekis, B. S., Ell, K., & Padgett, D. (2001). Educating social workers for health care's brave new world. *Journal of Social Work Education, 37,* 177–191.

Wallerstein, N. B., Yen, I. H., & Syme, S. L. (2011). Integration of social epidemiology and community-engaged interventions to improve health equity. *American Journal of Public Health, 101*(5), 822–830.

Watkins, E. L. (1985, June). The conceptual base for public health social work. In A. Gitterman, R. B. Black, & F. Stein (Eds.), *Public health social work in maternal and child health: A forward plan* (pp. 17-33). Proceedings of the working conference of the Public Health Social Work Advisory Committee of the Bureau of Health Care Delivery and Assistance. Rockville, MD: Division of Maternal and Child Health.

Wheeler, D. P., & Bragin, M. (2007). Bringing it all back home: Social work and the challenge of returning veterans. *Health and Social Work, 32*(4), 297–300.

Winslow, C.-E. A. (1920, January 9). The untilled fields of public health. *Science, 51*(1306), 23-33. doi:10.1126/science.51.1306.23. PMID 17838891. Retrieved March 5, 2012, from http://www.sciencemag.org/cgi/pmidlookup?view=long&mid=17838891

CHAPTER 2

Ethics for Public Health Social Workers

Elaine Congress

INTRODUCTION

*V*alues and ethics form the core of the social work and public health professions. Ethics related to public health care can be viewed as growing largely from three approaches: (1) values inherent in public health practice, (2) concepts and language, and (3) health and human rights (Slomka Quill, des Vignes-Kendrick, & Lloyd, 2008). These three approaches are compatible with the values and ethics set forth by the National Association of Social Workers (NASW) and the American Public Health Association (APHA). This chapter examines some of the values and ethics that guide public health social work practice, various ethical dilemmas public health social workers encounter and the methods used to resolve them, and the guidelines for ethical practice for public health social workers.

Although the public health and social work professions have similar values and ethical principles, there are differences in how each profession renders services. These differences have at times created tension between public health and public health social work professionals. The values as set forth by APHA are:

1. Humans have a right to the resources necessary for health.
2. Humans are inherently social and interdependent.
3. The effectiveness of institutions depends heavily on public trust.
4. Collaboration is a key element to public health.
5. People and their physical environment are interdependent.
6. Each person in a community should have an opportunity to contribute to public discourse.
7. Identifying and promoting the fundamental requirements for health in a community is of primary concern to public health.
8. Knowledge is important and powerful.

9. Science is the basis for much of our public health knowledge.
10. People are responsible to act on the basis of what they know.
11. Action is not based on information alone (Public Health Leadership Society, 2002).

The social work profession specifies its core values in the Code of Ethics (NASW, 2008). The following six are listed as core values and principles:

Value: Service

Ethical Principle: Social workers' primary goal is to help people in need and to address social problems.

Value: Social Justice

Ethical Principle: Social workers challenge social injustice.

Value: Dignity and Worth of the Person

Ethical Principle: Social workers respect the inherent dignity and worth of the person.

Value: Importance of Human Relationships

Ethical Principle: Social workers recognize the central importance of human relationships.

Value: Integrity

Ethical Principle: Social workers behave in a trustworthy manner.

Value: Competence

Ethical Principle: Social workers practice within their areas of competence and develop and enhance their professional expertise.

There is much congruity between the public health and social work professional values and ethics. Each stresses the dignity and worth of the individual and the importance of human relationships. The public health profession values collaboration, which is a cornerstone of the roles social workers perform daily.

HEALTHY PEOPLE 2020

Involving individuals in decision making regarding their health is very congruent with both social work and public health values. The U.S. Department of Health and Human Services sought consumer input while developing the *Healthy People 2020* report. *Healthy People 2020* was based on an "extensive stakeholder feedback process that is unparalleled in government and health" (*Healthy People 2020*, 2010, p. 1) and included the integration of professional public health experts, health organizations, and the general public. The U.S. Department of Health and Human Services received more than 8,000 comments regarding the selection of *Healthy People 2020* objectives. On the basis of these comments, a number of new topic areas were included:

- Adolescent Health
- Blood Disorders and Blood Safety
- Dementias, including Alzheimer's Disease
- Early and Middle Childhood
- Genomics
- Global Health
- Health-Related Quality of Life and Well-Being
- Health Care-Associated Infections
- Lesbian, Gay, Bisexual and Transgender Health
- Older Adults
- Preparedness
- Sleep Health
- Social Determinants of Health

An ongoing focus of both *Healthy People 2010* and *Healthy People 2020* has been the elimination of health disparities and inequities. Because of their commitment to promoting social justice this topic is of particular concern to public health social workers. Advocating for health equity is stressed both within public health codes that state that all humans have a right to health and the social work code of ethics that promotes social justice. Health disparities refers to the differences in illnesses, chronic health conditions, and mortality that occur across racial, ethnic, and economically oppressed groups, of which people of color are often the most at risk. Given that unequal access to health care based on race and ethnicity has been a contributing factor to health disparities (Smedley, Stith, & Nelson, 2003), working to overcome disparate health care access and to improve health outcomes for all people is an important area for public health social workers (Keefe, 2010).

Healthy People 2020 recognizes that the goal of reducing health inequities and disparities cannot be limited only to public health in the United States, but must include other countries as well. As a result, Global Health has become a new topic area and is listed as one of the *Healthy People 2020* core topics. Moreover, four of the United Nations Millennium Development Goals relate specially to health. For instance, Goal 1: eradicate extreme poverty; Goal 4: reduce child mortality; Goal 5: improve maternal health; and Goal 6: combat HIV/AIDS, malaria, and other diseases (United Nations, 2011) are all health concerns we face in the United States.

ETHICAL STANDARDS FOR SOCIAL WORKERS AND PUBLIC HEALTH PROFESSIONALS

While values are the underlying beliefs of an individual or of a profession, ethical standards are needed to provide guidance on implementing them. Both APHA and NASW have ethical codes to guide their members in ethical practice (NASW, 2008; Public Health Leadership Society, 2002). Although the NASW Code of Ethics does not specify "health care," the provision of service to clients without discrimination related to ethnicity, race, immigration status, and national origin is stressed. As a result, social workers must "strive to ensure access to needed information, services, and resources ... for all people" (NASW, 2008, p. 5), which includes health care. Similarly, the APHA states that "Public health programs should incorporate a variety of approaches that anticipate and respect diverse values, beliefs and cultures in the community" (Thomas, Sage, Dillenberg, & Guillory, 2002, p. 1958).

The NASW Code of Ethics has 167 standards divided into the following six categories: (1) social workers' ethical responsibilities to clients, (2) social workers' ethical responsibilities to colleagues, (3) social workers' ethical responsibilities in practice settings, (4) social workers' ethical responsibilities as professionals, (5) social workers' ethical responsibilities to the social work profession, and (6) social workers' ethical responsibilities to the larger society (NASW, 2008). Many of the NASW standards apply to direct practice and are primarily focused on work with individuals.

The APHA Social Work section has developed a set of standards to guide professional practice for public health social workers, which include:

Professional Standard #1. PHSW uses social epidemiology principles to assess and monitor social problems affecting the health status and social functioning of its risk populations within the context of family, community, and culture.

Professional Standard #2. PHSW uses social epidemiology principles to identify and assess the factors associated with resiliency, strengths, and assets that promote optimal health.

Professional Standard # 3. PHSW uses social epidemiology principles to identify, measure, and assess the social factors contributing to health issues, health hazards, and stress associated with ill health.

Professional Standard #4. PHSW uses social epidemiology principles to evaluate the effectiveness, accessibility, and quality of individual, family, and population-based health interventions.

Professional Standard #5. PHSW uses social planning, community organizational development, and social marketing principles to inform and educate individuals, families, and communities about public health issues.

Professional Standard #6. PHSW uses social planning, community organizational development, and social marketing principles to empower and mobilize individuals, families, and communities to become active participants in identifying and addressing public health concerns to improve individual, family, and societal well-being.

Professional Standard #7. PHSW uses social planning, community organizational development, and social marketing to promote and enforce legal requirements that protect the health and safety of individuals, families, and communities.

Professional Standard #8. PHSW uses social planning, community organizational development, and social marketing to assure public accountability for the well being of all, with emphasis on vulnerable and underserved populations.

Professional Standard #9. PHSW uses social planning, community organizational development, and social marketing to develop primary prevention strategies that promote the health and well-being of individuals, families, and communities.

Professional Standard # 10. PHSW uses social planning, community organizational development, and social marketing to develop secondary and tertiary prevention strategies to alleviate health and related social and economic concerns.

Professional Standard # 11. PHSW provides leadership and advocacy to assure the elimination of health and social disparities wherever they exist such as, but not limited to, those based on community, race, age, gender, ethnicity, culture, or disability.

Professional Standard # 12. PHSW provides leadership and advocacy to assure and promote policy development for providing quality and comprehensive public health services within a cultural, community, and family context.

Professional Standard #13. PHSW supports and conducts data collection, research, and evaluation.

Professional Standard #14. PHSW assures the competency of its practice to address the issues of public health effectively through a core body of social work knowledge, philosophy, code of ethics, and standards (Social Work Public Health Standards and Competencies, 2005).

There are many areas of similarities in that each profession stresses the competency of the professional, the promotion of social justice through combating inequities, and concern about vulnerable populations. A major difference between the two sets of ethical standards and competencies is public health's greater focus on the use of social epidemiology and prevention, while social work's code of ethics stresses greater focus on the individual clients and the clinical professional responsibilities. Another difference is public health's macro-level emphasis on social planning and community organizational development, while social work's focus is also on the individual, family, and group levels of direct practice.

In addition to cultural sensitivity and competence in work with diverse populations, both social workers and other public health professionals address the importance of advocacy for the most vulnerable members of our society. Social workers are advised to engage in "social and political action to insure that all people have equal access to the resources, employment, services and opportunities they require to meet their basic human needs" (NASW, 1999, p. 27), while the principles of the ethical practice in public health propose that "public health should advocate for, or work for the empowerment of, disenfranchised community members ensuring that the basic resources and conditions necessary for heath are accessible for all people in the community" (Thomas et al., 1958).

Another similarity between the public health and the social work ethical codes is the dual focus on individuals and communities. Public health providers look to healthy populations and communities as well as healthy individuals (Gebbie, Rosenstock, & Hernandez, 2003). Similarly, social workers define clients not only as individuals, but also families and communities (Congress, 1999). This is different from medical providers who primarily focus on interactions between an individual patient and a health care provider.

From Values to Ethics: Ethical Dilemmas

Values and principles have small worth unless they can be actualized in practice (Congress, 1999; Perlman, 1976). While the values and standards of public health and social work seem very clear and straightforward, dilemmas often arise when there are conflicts of values. For example, NASW cites self-determination as an important social work value only to be limited when "clients' actions or potential actions pose a serious, foreseeable and imminent risk to themselves or others" (NASW, 2008, p. 7). In general, public health professionals support individuals' rights to make their own health decisions about following healthy habits or pursuing a particular type of treatment for an illness. Public health, however, is also committed to protecting the health of the greatest number of individuals. This principle serves as the foundation of policies about immunization programs and the reporting of communicable diseases. While clients can exercise their right to self-determine their personal health decisions, their rights to self-determination may be limited if their decisions will expose others to illness.

Culturally Competent Practice Dilemmas

The NASW Code of Ethics stresses the importance of cultural competency. Social workers should "be able to demonstrate competence in the provisions of services that are sensitive to clients' cultures and to differences among people and cultural groups" (NASW, 2006, p. 9). In the Standards for Cultural Competence in Social Work Practice, competence is defined as "the process by which individuals and systems respond effectively to people of all cultures ... in a manner that recognizes, affirms, and values the worth of individuals, families, and communities and preserves the dignity of each" (Center for Cross Cultural Health, 1997, p. 11). Culturally competent practice involves more than speaking the client's language or having knowledge about a client's specific culture. It involves understanding and accepting how culture has shaped clients' health beliefs. Pursuant to these principles, a public health social worker should maximize the clients' self-determination, especially for clients who may have different cultural backgrounds than the worker. In working with clients from diverse backgrounds, the social worker needs to be continually aware of the power dynamics that enter into any social work relationship, especially when working with individuals who are from culturally diverse backgrounds, and how this power has been used to oppress vulnerable people.

An ethical challenge may arise when the cultural beliefs of clients may not seem to be promoting health and freedom from illness as perceived by the public health social worker. A social worker may promote self-determination in terms of cultural beliefs when a client elects to use an herbal remedy in addition to pursuing regular medical care. An ethical dilemma may emerge, however, if the client uses a folk remedy as the only form of treatment for a life-threatening illness. For example, consider the case of a 50-year-old female patient recently diagnosed with leukemia who told her social worker that she had decided not to pursue medical treatment. Instead, she believed that taking a special preparation her grandmother made would cure her. Using professional judgment, the social worker could argue that self-determination should be compromised because there is risk of "serious, foreseeable and imminent harm to a client or other identifiable person" (NASW, 2008, p. 10).

How direct should the social worker be in encouraging the client to follow prescribed medical treatment? Although most adults might have the right to make individual decisions about their health care, court proceedings can be initiated to declare clients incompetent to make their own health decisions. A court proceeding to declare a person incompetent is used most frequently for older people and people with mental and developmental disabilities. If self-determination regarding one's health care is an important value, public health social workers need to ensure that competency hearings are initiated only as a last resort and are not disproportionately used for vulnerable populations.

An even more challenging dilemma arises when the sick client is a child whose parents believe that only a specific folk remedy should be used. Goldberg (2000) sees a dilemma for social workers who strive to respect the beliefs of all cultures but also support basic human rights. Although social workers are respectful of differing health beliefs, a conflict can arise if the practice is potentially life threatening. For example, what is the appropriate ethical stance for a public health social worker to take if a parent chooses to consult a faith healer rather than a surgeon for a child with a brain tumor? Should the parents be referred to Child Protective Services because they did not pursue recommended medical treatment for their child?

Informed Consent Dilemmas

Another ethical concern and challenge for the public health social worker is enhancing informed consent for all clients. There are numerous examples in medical history of disadvantaged and vulnerable populations not being afforded informed consent. The often-cited Tuskegee Syphilis Experiment from 1932 to 1972 is a classic example of a minority group that was not given the option to exercise informed consent because information about effective treatment was withheld. The NASW Code of Ethics states that social workers are advised to "use clear and understandable language to inform clients of the purpose of the service, risks related to the services, limits to services because of the requirements of third party payer, relevant costs, reasonable alternatives, clients' right to refuse or withdraw consent, and the time frame covered by the consent" (NASW, 2008, pp. 7–8).

Informed consent requires three main elements: presumption of competence, voluntary action, and disclosure before consent. Presumption of competency implies that a client can gather diverse information, exercise judgment, and make a decision that may differ from that of the practitioner (Palmer & Kaufmann, 2003). Minors and individuals ruled incompetent by the courts are presumed unable to provide informed consent. This is not an inflexible policy, though, because minors, people with mental illnesses, individuals with disabilities, and individuals affected by dementia are increasingly given the option of exercising informed consent to the extent of their ability.

Ensuring that all people are deemed competent to make their own decisions is vitally important. There may be an erroneous perception that people who do not understand English and have limited education and ability to understand medical terms may not be competent to make their own decisions. The use of professional interpreters and explanations of medical conditions and procedures in simple vocabulary may help such individuals to make competent health care decisions. In order for patients to be ruled incompetent to make decisions, a court decision that is not based on an individual's diagnosis, education, or understanding of English must be made.

Another important aspect of informed consent involves voluntary action without duress or coercion. Voluntary action may be hampered when there are institutional pressures to prevent clients from making independent decisions. Vulnerable people with limited education may be overly influenced by the authority of the health care provider and thus not able to exercise independent judgment. This may be especially true for populations of individuals who have been stigmatized, oppressed, and excluded from making their own decisions. All too often clients are prescribed medications with serious side effects without being informed of the full extent of the medications' possible side effects. Care must be taken that clients are able to refuse taking medications without undue threats that doing so will be detrimental to their health.

A final condition for informed consent is that the consent must be preceded by the disclosure of adequate information. All possible risks and side effects must be reviewed and understood before clients can be expected to exercise their right to informed consent, even when such disclosure may lead clients to refuse treatment. For example, the American Psychiatric Association reported that nearly 50% of individuals with severe and persistent mental illnesses may develop permanent neurological symptoms, such as tardive dyskinesia, as a result of the medications they take (Swenson, 1997). Yet many psychiatric patients and their families are from disadvantaged populations and may be pressured to take very strong psychotropic medications without having had the possible risks made clear to them.

Ethical Dilemmas and Decision Making

Ethical dilemmas often arise from conflicting values. A study of 45 public health practitioners, who were not social workers, identified the following five areas as ethically challenging in public health: (1) adequately using public health authority, (2) making decisions related to resource allocation, (3) negotiating political interference in public health practice, (4) maintaining standards of quality of care, and (5) defining the scope of public health (Baum, Gollust, Goold, & Jacobson, 2009). The practitioners reported they often used a "social justice" value orientation and consultation with colleagues to guide their ethical decision making. Few of them knew about or relied on formal methods of decision making.

Kass (2001) developed the following ethical framework for public health practice to apply public health to actual practice: (1) What are the public health goals of the proposed program? (The articulated goals would stem from public health professional values.) (2) How effective is the program in achieving its stated goals? (3) What are the known or potential burdens of the program? (4) Are there ethical risks to confidentiality and privacy, liberty and self-determination, and justice when public health interventions are focused only on special populations? (5) Can burdens be minimized? (6) Are there alternative approaches that can be considered? (7) Is the program implemented fairly? and (8) How can the benefits and burdens of a program be fairly balanced?

Despite an increasing interest in bioethics, social work literature on ethical decision making in the public health field has been limited. Several models of social work ethical decision making have been developed (Congress, 2000; Lowenberg, Dolgoff, & Harrington, 2008; McAuliffe & Chenoweth, 2008). However, because of time constraints social workers do not often use a model of ethical decision making. To help social workers apply a simple but structured model for ethical decision making, Congress (2000) put forward a simple acronym (the ETHIC model) to be used: Examine values—personal, social, cultural, client, and professional. Think about the Code of Ethics, laws and regulations, and agency policies. Hypothesize about different scenarios. Identify who is most vulnerable and who will be harmed. Consult with supervisors and colleagues.

Competing Values

A continuing challenge in ethical decision making is deciding between two competing values. For example, there often is a conflict between self-determination and preservation of life. Some situations are very clear; for example, if a person expresses suicidal intent, then preservation of life trumps self-determination. But what if the person engages in health practices that are detrimental to one's well-being? For example, a public health social worker may have a patient with diabetes who insists on eating a rich dessert each night. Adults living in the community may be able to self-determine their dietary habits even if the preservation of life is threatened. Within an institution, however, people may be less able to exercise self-determination, especially if their behavior is life threatening.

Hierarchies of ethical principles have been developed to help social work in addressing these dilemmas. Harrington and Dolgoff (2008) researched how social workers order ethical principles used to resolve ethical dilemmas: (1) autonomy and freedom (self-determination), (2) equality and inequality, (3) least harm, (4) privacy and confidentiality, (5) protection of life, (6) quality of life, and (7) truthfulness and full disclosure. The authors indicated that there was little consistency about how social workers rank these often-competing principles. One example was the principle promoting right to self-determination versus the principle promoting preservation of life. The context in which the dilemma takes place is very important: A social worker working with a healthy 18-year-old with suicidal intent might approach the hierarchy very differently than a social worker working with a 75-year-old with a suicide plan who was recently diagnosed with terminal lung cancer. In the first example, the social worker might find that the fifth principle, "supporting the protection of life," is the most important, while in the second example the social worker might decide that Principle 1, "supporting self-determination," and Principle 6, "quality of life," are primary.

Although there seems to be much concurrence between public health and social work, there may be ethical dilemmas that arise in the focus of the two professional areas and produce conflict for the public health social worker. Public health social workers are committed to "the promotion of positive health behaviors in the development of lifestyles by individuals, families, and groups" (Social Work Public Health Standards and Competencies, 2005). The NASW Code of Ethics principle of self-determination states that clients have the right to make their own decisions except when there is a clear, foreseeable, and imminent possibility of risk to self and others (NASW, 2008).

Because of the primary focus on populations, public health may minimize individual self-determination. Both professions would agree that if an individual pursues a health belief that is dangerous to oneself or others the individual does not have a right to exercise the right to self-determination. An example might be a parent who refuses to have one's child receive immunizations against infectious diseases. Such a decision poses danger for the child as well as other children who might not yet be immunized. The discovery of various childhood vaccines is a major victory in public health within the past century. Public health professionals stress that all children should be immunized. Does the parent's decision not to immunize the child present a conflict for public health social workers who may be more receptive to the parent's individual beliefs that immunizations are not safe for the child or that immunizing a child goes against the parent's religious beliefs?

What if the health practice, however, is not threatening to others as, for example, an individual who does not want to follow a healthy diet? This choice might be dangerous to the individual, but not to society as a whole. Currently there are major public health campaigns to address obesity, especially among children. Is there a difference in how a public health professional and a public health social worker would work with a mother who feeds her obese child an unhealthy diet? Would a non–social work public health professional grant as much self-determination to clients as public health social workers grant?

Ethical Dilemmas: Limited Resources

Ethical challenges often arise during times of limited resources. While public health social workers have an ethical responsibility to provide equal treatment for everyone, the question arises, what if there are not enough health care resources to meet everyone's needs? Decisions are often made about distributing limited resources according to one of the following four principles of distributive justice (Congress, 1999). Principle 1: Each person should receive an equal share of the resources. This principle seems in accordance with public health social work values, but it is challenging and complex to administer in practice. For example, what if there is only one available bed in a nursing home, one heart available for a transplant, or a very limited amount of flu vaccine to be distributed? Some health care resources are not divisible, which makes equal distribution challenging for the public health social worker.

Principle 2: Resources should be distributed on the basis of need. This principle also seems to be in accordance with public health social work values. Given that social workers often work with and provide services to clients who are the most needy and vulnerable, if there are limited resources available, how are decisions to be made when there are competing needs? Often this becomes a generational debate; that is, should limited financial resources be used to fund a long-term care facility or adolescent recreational center? At times, decisions about need are determined by a health triage model, which originated during World War II when difficult decisions were often made not to treat the most severely injured, but rather those who had the best chance of survival. For many public health social workers with a professional commitment to help the most vulnerable this decision may not seem the right one. Yet in many health care settings social workers have very large caseloads and must make decisions daily about who will receive services and who will not. Often individuals with short-term needs are seen first, while those with longer term needs, are seen last.

Principle 3: Distributive justice is related to compensation based on past and present oppression. This principle has always been important to social work and is certainly a key issue with the current discussion about health disparities that are related to racial and ethnic differences. Social workers are frequently in support of special programs that address the needs of groups that are particularly affected by serious health conditions or who lack access to health resources. One example is the development of special health programs for undocumented immigrants who are not covered by federal health care plans.

Principle 4: Contribution based on one's means. This principle has frequently been the basis for how health services have been distributed in the United States. Individuals who are working and can pay for health care insurance receive coverage, while the unemployed, who cannot afford health care, do not pay. Most social workers find this principle troublesome, especially with our beliefs that everyone should have equal access to health care; however, this policy has long characterized how health care services are delivered in the United States.

Dilemmas: Employing Health Care Institutions

Social workers face various dilemmas between advocating for their clients' rights to choose various health care options and the needs of their employing institutions. The NASW Code of Ethics states that social workers have an ethical responsibility to their employer (NASW, 2008). A problem may emerge when working with a hospitalized immigrant patient whose behavior seems contrary to accepted medical practices. The dilemma for the social worker presents itself when a relative of the patient continues to bring in food that is antithetical to a prescribed diet. Another dilemma would be in the case of hospital policy that mandates a clear discussion about end-of-life decisions with terminal clients if such a client refuses to have this discussion, believing the discussion itself will bring bad luck. Gutheil and Heyman (2005) suggested that members of many minority groups are particularly wary of making end-of-life decisions.

Ethical Guidelines

The following guidelines may be helpful for ethical practice in public health social work:

1. Communication: The public health social worker should strive to improve communication between all participants in health care, especially for disadvantaged and other vulnerable populations. The "need to contour public health according to the cultural ways of different groups" has been well documented in public health literature (Gebbie et al., 2003, p. 80). Health care providers must work to ensure that clients' voices are heard in health care and seek to improve communication and understanding between consumers and health care providers.

2. Education: Many health care consumers lack basic understanding about medical conditions and available treatments, especially of preventive methods that can lead to improved health outcomes. Public health social workers can take responsibility to educate individuals about illness, treatment options, and prevention. Although some individuals, especially undocumented immigrants, may have limited access to services, social workers have a role in educating all people about available health benefits. Social workers also can serve as culture brokers by educating doctors and other

medical personnel about a patient's cultural beliefs, practices, and social and community environment.

3. Empowerment: Building on a patient's strengths, public health social workers can help empower the patient to take responsibility for one's health care. Mothers often neglect taking care of their own health needs because they are so occupied with assuring their child's health care needs are being taken care of. Public health social workers can work with mothers by empowering them to articulate their health needs with various health providers and seek available health care options.

4. Advocacy: Within health care settings social workers can advocate to ensure that their clients receive equal health care despite differing economic, social, and cultural backgrounds. Advocacy needs to take place not only within health care settings, but also in the larger health care community. On a local level, public health social workers can advocate for all residents to live in a safe and healthy environment. On state and national levels, social workers can advocate for the adoption of laws and policies that provide everyone with accessible and appropriate health care. On an international level, public health social workers can advocate that the Millennium Development Goals regarding health are achieved for people around the world.

DISCUSSION QUESTIONS

1. What are the principal values and ethical principles that guide social work practice?
   To answer this question, think about a particular group of individuals and the specific health issues they face. An example may be low-income gay men living with HIV who need health care but are uninsured and are unable to pay for services. Consider the ethical principles that would address your issues.
2. What are the principal values and ethical principles that guide public health practice?
   To answer this question, think about a larger population of individuals such as Somali refugee children who are unable to attend school unless they are properly immunized.
3. How are the principles similar?
4. Are there areas of difference?
5. What ethical challenges do public health social workers encounter in culturally competent practice?
6. What ethical challenges do public health social workers face while providing an opportunity for their clients to exercise informed consent?
7. How can a public health social worker resolve these ethical dilemmas?

INTERNET RESOURCES

American Public Health Association: Public Health Social Work

(www.apha.org/membergroups/sections/aphasections/socialwork/about/)

The Social Work section's website outlines standards and competencies for public health social work practice.

Healthy People 2020

(www.healthypeople.gov)

As discussed in this chapter, *Healthy People* is a set of health objectives released by the U.S. Department of Health and Human Services. *Healthy People* is published at the beginning of each decade. The document specifies goals and objectives designed to meet the health care needs of Americans and to guide public and private agencies.

International Federation of Social Workers (IFSW): Policy Statement on Health

(www.ifsw.org/p38000081.html)

This IFSW policy statement presents health as a fundamental human right, outlines health disparities, reports on the impact of globalization on health, discusses global issues that undermine the health of vulnerable populations, and puts forward guidelines for social workers.

Robert Wood Johnson Foundation

(www.rwjf.org/)

The Robert Wood Johnson Foundation website provides information about various federal initiatives related to key issues on health including health disparities, health policy, funding opportunities, and up-to-date news on health issues from around the country.

The Urban Institute: Health Policy

(www.urban.org/health/index.cfm)

The Urban Institute provides policy analyses on various health-related issues, including health care reform, third-party payment systems, health disparities, and immigrant health.

World Health Organization (WHO): World Millennium Goals

(www.who.int/topics/millennium_development_goals/en/)

The WHO collects data from around the world on issues related to health, disease surveillance, and access to health care. The site also provides information detailing health-related World Millennium Goals.

REFERENCES

Baum, N., Gollust, S., Goold, S., & Jacobson, P. (2009). Ethical issues in public health practice in Michigan. *American Journal of Public Health*, *99*(2), 369–374.

Center for Cross Cultural Health. (1997). *Caring across cultures: The provider's guide to cross cultural health care*. St. Paul, MN: Author.

Congress, E. (1999). *Social work values and ethics: Identifying and resolving professional dilemmas*. Pacific Grove, CA: Wadsworth.

Congress, E. (2000). What social workers should know about ethics: Understanding and resolving practice dilemmas. *Advances in Social Work*, *1*(1), 1–25.

Gebbie, K., Rosenstock, L., & Hernandez, L. (2003). *Who will keep the public healthy: Educating public health professionals for the 21st century*. Washington, DC: The National Academies Press.

Goldberg, M. (2000). Conflicting principles in multicultural social work. *Families in Society*, *81*(1), 12–33.

Gutheil, I., & Heyman, J. (2005). Working with culturally diverse adults. In E. Congress & M. Gonzalez (Eds.), *Multicultural perspectives in working with families* (pp. 111–127). New York: Springer Publishing.

Harrington, D., & Dolgoff, R. (2008). Hierarchies of ethical principles in ethical decision making. *Ethics and Social Welfare*, *2*(2), 183–196.

Healthy People 2020. (2010). Retrieved July 26, 2011, from http://www.healthypeople.gov/2020/default.aspx

Kass, N. (2001). An ethics framework for public health. *American Journal of Public Health*, *91*(11), 1776–1782.

Keefe, R. H. (2010). Health disparities: A primer for public health social workers. *Social Work in Public Health*, *25*(3), 237–257.

Lowenberg, F., Dolgoff, R., & Harrington, D. (2008). *Ethical decisions in social work practice* (8th ed.). Belmont, CA: Thomson/Brooks Cole.

McAuliffe, D., & Chenoweth, L. (2008). Leave no stone unturned: The inclusive model of decision making. *Ethics and Social Welfare*, *2*(1), 38–44.

National Association of Social Workers. (2008). *Code of ethics*. Washington, DC: Author.

Palmer, N., & Kaufmann, M. (2003). The ethics of informed consent: Implications for multicultural practice. *Journal of Ethnic and Cultural Diversity in Social Work*, *12*(1), 1–26.

Perlman, H. H. (1976). Believing and doing: Values in social work education. *Social Casework*, *57*(6), 381–390.

Public Health Leadership Society. (2002). *Principles of the ethical practice of public health*. Washington, DC: American Public Health Association.

Social Work Public Health Standards and Competencies. (2005). Retrieved July 29, 2011, from www.oce.sph.unc.edu/cetac/phswcompetencies_may05.pdf.

Slomka, J., Quill, B., des Vignes-Kendrick, M., & Lloyd, L. (2008). Professionalism and ethics in the public health curriculum. *Public Health Reports, 123*(2), 27-35.

Smedley, B. D., Stith, A. Y., & Nelson, A. R. (2003). *Unequal treatment: Confronting racial and ethnic disparities in health care.* Washington, DC: The National Academic Press.

Swenson, L. (1997). *Psychology and law for helping professions.* Pacific Grove, CA: Brooks/Cole.

Thomas, J. C., Sage, M., Dillenberg, J., & Guillory, V. J. (2002) A code of ethics for public health. *American Journal of Public Health, 92*(7), 1057-1059.

United Nations. (2011). *Millennium development goals.* Retrieved July 28, 2011, from http://www.un.org/millenniumgoals/bkgd.shtml

PART II

Life Span

*A*s public health social workers, we are always concerned about ensuring quality health care across the life span. Much literature has been published on factors that help predict positive maternal and child, adolescent, and adult health. We all know that adopting a healthy lifestyle that includes eating lean meat, fresh fruits and vegetables, and whole grains; exercising regularly; and maintaining a healthy weight will improve longevity and quality of life.

The chapters in this section focus on many of the health problems people face throughout their lives. Each chapter addresses the health needs of a particular age group. Chapter 3 is concerned with maternal and child health care. The authors of this chapter consider the goals of current U.S. legislation to address the growing health needs of this population, the ever-present disparities in health outcomes in maternal and child health care by race, and the roles public health social workers play to assure quality health care and positive health outcomes for mothers and children. Chapter 4 is devoted to the topic of adolescent health. The authors address the growing concerns surrounding obesity, sexually transmitted diseases, teenage violence, and school bullying. There has been a great deal of research published in recent years on these health problems as well as teenage tobacco and substance use, eating disorders, and mental health issues. The authors bring to light these and other issues, including motor vehicle injuries and teen suicide. Chapter 5 is dedicated to health care needs of the elderly. As our nation's elderly population continues to grow, public health social workers must be attuned to their direct-care needs as well as the health and social policies developed to address those needs. The chapter author focuses not only on the elderly but also on individuals who provide caregiving services, including spouses, family members, and the formal and informal service delivery system.

Adequately addressing health needs across the life span is a daunting task and goes beyond the scope of this book. As public health social workers, we all too often focus only on the services provided and the health needs these services address. While you read the chapters, think about other health needs your community faces and which age groups are most directly affected by them. Think about what services should be developed to address these problems, which departments within your community's social service delivery system should oversee the services, and what service outcomes you would like to see that would indicate the problems are being remedied.

CHAPTER 3

Maternal and Child Health

Chris Anne Rodgers Arthur, Whitney E. Mendel, and Theora A. Evans

MATERNAL CHILD HEALTH: DEFINED

*M*aternal and child health (MCH) is a long-standing, global public health concern. The Maternal and Child Health Bureau of the U.S. Department of Health and Human Services, defines MCH as the health and well-being of a mother from pregnancy to postpartum care, and the subsequent health and well-being of her child from infancy to age 18. Universal measures of MCH are maternal mortality (death of a mother during pregnancy, childbirth, or the postpartum period), infant mortality (death of a child during the first year of life), and child mortality (death of a child under the age of 5).

The context of MCH practice varies dramatically across the world and often reflects the economic, social, political, and environmental conditions in which the mother and child reside. To provide a glimpse at this variation across the globe, consider that in 2005 the rates of maternal mortality ranged from 900 deaths per 100,000 live births in Africa to 27 per 100,000 live births in Europe (The Henry J. Kaiser Family Foundation, 2009). Similarly, in 2007, the rate of death of a child under the age of 5 ranged from 145 per 1,000 live births in Africa compared to 15 per 1,000 live births in Europe.

More striking are the causes of child mortality globally. In 2008, 31% of child deaths were the result of neonatal complications. The remaining causes of death are of known preventable and treatable illnesses, such as diarrhea, pneumonia, malaria, and measles. In total, approximately 9 million children die each year as the result of largely preventable illnesses (The Henry J. Kaiser Family Foundation, 2009).

As mentioned above, a host of factors influence the health of the mother and child, not the least of which is the environment in which an expectant mother resides. The social determinants of health, the conditions in which

41

a mother lives, works, and plays, directly affect the health and development of her growing child (World Health Organization, 2011). Furthermore, her environment is not limited to the physical location of her residence but also includes the psychological, social, and economic climate that she experiences prior to and throughout her pregnancy and in which the child is raised.

As one might imagine, the specific conditions that contribute to the social determinants of health are not universal. As is evident in the global picture of MCH, the variation in social determinants of health within the United States is reflected in the differences in health and well-being among mothers and their children from state to state, city to city, even from one street to the next.

Disparities in health outcomes, including measures of MCH such as birth weight and gestational age of the infant upon delivery, are often discussed in terms of race and ethnicity. Although there is evidence to suggest that race and/or ethnicity contribute to health outcomes, many would argue that social class provides a more comprehensive understanding of health disparities (Adler & Rehkopf, 2008; Kawachi, Daniels, & Robinson 2005; Williams & Collins, 2001).

HEALTHY PEOPLE 2020 OBJECTIVES: THE GOAL

In the United States, the elimination/reduction of infant mortality has been one of the critical objectives of Healthy People since its inception (1979). *Healthy People 2020* lists 33 MCH objectives under seven topics (www.healthypeople.gov/2020/topicsobjectives2020/objectiveslist.aspx?to picid=26). Space limitations prohibit a comprehensive examination of all 33 objectives. However, given that researchers have identified low birth weight (LBW) as the leading indicator for infant mortality and morbidity, this chapter will explore the determinants and consequences of LBW, and public health social work (PHSW) practice employed to eliminate and remediate the known risk factors of LBW.

INFANT MORTALITY AND LBW: THE PRESENTING ISSUE

The infant mortality rate is a key public health indicator of health, access to health care services, and the well-being of a community. As per the Centers for Disease Control and Prevention report (2008), the U.S. infant mortality rate is higher than the rates of most other developed countries, and the gap is continually growing. In all, 46% of all infant deaths in the United

States are the result of LBW, sudden infant death syndrome, and congenital malformations, and 36.1% of the deaths were preterm related. Although rates stabilized and decreased slightly from 2005 to 2006, 54% of all infant deaths occurred among infants born at less than 32 weeks of gestation (Matthews & MacDorman, 2010).

High rates of infant mortality, LBW, and short gestational age often comprise the definition of poor birth outcomes as they are all indisputably linked. However, when extricated, the rates are not identical. In the Institute of Medicine report *Preterm Birth: Causes, Consequences, and Prevention* (2007), much of the discussion informed by research on LBW and its implications further evidences that the problems and populations (LBW and preterm) often overlap and, in some cases, interact.

The U.S. infant mortality rate generally declined throughout the 20th century, but has stagnated during the early 21st century (World Bank, World Development Indicators, 2009). Despite continuous federal and state funding, the creation of public MCH clinics nationwide, marketing campaigns, community outreach programs, media public service announcements, and the establishment of perinatal networks, the U.S. infant mortality rate did not decline significantly between 2000 and 2005, a fact that has generated concern for researchers and policymakers (Matthews & MacDorman, 2008). The aforementioned ratings are due primarily to disparities that continue to exist among various racial and ethnic groups in this country, particularly African Americans.

According to the Center for Health Statistics (2010), the average rate of infant mortality for White Americans was 5.7. The average rate of infant mortality for African Americans was 13.1—nearly double the overall national average and approximately 60% higher than for White Americans.

In the past 60 years the national rate of infant mortality has dropped significantly, from 38.2 percent in 1945 to 6.8 percent in 2006. However, the national average of infant mortality can be deceiving as it obscures the disparities in rates among different populations and within racial and ethnic groups. For example, in 2006, the infant mortality rate for the United States was 6.68 per 1,000 live births, ranging from 4.52 for mothers from Central and South America to 13.35 for non-Hispanic Black mothers. Overall, the infant mortality rate for non-Hispanic White mothers was 5.58 compared to 5.34 for Mexican mothers and 5.08 for Cuban mothers. The preterm-related infant mortality rate for non-Hispanic Black mothers was 3.4 times higher than the rate for non-Hispanic White mothers and almost 3 times the rate for mothers of either Central and South American origin or Asian and Pacific Islands origins (Matthews & MacDorman, 2010).

The infant mortality rate (29%) that exceeds the national rate among non-Hispanic Black women is attributable to infants of LBW. However, when comparing rates pertaining to only LBW, the disparity between non-Hispanic

Black mothers and Mexican mothers ranges from 14.0% to 6.6%, respectively (Matthews & MacDorman, 2010, p. 8).

SOCIAL DETERMINANTS OF HEALTH: PROTECTIVE OR RISK FACTORS

The World Health Organization established the Commission on Social Determinants of Health to facilitate awareness and movement toward policies addressing health inequalities. Social determinants can be defined as the aggregate of socially structured environments, inclusive of social networks, policies, physical, social, and political infrastructures and systems that provide the context for peoples' lives (Commission on Social Determinants of Health, 2007). The concept embraces a multilevel, multisector, multisystems approach to identifying causes and seeking solutions in which individuals and communities are empowered to organize, participate, and advocate for positive change. Critical to the process of addressing social determinants is identifying the underlying systemic and often-interrelated variables that impinge upon and support health.

Health disparities are often indicative of inequities in other aspects of society. It is well understood that biopsychosocial, emotional, environmental, and physical factors such as poor nutrition, alcohol consumption, adolescent pregnancy, toxic exposures, previous preterm and LBW deliveries, chronic illness, infections, and physical abuse are associated with poor birth outcomes (Hellerstedt et al., 1998; Martin et al., 2010; Wilkinson & Marmot, 2003). However, when these and other factors, such as income and behaviors, are accounted for, racial and ethnic differences remain significant. Although access to health services for pregnant women has improved, medical services alone can neither completely account for nor eradicate seemingly intransigent disparities. Therefore, in order to identify and address negative trends and patterns that are corollaries to negative birth outcomes, it is necessary to address the root causes or "causes of the causes" (Marmot, 2005, p. 22).

Lifestyle and personal decision making inarguably play a key role in the health of the individual, yet they, too, are under the influence of social determinants (Minkler, 1999). The relationship between the social context in which individuals and populations operate and their health-related choices are associated with proximal influences, many of which are outside the spheres of awareness or control. Poverty is at the core of negative health outcomes across the life course, and it exerts its influence, as indicated by the direct relationship between socioeconomic status (SES) and health status. SES and its influences are greater than income alone. Inherently, SES encompasses social gradient and social networks that dictate place and quality of residence, availability of physical resources, and degree of control over the material environment. Social determinants co-occur, are interactive (Behrman & Butler, 2007), and influence social positioning and access to information, goods, services, and economic opportunities.

Similarly, access to health is also much more than a medical phenomenon. Larsen and Halfon (2009) found that health insurance alone does not account for all disparities. Financial and nonfinancial barriers, such as time constraints and the amounts of co-pay and transportation, may need to be considered. For example, families that receive hourly wages may not have the benefit of medical leave and are unable to schedule medical appointments.

Fundamentally, the problems associated with disparities are "social," such that they are constructed by humans and can be deconstructed by systematic change and attention to specific outcomes. Environmental exposure to toxins is "social" to the extent that human decisions, the distribution of power, and discriminatory practices by institutional and policymakers (who establish levels of exposure) determine the proximity of industries that produce toxic substances from residential communities.

Through advocacy, community education, and empowerment, individuals can collectively take action to affect change on the environments that shape their lives (Table 3.1).

TABLE 3.1   Social Determinants of Low Birth Weight Infant

INDIVIDUAL	INTERPERSONAL	COMMUNITY	SYSTEMS	POLICY
Genetic	Familial	Environmental exposures	Economic systems	Health insurance
Race/ethnicity	Marital relationship	Presence/absence of physical violence	Safe workplace	Expansion of eligibility for medical and support services
Health-related behaviors	Presence/absence of physical violence	Viable community participation in planning and delivery of services	Quality of schools	Funding for preconception and interpregnancy care
Physical health status	Patient–provider relationships	Community empowerment	Health insurance	Safe and equitable workplace
Mental health status	Social support	Social support	Quality health care	
Literacy/ Information seeking	Marital status	Safe and secure food and water sources	Transportation	
Stress		Healthy physical environment	Mental health and addiction services	

PUBLIC HEALTH SOCIAL WORK AND MCH: THE JOURNEY

MCH was a point of convergence for public health and social work. In 1880 (a century prior to the introduction of Healthy People Objectives), the infant mortality rate was 288 per 1,000 live births (Bremner, 1971). The maternal and infant mortality rates were second only to those related to loss of life due to communicable diseases such as TB, diphtheria, and syphilis. Infectious diseases had a direct impact on the health status of women and children.

The first comprehensive analysis of TB in the United States was conducted by social workers in 1903 (Trattner, 1994). Jane Addams, Julia Lathrop, and Edith and Grace Abbott initially employed qualitative research methods as the means to generate data to support social action and policy formulation. With the institution of sanitation practices, control of infectious disease (Starr, 1982), and advances in medical education and the passage of social/health policies, infant mortality rates began to decline. In 1900, the U.S. infant mortality rate was approximately 100 infant deaths per 1,000 live births.

The 20th century was dubbed the "Century of the Child" (Costin, 1985, p. 52). In 1909, children's services exploded onto the national scene as an outcome of the first White House Conference on the Care of Dependent Children. The Children's Bureau (CB) was the brainchild of Lillian Wald, head of the Henry Street Settlement House, in 1903. The establishment of the CB within the Labor Department in 1912 was one of several resulting milestones linked to the White House Conference on Children. The mission of the CB was restricted to the investigation and reporting of information affecting the welfare of children. Homer Folks is credited with strongly suggesting that Julia Lathrop focus on infant and maternal mortality versus child labor issues (Parker & Carpenter, 1981).

The Sheppard-Towner Act of 1921 (also referred to as the Maternity-Infancy Act), initially introduced by Jeanette Rankin of Montana in 1917, was the first legislation to emerge from the work of the CB. Rankin was a social worker and the first woman elected to Congress: her bill failed but was later reintroduced (Pond, 1982). The Sheppard-Towner Act was a federal-state-municipality partnership for the provision of community health services to children, administered by the CB. The act was the outgrowth of statistical data collected by the bureau documenting the state of the child. Demographics, including birth and death registrations, had not been collected, reported, and/or maintained uniformly on a national basis, prior to the CB's creation. The information garnered indicated a positive correlation among poverty, poor health, and infant mortality (Chambers, 1963).

The Sheppard-Towner legislation established clinics, primarily in rural communities, to provide prenatal and postnatal care for all pregnant women. There was neither a means test nor was stigma attached to service utilization (Pond, 1982). With the funds allocated to this program, physician–nurse teams and midwives provided obstetrical care, performed well-child exams, and instructed parents regarding normal growth and development patterns (Costin, 1985). Funding for the Sheppard–Towner Act ended in 1929, but federal fiscal assistance for MCH was subsequently supported by the passage of the Social Security Act (Title V) 1935 and other recent legislation. A number of prominent social workers sat on the committee that formulated the Social Security Act. The U.S. government has continued to invest in maternal child health through programs, such as WIC (a supplemental food program for women, infants, and children), developed in 1972, the Healthy Start Program in 1991, and the federal program providing health insurance to children living below the poverty level, known as SCHIP (the State Children's Health Insurance Program), in 1997 (Alexander, Richman, Rim, & Lane, 2009).

PRACTICE THEORY: THE CONCEPTS

Instrumental to public health social work practice are the principles of social epidemiology and the theory of empowerment. Applying the principles of social epidemiology sets public health social work apart from generalized social work practice. As the leading social epidemiologist Nancy Krieger (2001) suggests, our bodies and consequently our health are affected by our living conditions ranging from lead paint exposure to structural or systemic discrimination. Although this approach is similar to the notion of the Person-In-Environment (Hare, 2004; Karls & Wandrei, 1995) construct often taught in generalized practice, social epidemiology specifically looks at the ramifications of one's environment on one's health. This lens is also referred to as the *socioenvironmental approach*. Regardless of the name, the underlying current in all public health social work interventions is movement toward social justice.

The theory of empowerment lies at the core of all social work practice and social justice. Empowerment is not clearly defined. According to Werner (1988), empowerment is a process whereby individuals or communities work together in an effort to gain control over events and conditions that determine their lives. Empowerment, in the context of public health, implies building upon existing strengths and resources to improve the quality of life of an individual, population, or community. It is important to understand that one person cannot empower another; empowerment is not a gift to be bestowed on another. Empowerment comes from within an individual or community. Social justice is a structural issue that is actualized through changes in social/health policies and attitudes of controlling forces within the larger society.

As one might imagine, empowerment looks different from one community to the next and is dependent on the needs of the at-risk cohort. To be empowered is not a linear function where one moves from Point A to Point B but a process allowing progress and backtracking when needed. Laverack (2004) suggested that there is a continuum of empowerment and cautioned that social workers and other community workers be careful to "check our interpretation of empowerment to ensure it is relevant to the cultural context of the people involved" (p. 13).

A social epidemiological lens, with its push for social justice, broadens the scope of public health social work practice and warrants a focus on micro/individual interventions and macro/societal interventions. Utilizing the theory of empowerment to fuel this spectrum of interventions helps to encourage and facilitate a more cohesive and sustainable community for the mother and her child.

Another fundamental element of public health practice is prevention: primary, secondary, and tertiary. Public health social work engages at all three levels; however, the overall goal is to work toward primary prevention, or the prevention of the development of disease or health conditions. This prevention focus necessitates a multifaceted approach to public health social work, improving social determinants of health to foster equitable distribution of resources and the promotion of health equity.

According to Grason and Guyer (1995), among the essential public health functions to promote MCH in America are to

1. Assess and monitor MCH status to identify and address problems.
2. Diagnose and investigate health problems and health hazards affecting women, children, and youth.
3. Inform and educate the public and families about MCH issues.
4. Mobilize community partnerships among policymakers, health care providers, families, the general public, and others to identify and solve MCH problems.
5. Provide leadership for priority setting, planning, and policy development to support community efforts to assure the health of women, children, youth, and their families.
6. Promote and enforce legal requirements that protect the health and safety of women, children, and youth, and ensure public accountability for their well-being.
7. Link women, children, and youth to health and other community and family services and assure access to comprehensive, quality systems of care.
8. Assure the capacity and competency of the public health and personal health workforce to effectively address MCH needs.

9. Evaluate the effectiveness, accessibility, and quality of personal health and population-based MCH services.
10. Support research and demonstrations to gain new insights and innovative solutions to MCH-related problems.

PUBLIC HEALTH SOCIAL WORK PRACTICE IN MCH: THE PROCESS

The perpetual disparities in infant birth weight, a fundamental barometer of MCH, speak to the pressing need for informed and effective public health social work. As is defined by the World Health Organization (2007, p. 41), health is a state of complete physical, social, and mental well-being, and not merely the absence of disease or infirmity. In other words, health is truly a matter of wellness in mind, body, and spirit. This holistic perception of health warrants an interdisciplinary team of health professionals, including public health social workers, to address the spectrum of needs of individuals and communities. As delineated in the public health social work Standards and Competencies (2005), public health social workers in MCH engage at all levels of public health (micro, mezzo, and macro), with a focus on primary prevention. The role of an MCH public health social worker includes but is not limited to health educator, policy developer, researcher, advocate, consultant, community organizer, and direct service provider.

PERINATAL NETWORKS: CORE FUNCTIONS OF PUBLIC HEALTH: ASSESSMENT AND ASSURANCE

Public health social work in MCH and the above-mentioned key functions are best illustrated by the work and role of Perinatal Networks. Perinatal Networks have been established in numerous states across the country in response to the need of women and children at risk due to poverty. These networks are sponsored by the Department of Health, which offers funding based on the need of the locality while concentrating funding in areas at greatest risk based on rates of LBW, infant mortality, late entry into prenatal care, and teen pregnancy. According to the New York State Department of Health (2003), the purpose of a Perinatal Network is to work at a community level to improve perinatal health, which includes preconception health of women through pregnancy and postpartum care to reduce poor birth outcomes.

Perinatal Networks collaborate with area health care providers to identify gaps in access in their community perinatal services and help to fill those gaps through community outreach, education, and advocacy. As members of an interdisciplinary team, public health social workers are an essential force behind the maintenance, facilitation, and progression of Perinatal Networks; playing vital roles in case management, community outreach, education, and health promotion. As is the case in many social work settings, these various roles are not mutually exclusive and are often combined to best meet the needs of the individual client or subpopulation.

One of the integral functions of a Perinatal Network is to reach out to and draw in mothers most in need of services. As one might imagine, connecting with an at-risk population such as drug-addicted pregnant women is a difficult task. Perinatal networks strive to meet a woman where she is, whether at her church, her beauty shop, or creating a health fair in her neighborhood. Simply providing information about services would be insufficient in engaging a mother at risk. Helping her meet immediate needs, such as food or shelter, will not only improve her well-being and that of her unborn child, it will also help to establish a level of trust. It is often trust that opens the door for a relationship between the client and the worker and may allow the client to feel more inclined to engage in other services. This approach to outreach, often referred to as *enhanced outreach*, differs from outreach of the past, which simply involved canvassing a neighborhood and distributing pamphlets of information.

An approach to engaging and interacting with an at-risk mother in the community that is growing in evidence and popularity is referred to as *Trauma-Informed Care* (TIC; Elliot, Bjelajac, Fallot, Markoff, & Reed, 2005). TIC assumes that each individual has been exposed to trauma in one's lifetime. This concept encourages the worker to consider what has happened to the client and how previous traumatic experiences may be affecting one's current situation. In conjunction with TIC, Solution-Focused Therapy (SFT; Gingerich & Eisengart, 2000) is also being utilized when working with this population. SFT shifts the focus of therapy (or engagement) from what is wrong to what is working. This approach acknowledges strengths and resources in a client and recognizes the client as the true expert in one's life. Both TIC and SFT are not unique to MCH public health social work but are proving helpful in reaching out and empowering young mothers to improve their lives and that of their children.

CURRENT LEGISLATIVE THREATS TO MCH: POLICY DEVELOPMENT

The most recent health care reform, The Patient Protection and Affordable Care Act of 2010, made $1.5 million available to states, tribes, and territories to expand Title V in an effort to develop and implement evidence-based home visiting programs (Association of Maternal Child Health Programs, 2011). Despite the infusion of monies into maternal child home visiting programs and the maintenance of funding to the Maternal Child Health Block

Grant, recent federal budget cuts stripped $504 million from WIC, $660 million from community health centers, and $260 million from biomedical research through the National Institutes of Health (March of Dimes, 2011).

These dramatic cuts in the federal budget directly impact the availability, access, and quality of perinatal, infant, and child health services across the nation. The diminished funds impede research efforts to determine the causes of preterm labor, limit direct services through the loss of social workers and health care providers, and curtail the capacity to reach and serve women and children most in need.

Despite good intentions, it is becoming increasingly difficult for children covered under Medicaid-SCHIP to access some medical and mental health services. Bisgaier and Rhodes (2011) suggested that access to outpatient specialty care is denied more frequently to Medicaid-SCHIP children than those covered by private insurers. In essence, appointments for public versus private pay patients are delayed or not available. The latter reflects the difference in payer reimbursement; Medicaid-SCHIP reimburses at a lower rate than private insurers and requires more paperwork for reimbursement. The reimbursement issue is not a new phenomenon; it merely highlights the continuing need for public health social work to advocate and facilitate the advocacy of other stakeholders on behalf of our youngest and least politically powerful citizens.

EVIDENCE-BASED PUBLIC HEALTH SOCIAL WORK PRACTICE AND NEUROSCIENCE: NEW HORIZONS

The *Merriam-Webster Dictionary* (2011) defines *neuroscience* as a life science focusing on the anatomy, physiology, biochemistry, or molecular biology of nerves and nervous tissue relating to behavior and learning. Neuroscience is opening avenues of knowledge with empirical data regarding the intersection of mind, body, and environment. Evidence-based research permits public health social work to anticipate risks associated with being a LBW or preterm infant and neurobehavioral impairments throughout the life span (Bhutta, Cleves, Casey, Cradock, & Arnand, 2002; Valsmakis, Kanaka-Gantenbein, Malamtisi-Puchner, & Mastorakos, 2006).

Magnetic resonance imaging comparing toddlers (18–24 months of age) born with very LBW and those born full-term indicated that there are regional brain structure differences between the respective groups (Lowe et al., 2011). Previous studies confirmed brain structure differences in adolescents and young adults who were LBW infants in comparison to full-term infants (Narberhaus et al., 2009; Nosarti et al., 2008). Additional data suggest that pain and stress experienced by fetuses in utero and by neonates may be linked to emotional and behavioral differences in childhood and adolescence for LBW or preterm versus full-term infants with average birth weight.

On the basis of available data, public health social workers as members of interdisciplinary teams have successfully initiated multimodal and multisystemic empirically supported interventions (Weissberg, Kumpfer, & Seligman, 2003). The latter includes but is not limited to anticipatory interventions such as early parenting training, community-based prevention programs, and special education in-school services designed to ensure that basic learning skills are available to the aforementioned population of at-risk children and youth.

SUGGESTED LEARNING ACTIVITIES: MCH CHAPTER

1. Social Determinants of Health

Public health social work is a matter of social justice. Public health social workers, in all fields, must consider social determinants of health (SDOH) and where and how to intervene. This exercise will help to raise awareness of the underlying systemic struggles that create and sustain health disparities and help to pinpoint the role of public health social workers in improving SDOH impacting MCH. As a class, list and define what you consider to be the SDOH that affect MCH. Break into small groups and assign each group one or two of the SDOH previously defined. Within the small groups, discuss what the assigned determinants look like within your community. Brainstorm ideas about how, as public health social workers in the field of MCH, you might address improving upon your communities SDOH. Consider the various levels of engagement (micro, mezzo, macro), public health social work roles, and potential community collaborators/stakeholders. (Do not forget the community members themselves!)

2. Defining Empowerment

Empowerment comes in many shapes and sizes and is a process, not a singular action. This exercise will highlight the diversity of empowerment and the importance of thoughtful and collaborative practice with individuals and communities around empowerment in MCH. In preparation for class, ask students to write down their personal definition of empowerment, including what it means to be empowered and how empowerment is achieved. In addition, ask the students to include a case example in which a public health social work practitioner facilitated a client or client system's empowerment process. Provide data that delineate how the practitioner and the client or client system defined and evaluated empowerment. Last, ask students to bring in a peer-reviewed article regarding empowerment that they can incorporate into their practice in MCH. As a class, discuss personal definitions and professional experiences, and create a reference list of journal articles.

3. Evidence-Based Practice in MCH

A public health social worker in MCH wears many hats, including case manager, counselor, health educator, and public policy advocate. Another crucial role, although often understated, is researcher. Not all public health social work will facilitate research, but all social workers can participate in the research process. In preparation for class, ask students to find a peer-reviewed journal article regarding public health social work practice in MCH or to bring in information (program manuals or program evaluation write-ups) from their internship placement or other practice setting. As a class, discuss the relevance of evidence-based practice and brainstorm ways in which students, as practitioners, can become evidence builders in the field. In addition, discuss areas of MCH that are in particular need of evaluation and research and how research may help issues plaguing MCH, such as poor birth outcomes and federal budget cuts in Medicaid. As before, create a reference list for the class in an effort to add to their "toolkit" of practice resources.

4. Health Promotion, Empowerment, and Advocacy

Low-income women of childbearing age who engage in unprotected sex are at risk for pregnancy and the delivery of a LBW/preterm infant. You (a public health social worker) are engaged in community-based health promotion and advocacy.

(a) Develop a fact sheet addressing the threats of LBW/preterm delivery to neonates and infants.
(b) Employing an empowerment framework and cognitive behavioral theory, outline elements of a curriculum for a teen–parent group. The curriculum should target the importance of caring for an LBW/preterm neonate.
(c) Formulate culturally appropriate public service announcements. Be sure that the public service announcement to sexually active women addresses the need for early, regular, and ongoing prenatal care for each and every pregnancy.
(d) Using a social media network, demonstrate how you would disseminate your culturally appropriate messages.

INTERNET RESOURCES

Children's Bureau History

(www.acf.hhs.gov/programs/cb/aboutcb/history_cb_transcript.htm)

March of Dimes: Peristats

(www.marchofdimes.com/peristats/)

Federal Children's Bureau History

(www.larrydewitt.net/SSinGAPE/fedchildren.htm)

FUNCTIONS FRAMEWORK: Essential Public Health Services to Promote Maternal and Child Health in America

(www.jhsph.edu/bin/i/j/pubmchfx.pdf)

Julia Lathrop

(www.nwhm.org/education-resources/biography/biographies/julia-lathrop/)

MCH Timeline: History, Legacy, and Resources for Education and Practice. (2009). Health Resources and Services Administration: Maternal and Child Health Bureau

(http://mchb.hrsa.gov/timeline/index.shtm)

National Center for Education in Maternal and Child Health

(www.ncemch.org/)

World Health Organization

(www.who.int/suggestions/faq/en/)

REFERENCES

Adler, N. E., & Rehkopf, D. H. (2008). U.S. disparities in health: Descriptions, causes, and mechanisms. *Annual Review of Public Health, 29*, 235–252.

Alexander, G., Richman, A. R., Rim, S. H., & Lane, B. M. (2009). *MCH timeline: History, legacy, and resources for education and practice.* HRSA: Maternal and Child Health Bureau. Retrieved from: http://mchb.hrsa.gov/timeline/index.shtml

Association of Maternal and Child Health Programs. (2011). *The Patient Protection and Affordable Care Act: Maternal and child health related highlights.* Retrieved from http://www.amchp.org/Advocacy/healthreform/Documents/Senate%20Bill%20-%20MCH%20Highlights%203%2022%2010.pdf

Behrman, R. E., & Butler, A. S. (Eds.). (2007). *Preterm birth: Causes, consequences, and prevention.* Washington, DC: National Academies Press.

Bhutta, A. T., Cleves, M. A., Casey, P. H., Cradock, M. M., & Arnand, K. J. S. (2002). Cognitive and behavioral outcomes of school-aged children who were born pre-term: A meta-analysis. *Journal of the American Medical Association, 288*(6), 728–737.

Bisgaier, J., & Rhodes, K. V. (2011). Auditing access to specialty care for children with public insurance. *New England Journal of Medicine, 364*(24), 2324–2333.

Bremner, R. H. (1971). *American social history since 1860.* New York: Appleton-Century-Croft.

Center for Health Statistics. (2010). *March of Dimes: Perinatal statistics.* Retrieved from http://www.marchofdimes.com/peristats/level1.aspx?reg=99&top=5&stop=23&lev=1&slev=1&obj=1

Chambers, C. A. (1963). *Seedtime of reform: American social service and social action 1918-1933.* Minneapolis, MN: University of Minnesota Press.

Commission on Social Determinants of Health. (2007). *Achieving health equity: From root causes to fair outcomes: Commission on Social Determinants of Health interim statement.* Geneva, Switzerland: World Health Organization.

Costin, L. B. (1985). The historical context of child welfare. In J. Laird & A. Hartman (Eds.), *A handbook of child welfare: Context, knowledge and practice* (pp. 34–76). New York: Free Press.

Elliot, D. E., Bjelajac, P., Fallot, R. D., Markoff, L. S., & Reed, B. G. (2005). Trauma-informed or trauma-denied: Principles and implementation of trauma-informed services for women. *Journal of Community Psychology, 3*(4), 461–477.

Gingerich, W. J., & Eisengart, S. (2000). Solution-focused brief therapy: A review of the outcome research. *Family Process, 39*(4), 477–498.

Grason, H. A., & Guyer, B. (1995). *Public MCH program functions framework: Essential public health services to promote maternal and child health in America.* Retrieved from http://www.jhsph.edu/bin/i/j/pubmchfx.pdf

Hare, I. (2004). Defining social work for the 21st century. The International Federation of Social Workers' revised definition of social work. *International Social Work, 47,* 407–424.

Hellerstedt, W. L., Pirie, P. L., Lando, H. A., Curry, S. J., McBride, C. M., Grothaus, L. C., et al. (1998). Differences in preconception and prenatal behaviors in women with intended and unintended pregnancies. *American Journal of Public Health, 88,* 663–666.

The Henry J. Kaiser Family Foundation. (2009). *U.S. and global maternal child health fact sheet.* Retrieved from http://www.kff.org/globalhealth/upload/7963-02.PDF

Karls, J. M., & Wandrei, K. E. (1995). Person-in-environment. In R. L. Edwards (Ed.-in-Chief), *Encyclopedia of social work* (19th ed., Vol. 3, pp. 1818–1827). Washington, DC: NASW Press.

Kawachi, I., Daniels, N., & Robinson, D. E. 2005. Health disparities by race and class: Why both matter. *Health Affairs 24,* 343–352.

Krieger, N. (2001). Theories for social epidemiology in the 21st century: An ecosocial perspective. *International Journal of Epidemiology, 30,* 668–677.

Larsen, K., & Halfon, N. (2009). Family income gradients in the health and health care access of US children. *Maternal and Child Health Journal, 14*(3), 332-342.

Laverack, G. (2004). *Health promotion practice: Power and empowerment.* London: Sage Publications.

Lowe, J., Duvall, S. W., Maclean, P. C., Caprihan, A., Ohis, R., Qualls, C., et al. (2011). Comparison of structural magnetic resonance imaging and development in toddlers born very low birth weight and full-term. *Journal of Child Neurology, 26*(5), 586-592.

March of Dimes. (2011). *Working to improve the health of women and children.* Retrieved from http://www.marchofdimes.com/advocacy/actioncenter.html

Marmot, M. (2005). Social determinants of health inequalities. *The Lancet, 365,* 1099-1104.

Martin, K. S., Hamilton, B. E., Sutton, P. D., Ventura, S. J., Mathews, T. J., & Osterman, M. J. (2010). Births: Final data for 2008. *National Vital Statistics Reports, 59*(1), 1-72.

Matthews, T. J., & MacDorman, M. F. (2008). Recent trends in infant mortality in the United States (*NCHS Data Brief,* Number 9). Atlanta, GA: National Center for Health Statistics.

Matthews, T. J., & MacDorman, M. F. (2010). Infant mortality statistics from the 2006 period linked birth/infant death data set. *National Vital Statistics Reports, 58*(17), 1-32.

Merriam-Webster Dictionary. (2011). Retrieved from http://www.merriam-webster.com/dictionary/neuroscience?show=0&t=1308630031

Minkler, M. (1999). Personal responsibility for health? A review of the arguments and the evidence at the century's end. *Health Education and Behavior, 26*(1), 121-140.

Narberhaus, A., Lawrence, E., Allin, M. P., Walshe, M., McGuire, P., Rifkin, L., et al. (2009). Neural substrates of visual paired associates in young adults who were born very young pre-term birth: Alternations in fronto-parieto-occipital networks and caudate nucleus. *Neuroimage, 47,* 1904-1913.

New York State Department of Health. (2003). *Comprehensive prenatal–perinatal services network.* Retrieved from http://www.health.state.ny.us/community/pregnancy/health_care/prenatal/comprehensive_services_network/

Nosarti, C., Giouroukou, E., Healy, E., Rifkin, L., Walshe, M., Reichenberg, A., et al. (2008). Grey and white matter distribution in very preterm adolescents mediates neurodevelopmental outcome. *Brain, 131,* 205-217.

Parker, K. J. K., & Carpenter, K. E. M. (1981). Julia Lathrop and the Children's Bureau: The emergence of an institution. *Social Service Review, 55*(1), 60-77.

Pond, M. A. (1982). Block grants for health: A brief history of presidential initiatives. *Health Policy Quarterly, 2*(3/4), 180-198.

Public health social work practice project at the UNC School of Social Work. (2005). *Public health social work standards and competencies.* Columbus, OH: Ohio Department of Health. Retrieved March 5, 2012, from http://oce.sph.unc.edu/cetac/phswcompetencies_May05.pdf.

Starr, P. (1982). *The social transformation of American medicine: The rise of a sovereign profession and the making of a vast industry.* New York: Basic Books.

Trattner, W. I. (1994). *From poor law to welfare state: A history of social welfare in America* (5th ed.). New York: Free Press.

Valsmakis, G., Kanaka-Gantenbein, C., Malamtisi-Puchner, A., & Mastorakos, G. (2006). Causes of intrauterine growth restriction and the postnatal development of the metabolic syndrome. *Annals of the New York Academy of Sciences, 1092*, 138–147.

Weissberg, R. P., Kumpfer, K. L., & Seligman, M. E. P. (2003). Prevention that works for children and youth. *American Psychologist, 58*(6/7), 425–432.

Werner, D. (1988). Empowerment and health. Contact. *Christian Medical Commission, 102*, 1–9.

Wilkinson, R., & Marmot, M. (Eds.). (2003). *Social determinants of health: The solid facts* (2nd ed.). Copenhagen, Denmark: International Centre for Health and Society, WHO Regional Office for Europe.

Williams, D. R., & Collins, C. (2001). Racial residential segregation: A fundamental cause of racial disparities. *Public Health Reports, 116*, 404–416.

World Bank. (2009). *World development indicators*. Retrieved from http://data.world bank.org/indicator/SP.DYN.IMRT.IN

World Health Organization (2007). Commission of social determinants of health conceptual framework for action on social determinants of health. Retrieved from http://www.who.int/social_determinants/resources/csdh_framework_action_05_07.pdf.

CHAPTER 4

Adolescent Health

William J. Hall and Kathleen Rounds

INTRODUCTION

*A*dolescence is a particularly important transitional period for healthy development. During this period, youth begin to establish not only their self-identity, but also patterns of behavior that affect current and future health status. Many health conditions occurring in adolescence develop into chronic health problems during adulthood (e.g., obesity and type 2 diabetes). Also, the leading causes of death for adolescents (i.e., motor vehicle accidents, homicide, and suicide) are highly preventable. Therefore, in terms of public health interventions, adolescence is an opportune time not only to address the health problems that youth face, but also to prevent the onset of diseases and disorders that plague many Americans in their adulthood.

Although adolescence is generally a healthy period of life, a number of health problems begin, peak, or escalate during this period including obesity, unplanned pregnancy, sexually transmitted diseases (STDs), bullying and violence, psychological disorders, suicide, substance use, and motor vehicle injury. Adolescence is a vulnerable period of development for many youth. National mortality data show that from early adolescence (aged 10–14) to young adulthood (aged 20–24), the mortality rate increased by more than 400% (Xu, Kochanek, Murphy, & Teiada-Vera, 2010).

In this chapter, we provide an overview of major risks to adolescent health. Because adolescent health is significantly influenced by social and environmental factors, including family, peers, school, community, and culture, we examine health conditions emphasizing context. We also present the *Healthy People 2020* objectives that relate to youth for each health issue and discuss adolescent health disparities. We use a case study to illustrate how a public health social worker could use the core public health functions of assessment, policy development, and assurance to address an adolescent health problem at the community level. Finally, we conclude with a brief discussion of several emerging issues for public health social work practice with adolescents.

AN OVERVIEW OF MAJOR ADOLESCENT HEALTH PROBLEMS

Assessment, one of the core public health functions, requires that public health social workers understand the epidemiology of health problems and be able to identify protective and risk factors associated with these problems. The following section provides an overview of major adolescent health problems that public health social workers are likely to address in their practice with adolescents.

Overweight and Obesity

The proportion of adolescents who are overweight or obese has increased dramatically in recent decades and represents a serious public health threat for the 21st century. Since the late 1960s, the proportion of obese adolescents in the United States has more than tripled (Ogden & Carroll, 2010). Overweight is defined as a body mass index (BMI) at or above the 85th percentile and lower than the 95th percentile, and obesity is defined as a BMI at or above the 95th percentile for youth of the same age and sex (Barlow & Expert Committee, 2007). Recent national findings evidence that 16% of adolescents aged 12 to 19 are overweight, and an additional 18% are obese (Ogden, Carroll, Curtin, Lamb, & Flegal, 2010). Obesity can negatively affect youth in several ways as obese youth are more likely to have high blood pressure, high cholesterol, impaired glucose tolerance, type 2 diabetes, sleep apnea, asthma, bone and joint problems, fatty liver disease, gallstones, heartburn, and low self-esteem (Han, Lawlor, & Kimm, 2010). Obese youth are also more likely to be obese during adulthood (Biro & Wien, 2010).

Eating and drinking habits involving high-calorie, low-nutrient foods, as well as sedentary lifestyles, contribute to overweight and obesity. According to a national survey of dietary and activity behaviors, almost 30% of youth drank a nondiet soda at least once per day (Centers for Disease Control and Prevention [CDC], 2010). Additionally, 78% of youth did not eat fruits and/or vegetables 5 or more times per day. Likewise, 63% of youth did not engage in 60 minutes of physical activity per day for most days of the week (CDC, 2010). Conversely, adolescents spent an average of 7 hours and 38 minutes a day watching television, playing video games, using a computer, and talking on the phone (Rideout, Foehr, & Roberts, 2010).

Environmental factors play a role in adolescent obesity. Youth from low-income families and neighborhoods are at greater risk for obesity as healthy foods and opportunities for physical activity require financial resources (Lee, Harris, & Gordon-Larsen, 2009). Moreover, many youth live in neighborhoods without sidewalks, trails, parks, and recreation centers for physical activity (Singh, Siahpush, & Kogan, 2010). Likewise, only 22% of middle schools and 9% of high schools provided 45 minutes of physical education each day for at least 18 weeks of the school year (Lee, Burgeson, Fulton, & Spain, 2007). Similarly, only 4% of states required schools offer multiple servings of fruit and nonfried vegetables during lunch; 14% of states required that schools limit the availability of deep-fried foods; and 18% of states required that schools make healthy beverages, such as water or low-fat milk, available to students (O'Toole, Anderson, Miller, & Guthrie, 2007). Finally, portion sizes in vending machines, restaurants, grocery stores, and homes have increased significantly in recent decades (Rolls, 2003).

The *Healthy People 2020* objectives to reduce adolescent obesity and overweight focus on improving diet via more fruits, vegetables, and whole grains, as well as less fat and added sugar (U.S. Department of Health and Human Services [DHHS], 2011). In addition, the objectives encourage more physical activity and muscle strengthening exercise, daily school-based physical education, and limited sedentary screen time.

Sexual and Reproductive Health Issues

Puberty, sexual identity development, and the expression of sexual feelings are hallmarks of adolescence. Rates of sexual activity increase significantly during adolescence. A national survey of high school students found that approximately 20% of 9th graders reported having sexual intercourse, whereas 50% of 12th graders reported having sexual intercourse (CDC, 2010). The median age at first sexual intercourse is 17 (Alan Guttmacher Institute, 2002).

Sexual behavior during adolescence can have lifelong implications in terms of pregnancy and STDs. Risky sexual behaviors include having unprotected sex, not using contraception, having multiple sexual partners, and using alcohol or drugs before sex. Among sexually active high school students, nearly 40% did not use a condom during last sexual intercourse, and 80% had not used birth control pills before last sexual intercourse (CDC, 2010). In addition, 21% of 12th graders had sexual intercourse with four or more partners (CDC, 2010). Though abstinence from sexual intercourse is the only 100% effective way to prevent pregnancy and STDs, research concludes that approximately 90% of youth have had sexual intercourse by the time they reach adulthood (aged 22–24; Mosher, Chandra, & Jones, 2005).

A sexually active female adolescent who is not using contraception has a 90% chance of getting pregnant (Harlap, Kost, & Forrest, 1991).

The unintended pregnancy rate is higher among adolescents than other age groups (Finer & Henshaw, 2006). Approximately 34% of female youth become pregnant before they reach age 20 (Henshaw, 2003). Teenage pregnancy is a problem because adolescent parents are often emotionally and financially unprepared for parenthood. Adolescent pregnancy and childbirth are linked to poor outcomes, such as inadequate prenatal care, low birth weight, single parenthood, poverty, and child maltreatment and neglect (Martin et al., 2010).

Researchers found that a majority of sexually active adolescents reported using some method of contraception at first sexual intercourse (79% for female adolescents and 87% for male adolescents) and at last sexual intercourse (84% for female adolescents and 93% for male adolescents; Abma, Martinez, & Copen, 2010). Methods of contraception varied as 95% of sexually experienced adolescents used condoms, 58% used withdrawal, 55% used the birth control pill, 17% used hormonal contraceptive injections, 17% used the calendar rhythm method, 11% used the transdermal contraceptive patch, 11% used the morning-after pill, and 7% used the vaginal contraceptive ring (Abma et al., 2010). In reality, most unintended teenage pregnancies occur because of inconsistent or incorrect use of contraception. Researchers found that the decline in the adolescent pregnancy rate since the 1990s was primarily due to increasing and consistent use of effective contraceptives as well as usage of multiple methods of contraception (e.g., condoms and birth control pills; Santelli, Lindberg, Finer, & Singh, 2007). Delaying sexual activity accounted for a small proportion of the reduction in adolescent pregnancy.

Adolescents are also disproportionately affected by STDs. Researchers have estimated that there are about 19 million new STD infections each year in the United States, and about half of them are among youth (Weinstock, Berman, & Cates, 2004). The most common STDs among youth are human papillomavirus (HPV), trichomoniasis, chlamydia, herpes, gonorrhea, HIV, syphilis, herpes, and hepatitis (Weinstock et al., 2004). STDs often go undiagnosed as many infections are asymptomatic. Nonetheless, infections can still be spread despite the absence of symptoms.

Adolescents are at increased risk of acquiring STDs because of barriers to accessing sexual and reproductive health services, including counseling on risky sexual behavior, contraception and STD prevention services, and STD testing (Rounds, 2004). Barriers to accessing care are due to lack of health insurance coverage, inability to pay, lack of transportation, discomfort with facilities and services designed for adults, fear of seeking care, concerns about confidentiality, and lack of information about services available (Hock-Long, Herceg-Baron, Cassidy, & Whittaker, 2003). In addition, female adolescents are at higher risk for certain STDs because of physiologically increased susceptibility to infection.

Schools play a major role in adolescent sexual and reproductive health. While almost all adolescents in the United States receive formal sex education before 18 years of age, 32% had not received instruction on methods of contraception, 7% had not been taught about STDs, and 11% had not learned how to prevent HIV/AIDS (Martinez, Abma, & Copen, 2010). A national survey of school-based health education courses found that 76% of middle schools and 87% of high schools taught abstinence as the most effective way to avoid pregnancy, HIV, and other STDs; 42% of middle schools and 65% of high schools taught about condom efficacy; and 21% of middle schools and 39% of high schools taught how to use a condom (Kann, Telljohann, & Wooley, 2007). Most schools do not provide sexual and reproductive health services, and only 5% of high schools made condoms available to students (Jones, Purcell, Singh, & Finer, 2005).

The *Healthy People 2020* objectives to reduce the adolescent pregnancy rate focus on increasing access to sexual/reproductive health care services, abstinence among adolescents, use of condoms and hormonal or intrauterine contraception, receipt of formal education on reproductive health, and discussion of sexual/reproductive health topics with parents or caregivers (DHHS, 2011). The STD objectives aim at reducing youth infections of chlamydia, pelvic inflammatory disease, gonorrhea, HPV, and herpes. Finally, the objectives to reduce HIV/AIDS among adolescents relate to increasing usage of condoms, encouraging testing for HIV, and increasing receipt of health care and treatment for adolescents with HIV.

Bullying and Violence

Youth violence involves a range of harmful behaviors, such as harassment and homicide, which can result in physical injury, psychological distress, and death. Youth are most frequently victimized by their peers. According to data from the National Survey on Health Youth Risk Behavior Survey, 20% of high school students reported being bullied at school, and 5% missed at least one day of school in the past month because they felt unsafe (CDC, 2010). Bullying or harassing behaviors can be physical (e.g., hitting or pushing), verbal (e.g., name calling or threatening), social/relational (e.g., spreading rumors or excluding others), or sexual (e.g., unwanted touching or offensive gesturing). One of the fastest growing forms of bullying is cyberbullying, in which electronic communication technologies such as e-mail, instant messaging, text messaging, and websites are used to harm others (Kowalski, Limber, & Agatston, 2008).

Violence-related behaviors are not confined to schools. Approximately one-third of youth had been in a physical fight in the past year, and 4% of these youth required medical attention (CDC, 2010). In 2009, over

650,000 youth aged 10 to 24 were treated in emergency departments in the United States for injuries caused by violence (National Center for Injury Prevention and Control [NCIPC], 2010). Injuries due to violence frequently involve weapons. Approximately 18% of youth reported carrying a weapon such as a gun or knife at least once in the past month (CDC, 2010). Homicide due to gun violence ranks as the second leading cause of death among adolescents (NCIPC, 2010).

Research demonstrates that environmental factors associated with youth violence include family, peer, school, and community factors (DHHS, 2001; Resnick, Ireland, & Borowsky, 2004). Family risk factors include low parental socioeconomic status, poor family functioning, low parental involvement and attachment, and exposure to family conflict and violence. Being socially rejected by peers, associating with delinquent peers, and gang involvement are also risk factors for violence. Educational risk factors include low academic achievement and school failure. Youth living in socially disorganized neighborhoods, high poverty communities, and areas with limited economic opportunities are at increased risk for violent behavior.

The *Healthy People 2020* objectives related to youth violence focus on improving school safety as well as reducing bullying, fighting, and weapon-carrying (DHHS, 2011). Because youth who are lesbian, gay, bisexual, transgender, or queer (LGBTQ) are frequently harassed, one objective advocates that schools prohibit bullying and harassment based on sexual orientation and gender identity.

Mental Health Problems

Adolescence is a stressful stage with many psychosocial challenges. Although most youth are able to successfully navigate these challenges and effectively cope, many others experience mental health disorders. Lifetime prevalence data from a nationally representative survey showed that 28% of adolescents aged 13 to 18 had a mental health disorder that severely impaired functioning (Merikangas et al., 2010). Psychological disorders rank as the most costly health problem among youth in the United States (Soni, 2009). If left untreated, mental health problems can lead to school failure, violence, juvenile incarceration, family dysfunction, social isolation, and suicide. Mental health disorders that are of special concern during adolescence include depression, suicide, anxiety, eating disorders, attention-deficit/hyperactivity disorder (ADHD), disruptive behavior disorders, and schizophrenia.

Depression

Many youth experience some symptoms of depression. However, depression is not a normal part of adolescents' psychological experience. Research shows that 12% of adolescents aged 13 to 18 experienced a depressive disorder (Merikangas et al., 2010). The age of onset for adolescent depression ranges from 11 to 14 years, and rates of depression increase significantly from early to late adolescence (Lewinsohn, Rohde, & Seeley, 1998; Merikangas et al., 2010). The course of depressive disorders varies; some youth may only experience one episode of major depression, while others experience chronic low-grade depression or recurrent depressive episodes into adulthood.

Suicide

Mental illness is the leading risk factor for youth suicide, with depressive disorders being the most common (Achilles, Gray, & Moskos, 2004). Data indicate that between early adolescence (aged 10–14) and young adulthood (aged 20–24) the suicide rate increased by 10-fold (NCIPC, 2010). Data from the CDC's Youth Risk Behavior Surveillance 2009 study found that approximately 14% of high school aged adolescents had seriously considered attempting suicide (CDC, 2010). In 2009, over 130,000 youth aged 10 to 24 intentionally harmed themselves to the point that they needed medical attention (NCIPC, 2010). Suicide is the third leading cause of death for youth (NCIPC, 2010).

Anxiety disorders

Momentary experiences of fear, worry, shyness, nervousness, and anxiety are normal during adolescence; however, excessive and debilitating anxiety is a symptom of an anxiety disorder. Anxiety disorders are the most prevalent mental health problem among adolescents; 32% of youth aged 13 to 18 have an anxiety disorder (Merikangas et al., 2010). The most common anxiety disorders among adolescents include a specific phobia (e.g., fear of heights), social anxiety disorder, separation anxiety disorder, and posttraumatic stress disorder. Most cases of anxiety disorders during adolescence began during childhood and often persist into adulthood, as anxiety disorders tend to be chronic.

Eating disorders

The average age of onset for eating disorders (i.e., anorexia and bulimia) occurs during late adolescence (Hudson, Hiripi, Pope, & Kessler, 2007). Research also shows that 3% of youth aged 13 to 18 have an eating disorder, and female youth are disproportionally affected (Merikangas et al., 2010). If left untreated, eating disorders can become chronic and pose serious threats to health and well-being. Anorexia has the highest mortality rate of any psychological disorder (Hudson et al., 2007).

ADHD

ADHD is often viewed as a childhood disorder; however, a majority of youth diagnosed with ADHD in childhood will continue to meet diagnostic criteria into adolescence (Wolraich et al., 2005). ADHD is characterized by (1) inattention, poor concentration, and disorganization, and/or (2) hyperactivity and impulsive behavior. A nationally representative survey reported that 9% of youth aged 13 to 18 had ADHD (Merikangas et al., 2010).

Although most mental health disorders entail a genetic predisposition, environmental stressors often trigger their onset. Environmental risk factors for adolescent mental health problems include family, peer, school, and situational factors (DHHS, 2000a). Family risk factors include family dysfunction and conflict, poor parent–child relationship, parental history of psychopathology or criminality, and coming from a low socioeconomic background. Peer and school risk factors include bullying or peer harassment, peer rejection, association with delinquent peers, frequent change in school, and low academic achievement. Exposure to traumatic and/or acute stressful life events, such as the death of a family member or friend, divorce, child abuse/maltreatment, exposure to violence, and natural disasters also put youth at risk for mental illness.

The *Healthy People 2020* objectives related to adolescent mental health problems aim at reducing depressive episodes, disordered eating behavior, and suicide attempts (DHHS, 2011).

Substance Use

Experimentation with alcohol, tobacco, and drugs is fairly common among adolescents. However, while some youth only experiment with or occasionally use various substances, others use substances on a regular basis and may develop dependence or addiction. Rates of drinking alcohol, smoking cigarettes, and using illicit drugs more than double between 8th and 12th grade (Johnston, O'Malley, Bachman, & Schulenberg, 2011). Indeed, substance use rates climb dramatically during adolescence and peak between late adolescence and early adulthood (aged 18 to 25; Substance Abuse and Mental Health Services Administration [SAMHSA], 2008).

Alcohol

Alcohol is the most commonly used substance among adolescents. According to a national survey of high school aged youth, 73% had drunk alcohol and 24% reported binge drinking (i.e., consumed five or more drinks of alcohol during a single occasion; CDC, 2010). Alcohol use among youth is associated with accidental injuries, academic problems, delinquency, and violence (SAMHSA, 1999).

Tobacco

Every day in the United States, about 4,000 adolescents try their first cigarette (SAMHSA, 2007). Among high school students, 46% had tried cigarette smoking, 14% had smoked cigars, and 9% had used smokeless tobacco (i.e., chewing tobacco, snuff, or dip; CDC, 2010). Youth make up the largest proportion of new smokers, and the younger people begin smoking, the more likely they are to become addicted to nicotine (DHHS, 2000b).

Drugs

Many adolescents experiment with and use drugs. Marijuana is the most commonly used illicit drug among youth. Among high school aged youth, 37% had used marijuana, 7% had used ecstasy, 6% had used cocaine, 4% had used methamphetamines, 3% had used heroin, and 3% had used steroids not for medical reasons (CDC, 2010). Nearly one-quarter (23%) of high school students were offered, sold, or given illegal drugs by someone at school (CDC, 2010). While rates of illicit drug use among youth have dropped slightly in the past decade, illicit use of prescription drugs increased slightly (Johnston et al., 2011). Approximately 15% of adolescents reported that they had used a prescription drug without a doctor's permission. The most commonly abused prescription medications among youth include pain relievers, sedatives, tranquilizers, amphetamines, narcotics, stimulants, and depressants. Adolescents also misuse over-the-counter medications, such as cold and cough medicines (National Institute on Drug Abuse, 2005).

The *Healthy People 2020* objectives related to adolescent drug use aim at reducing use of illicit drugs, prescription drugs, steroids, and inhalants as well as broadening perceptions about the risks of substance abuse and increasing disapproval of substance abuse among adolescents (DHHS, 2011). The alcohol objectives focus on reducing binge drinking and riding with drivers who had been drinking. The tobacco-related goals for adolescents intend to reduce tobacco use, initiation of tobacco use, exposure to secondhand smoke, exposure to tobacco advertisements, and sale of tobacco products to minors. Objectives concerning schools advocate for tobacco-free schools and reducing drug exchanges at school.

Motor Vehicle Injury

Motor vehicle accidents are the leading cause of death for adolescents (NCIPC, 2010). The risk of having a motor vehicle accident is higher among adolescents than any other age group (Insurance Institute for

Highway Safety [IIHS], 2009). In 2009, over 430,000 youth aged 15 to 20 were treated in emergency departments in the United States for injuries caused by motor vehicle accidents (NCIPC, 2010). In addition, recent mortality data indicate that every day in the United States there are about a dozen motor vehicle-related deaths among adolescents.

High rates of motor vehicle injury among youth are attributed to lack of driving experience and lack of maturity. Adolescents' lack of driving experience makes it difficult for them to recognize, assess, and respond to dangerous or hazardous situations (McCartt, Mayhew, Braitman, Ferguson, & Simpson, 2009). The risk of motor vehicle crash is particularly high during the first months that adolescents are licensed to drive (Mayhew, Simpson, & Pak, 2003; McCartt, Shabanova, & Leaf, 2003). Peer influences are also significant: Research shows that the presence of other adolescent passengers increases the risk of motor vehicle accident, and risk increases with the number of adolescent passengers (Chen, Baker, Braver, & Li, 2000). Finally, motor vehicle–related injury and death among youth are highest during the summer months, the weekend (Friday, Saturday, and Sunday), and nighttime (6:00 p.m. to 3:00 a.m.; IIHS, 2009).

Risky driving behaviors are also associated with motor vehicle accidents. Compared to other age groups, adolescents have the lowest rate of seat belt use; in one survey, 20% of drivers aged 16 to 24 were observed not wearing a seat belt (National Highway Traffic Safety Administration [NHTSA], 2009). Similarly, 10% of high school-aged youth never or rarely wore a seat belt when riding in a car (CDC, 2010). Adolescent drivers are also more likely to speed and tailgate (McCartt et al., 2009). Emerging research on distracted driving among youth showed that cell phone use increased the likelihood of motor vehicle injury (Neyens & Boyle, 2008), and 82% of adolescent drivers surveyed reported driving while using a cell phone (Allstate Foundation, 2009). There is also a strong connection between alcohol use and motor vehicle injury. In 2009, approximately one-quarter of adolescent drivers aged 15 to 20 involved in fatal car crashes had been drinking alcohol (NHTSA, 2011).

The *Healthy People 2020* objectives related to motor vehicle accidents intend to reduce injuries and deaths as well as increase use of restraints (DHHS, 2011). The objectives also advocate for effective statewide graduated drivers' licensing programs.

Comorbidity

Health risk behaviors and problematic outcomes are not isolated phenomena in the lives of adolescents. Researchers have demonstrated the interrelatedness of many adolescent health problems. For example, adolescent obesity is associated with both depression and oppositional defiant disorder (Mustillo et al., 2003). Risky sexual behavior among youth is associated with psychological problems and substance use (Elkington, Bauermeister, & Zimmerman, 2010). Approximately 22% of sexually active youth had used alcohol or drugs before last sexual intercourse (CDC, 2010). There are also relationships between violence and sexual/reproductive health. For one, sexual assault is a form of violence, and 11% of young women and 5% of young men reported that they had been forced to have sexual intercourse (CDC, 2010). Violence also often occurs in the context of a romantic relationship, as 10% of youth reported that their boyfriend or girlfriend had physically abused them (CDC, 2010). Youth violence is associated with psychological problems, risky sexual behavior, substance use, and risky driving behavior (DHHS, 2001). The co-occurrence of mental health disorders and substance use is also common. It is also not uncommon for youth to have co-occurring psychological disorders, as 40% of adolescents with a psychological disorder reported more than one class of disorder (Merikangas et al., 2010). Finally, the causal relationship between substance use and motor vehicle injury is substantial. Understanding the relationships among adolescent health problems and shared risk factors will assist public health social workers in the development of comprehensive and effective prevention and intervention programs.

ADOLESCENT HEALTH DISPARITIES

Health disparities are significant differences in health risk factors, rates of disease prevalence, and mortality among population groups. These disparities may vary by many factors. By understanding health disparities, public health social workers can design and target interventions that are evidence based and culturally appropriate for those who are most at risk.

Although biological factors may account for some differences in health conditions for certain population groups, the socioecological systems model emphasizes understanding the interactions among individual and environmental factors in determining health status. Health disparities among minority groups, including racial/ethnic minorities, women, sexual minorities, and gender minorities may be due to sociocultural forces such as historical and continuing patterns of disenfranchisement and institutional discrimination. Minority groups not only systems of oppression not only at the societal level, such as racism, ethnocentrism, classism, sexism, and heterosexism, but also prejudice, biases, and stereotypical assumptions held by individuals, including health providers. In addition, the stress of belonging to a socially stigmatized group may affect well-being.

American Indians, African Americans, and Hispanic/Latino Americans are disproportionately at risk for obesity, STDs, teen pregnancy and childbirth, violence, mental health problems, substance use, and motor vehicle injury. Many of these youth live in communities with few resources but numerous environmental hazards. Disparate health outcomes exist for refugee and immigrant youth, which may be due to stressful migration journeys, acculturation, citizenship status, poverty, and lack of culturally sensitive services.

Differences in health outcomes among population groups are often mediated by socioeconomic status. Youth from families and communities with low socioeconomic status likely have more limited access to health insurance, preventive services, and treatment. In addition, the stress associated with living in poverty and in unsafe and hazardous environments likely threatens well-being.

In terms of gender, young women are disproportionately at risk for sexual and reproductive health issues, as well as internalizing psychological problems. This may be due to sociocultural gender stereotypes. On the other hand, male youth experience disparate levels of violence, externalizing psychological problems, and motor vehicle injury, which may be due to higher levels of risk taking among male youth and sociocultural gender expectations.

Geographic differences in health outcomes also exist which may be related to regional culture or to state-level policies and programs. For example, youth living in rural and urban areas often experience more health problems than their suburban counterparts. These disparities may be attributed to poverty, environmental hazards, and barriers to accessing health care services. Health disparities exist among states as well as geographic regions (i.e., the North, South, Midwest, and West), which may be due to state-level policies and programs impacting health as well as sociocultural factors. Indeed, one's culture has a significant influence on health in terms of sociocultural ideals and preferences, as well as normative behaviors and activities.

PUBLIC HEALTH SOCIAL WORK PRACTICE IN ADDRESSING ADOLESCENT HEALTH PROBLEMS

Public health social workers use a preventive, evidence-based, socioecological systems approach to develop, deliver, and evaluate interventions at the program, community, and policy levels to address adolescent health problems. This approach aligns with the core public health functions of assessment, policy development, and assurance (Institute of Medicine, 2002). In order to fulfill these functions, public health social workers perform the following services (Core Public Health Functions Steering Committee, 1994): (1) monitor, identify, and investigate community health problems; (2) mobilize community partnerships to understand and solve health problems; (3) advocate for policies that promote health and well-being; (4) provide health services and implement intervention programs; (5) promote access to health care services; (6) inform, educate, and empower individuals, groups, and communities about health issues; and (7) evaluate the efficacy, accessibility, compatibility, and quality of health services, programs, and policies. Social workers participating in core public health functions need to master a range of competencies. These include having knowledge and skills in collecting, analyzing, and interpreting epidemiology and other data; designing and conducting needs assessments; program planning, implementation, and evaluation; and critically assessing the impact of policies and developing and advocating for policies that promote the health of the public. Equally important are competencies in leading, partnering, and communicating with multiple disciplines and community stakeholders, working in a culturally competent manner, and building coalitions among diverse groups. Public health social workers are guided in their practice by the National Association of Social Workers' Code of Ethics and the American Public Health Association Creed.

The following case study illustrates how a social worker could use the public health social workers standards and competencies to actualize core public health functions to address teen pregnancy. Discussion questions are listed at the end of the case study. A number of websites that provide current data and statistics on adolescent health as well as effective, evidence-based health interventions for youth are listed in Appendix B at the end of this book.

Case Study

The health director at the Sunny County public health department has asked the lead public health social worker to develop a project to address the county's teen pregnancy problem. The county reportedly has one of the highest teen pregnancy rates in the state. To initiate this project the public health social worker examines the most recent teen pregnancy statistics for the county and finds that in 2010 there were 110 pregnancies for every 1,000 young women aged 15 to 19, that the county had the third highest teen pregnancy rate in the state, and that the rate has been trending upward. Through her initial fact finding, she discovers that for the past 3 years, the county public health department has missed the opportunity to apply for and receive $225,000 of funding ($75,000 per year) from the state department of health and human services. These grants could have been used for pregnancy prevention awareness campaigns, as well as programs to deliver direct services to prevent teenage pregnancy. In addition, she learns that the school district for the county has an abstinence-only until marriage sex education policy.

The public health social worker creates a teen pregnancy prevention task force composed of colleagues at the health department and community stakeholders who provide services to teens. She contacts a number of community-based organizations that work with teens to ask for representatives to serve on the task group. These organizations include a youth development organization serving at-risk teens, a nonprofit organization that provides family planning and reproductive health care services, parent–teacher associations and the school board, the department of social services, the local association of family and pediatric physicians, and faith-based organizations in the area. The group is tasked with investigating the problem and developing a plan for reducing adolescent pregnancy in the county. The public health social worker's role is to facilitate meetings, staff the task force, and keep the health department director and board updated on the group's findings and progress.

In the initial meetings of the task force, members produce a plan to systematically collect data to better understand the underlying risk factors contributing to the rate of teen pregnancy, as well as protective factors that may prevent teen pregnancy in their community. The task force decides to conduct a needs and resource assessment with the community. Given the resources available and the sensitive nature of the problem, the task force decides to design a series of focus groups composed of stakeholders to assess needs and resources. For maximum participation, stakeholders are invited to attend groups based on commonality (e.g., there is a focus group for youth, one for parents, one for educators, health care providers). Participants in the focus groups are asked about their concerns regarding the high teen pregnancy rate; the effects of teen pregnancy on teens, families, and their community; their theories about causes of the high teen pregnancy rate; ideas as to how to reduce the teen pregnancy rate; and strengths and resources in the community for designing interventions to address this problem.

Following the conclusion of the focus groups, the public health social worker analyzes and summarizes the data and presents them to the task force. After several meetings, during which the task force members discuss and interpret the findings, the public health social worker leads the group in identifying intervention targets. The task force members decide to focus on advocating for changes in policy on sex education in the schools, developing a community awareness campaign, and seeking funds for a pilot program targeted at teens at high risk for becoming pregnant. Because the task force has identified the school district's outmoded abstinence-only sex education policy as one of the risk factors, the public health social worker researches laws and policies related to school-based sex education in the state. She contacts the statewide adolescent pregnancy prevention coalition to learn about existing efforts to advocate for comprehensive sex education policies for schools. She invites the coalition to meet with the task force to present available resources for a community awareness campaign and to discuss ways that the two groups might partner to maximize resources.

The public health social worker researches and identifies effective, feasible, and compatible evidence-based program interventions to prevent adolescent pregnancy, which she presents to the group. To identify intervention programs, the public health social worker searches a number of websites cataloging effective adolescent pregnancy prevention programs: Advocates for Youth, National Campaign to Prevent Teen and Unplanned Pregnancy, Teen Pregnancy Prevention Programs for Replication, and Resource Center for Adolescent Pregnancy Prevention. The public health social worker facilitates meetings and works with the task force to come to a group consensus concerning programmatic recommendations for implementation.

After considering several intervention programs, the task group decides that a community-based health center intervention that is educational, behavioral, and psychosocial would be best for the county given the nature of the community, resources available, and level of intervention. The public health social worker recommends adapting the program slightly so that it is developmentally and culturally appropriate for the target population in the county. The task force decides to implement the program as a pilot for 1 year, with the possibility of extension if it is feasible and effective. Once the task force has agreed upon an approach, the public health social worker takes the lead in writing a teen pregnancy prevention grant proposal to obtain funding from the state department of health and human services. If funded, the public health social worker will take the lead in coordinating the design, implementation, and evaluation of the program. This will involve extensive partnering with community partners and stakeholders, many of whom serve on the task force or have been involved in the initial focus groups.

Questions for Discussion:

1. Identify the core public health functions and services that the public health social worker in the above case is involved in providing.
2. What public health social workers competencies (knowledge, skills, and values) does the public health social worker need to successfully engage the community in addressing the rising teen pregnancy rates in the county?

3. Select another adolescent health issue discussed in this chapter. Using websites listed at the end of the chapter, describe the prevalence of the problem nationally and in your geographic area. Are there disparities among groups in the prevalence of this problem? If so, describe what they are. What *Healthy People 2020* objectives address this problem? If you were the public health social worker assigned to address this problem in your community, what steps would you take? Be specific in identifying community stakeholders that you would involve and how you would partner with these groups; how you would collect data to adequately describe the problem and the risk and protective factors associated with the problem; and sources for evidence-based interventions at the policy, community, and programmatic level.

EMERGING ISSUES IN ADOLESCENT HEALTH

There are a number of unfolding issues that will affect adolescent health in the coming decades. Unlike previous generations, today's youth are growing up in a media-saturated age. While traditional forms of media (i.e., television, video games, movies, and magazines) will continue to influence adolescents, newer forms of media (i.e., smartphones and the Internet) increasingly play a major role in the everyday lives of youth in the United States. These technologies will affect the physical, mental, social, and sexual health of adolescents. In terms of health promotion, public health social workers can use these technologies to provide health education and to design interventions that are innovative and appealing to youth.

The adolescent population is also becoming increasingly diverse, underscoring the importance of culturally competent health professionals and interventions. According to population projections, Hispanic/Latino, African American, Asian, and multicultural populations will increase their proportions of the total population in the coming decades (U.S. Census Bureau, 2008). In addition, the decrease in sexual stigma in the United States has corresponded with more youth coming out as LGBTQ. Also, research findings report that the average age of coming out as gay or lesbian has fallen in recent decades, from 16 to 21 years of age (Savin-Williams, 2006). Recently, there has been growing attention focused on transgender and intersex youth. Although the research literature on these populations is scant, evidence exists that these youth face a number of problematic physical and mental health challenges.

Finally, there has been a dramatic increase in the rate of autism since the 1990s. Research shows that on average one in 110 children has an autism spectrum disorder (Autism and Developmental Disabilities Monitoring

Network Surveillance Year 2006 Principal Investigators, 2009). After completing high school, support services for many adolescents with autism are dropped (Taylor & Seltzer, 2011). Public health social workers can help ensure that this growing population receives needed services to transition from adolescence into adulthood, including case management, mental health and medical services, and vocational and housing support.

SUMMARY

In this chapter we provided an overview of critical health problems and issues that public health social workers need to know in order to effectively promote adolescent health in their communities. For each critical health issue, we examined the prevalence, health disparities, and risk factors and discussed *Healthy People 2020* objectives that address the health problem or issue. We presented a case study that illustrates the use of core public health functions by a public health social worker addressing an adolescent health issue at the county level. We concluded by presenting emerging issues, such as the influence of new media technologies on adolescent health behavior and the growing diversity in the adolescent population that are shaping public health social workers practice with adolescents.

INTERNET RESOURCES FOR EFFECTIVE ADOLESCENT HEALTH INTERVENTIONS

Advocates for Youth

(www.advocatesforyouth.org/for-professionals/programs-that-work)

Center for Mental Health in Schools

(http://smhp.psych.ucla.edu/)

Centers for Disease Control and Prevention Violence Prevention

(www.cdc.gov/ViolencePrevention/suicide/prevention.html)

Guide to Community Preventive Services

(www.thecommunityguide.org/adolescenthealth/index.html)

Konopka Institute for Best Practices in Adolescent Health

(www.med.umn.edu/peds/ahm/programs/konopka/konopkapubs/home.html)

National Campaign to Prevent Teen and Unplanned Pregnancy

(www.thenationalcampaign.org/resources/programs.aspx)

National Institute on Drug Abuse

(www.nida.nih.gov/Prevention/index.html)

Office of Adolescent Health

(www.DHHS.gov/ash/oah/prevention/research/programs/index.html)

Office of Juvenile Justice and Delinquency Prevention

(www.ojjdp.gov/mpg/)

REFERENCES

Abma, J. C., Martinez, G. M., & Copen, C. E. (2010). Teenagers in the United States: Sexual activity, contraceptive use, and childbearing, National Survey of Family Growth 2006–2008. *Vital and Health Statistics, 23,* 1–47.

Achilles, J., Gray, D., & Moskos, M. (2004). Adolescent suicide myths in the United States. *Crisis: The Journal of Crisis Intervention and Suicide Prevention, 25,* 176–182.

Alan Guttmacher Institute. (2002). *In their own right: Addressing the sexual and reproductive health needs of American men.* New York, NY: Author.

Allstate Foundation. (2009). *Shifting teen attitudes: The state of teen driving.* Northbrook, IL: Author.

Autism and Developmental Disabilities Monitoring Network Surveillance Year 2006 Principal Investigators. (2009). Prevalence of autism spectrum disorders—Autism and Developmental Disabilities Monitoring Network, United States, 2006. *Morbidity and Mortality Weekly Report Surveillance Summaries, 58*(SS10), 1–20.

Barlow, S. E., & Expert Committee. (2007). Expert Committee recommendations regarding the prevention, assessment, and treatment of child and adolescent overweight and obesity: Summary report. *Pediatrics, 120,* S164–S192.

Biro, F. M., & Wien, M. (2010). Childhood obesity and adult morbidities. *American Journal of Clinical Nutrition, 91,* 1499S–1505S.

Centers for Disease Control and Prevention. (1994). Preventing tobacco use among young people: A report of the Surgeon General. *Morbidity and Mortality Weekly Report, 43,* 1–10.

Centers for Disease Control and Prevention. (2010). Youth Risk Behavior Surveillance—United States, 2009. *Morbidity and Mortality Weekly Report, 59*(SS5), 1–142.

Chen, L., Baker, S. P., Braver, E. R., & Li, G. (2000). Carrying passengers as a risk factor for crashes fatal to 16- and 17-year old drivers. *Journal of the American Medical Association, 283,* 1578–1582.

Core Public Health Functions Steering Committee. (1994). *Public health in America.* Retrieved from http://www.health.gov/phfunctions/public.htm

Elkington, K. S., Bauermeister, J. A., & Zimmerman, M. A. (2010). Psychological distress, substance use, and HIV/STI risk behaviors among youth. *Journal of Youth and Adolescence, 39*, 514-527.

Finer, L. B., & Henshaw, S. K. (2006). Disparities in rates of unintended pregnancy in the United States, 1994 and 2001. *Perspectives on Sexual and Reproductive Health, 38*, 90-96.

Han, J. C., Lawlor, D. A., & Kimm, S. Y. (2010). Childhood obesity. *Lancet, 375*, 1737-1748.

Harlap, S., Kost, K., & Forrest, J. D. (1991). *Preventing pregnancy, protecting health: A new look at birth control choices in the United States.* New York, NY: Alan Guttmacher Institute.

Henshaw, S. K. (2003). *U.S. Teenage pregnancy statistics with comparative statistics for women aged 20-24.* New York, NY: Alan Guttmacher Institute.

Hock-Long, L., Herceg-Baron, R., Cassidy, A. M., & Whittaker, P. G. (2003). Access to adolescent reproductive health services: Financial and structural barriers to care. *Perspectives on Sexual and Reproductive Health, 35*, 144-147.

Hudson, J. I., Hiripi, E., Pope, H. G., & Kessler, R. C. (2007). The prevalence and correlates of eating disorders in the National Comorbidity Survey Replication. *Biological Psychiatry, 61*, 348-358.

Institute of Medicine. (2002). *The future of public's health in the 21st century.* Washington, DC: National Academies Press.

Insurance Institute for Highway Safety. (2009). *Fatality facts 2009: Teenagers.* Retrieved from http://www.iihs.org/research/fatality_facts_2009/teenagers.html

Johnston, L. D., O'Malley, P. M., Bachman, J. G., & Schulenberg, J. E. (2011). *Monitoring the Future, national results on adolescent drug use: Overview of key findings, 2010.* Ann Arbor, MI: Institute for Social Research at the University of Michigan.

Jones, R. K., Purcell, A., Singh, S., & Finer, L. B. (2005). Adolescents' reports of parental knowledge of adolescents' use of sexual health services and their reactions to mandated parental notification for prescription contraception. *Journal of the American Medical Association, 293*, 340-348.

Kann, L., Telljohann, S. K., & Wooley, S. F. (2007). Health education: Results from the School Health Policies and Programs Study 2006. *Journal of School Health, 77*, 408-434.

Kowalski, R. M., Limber, S. P., & Agatston, P. W. (2008). *Cyber bullying: Bullying in the digital age.* Malden, MA: Blackwell Publishing.

Lee, H., Harris, K. M., & Gordon-Larsen, P. (2009). Life course perspectives on the links between poverty and obesity during the transition to young adulthood. *Population Research and Policy Review, 28*, 505-532.

Lee, S. M., Burgeson, C. R., Fulton, J. E., & Spain, C. G. (2007). Physical education and physical activity: Results from the School Health Policies and Programs Study 2006. *Journal of School Health, 77*(8), 435-463.

Lewinsohn, P. M., Rohde, P., & Seeley, J. R. (1998). Major depressive disorder in older adolescents: Prevalence, risk factors, and clinical implications. *Clinical Psychology Review, 18*, 765-794.

Martin, J. A., Hamilton, B. E., Sutton, P. D., Ventura, S. J., Mathews, T. J., & Osterman, M. J. K. (2010). Births: Final data for 2008. *National Vital Statistics Reports, 59*, 1-72.

Martinez, G., Abma, J., & Copen, C. (2010). *Educating teenagers about sex in the United States.* Retrieved from http://www.cdc.gov/nchs/data/databriefs/db44.pdf

Mayhew, D. R., Simpson, H. M., & Pak, A. (2003). Changes in collision rates among novice drivers during the first months of driving. *Accident Analysis and Prevention, 35,* 683–691.

McCartt, A. T., Mayhew, D. R., Braitman, K. A., Ferguson, S. A., & Simpson, H. M. (2009). Effects of age and experience on young driver crashes: Review of recent literature. *Traffic Injury Prevention, 10,* 209–219.

McCartt, A. T., Shabanova, V. I., & Leaf, W. A. (2003). Driving experience, crashes, and teenage beginning drivers. *Accident Analysis and Prevention, 35,* 311–320.

Merikangas, K. R., He, J., Burstein, M., Swanson, S. A., Avenevoli, S., Cui, L., et al. (2010). Lifetime prevalence of mental disorders in U.S. adolescents: Results from the National Comorbidity Survey Replication—Adolescent Supplement (NCS-A). *Journal of the American Academy of Child and Adolescent Psychiatry, 49,* 980–989.

Mosher, W. D., Chandra, A., & Jones, J. (2005). Sexual behavior and selected health measures: Men and women 15–44 years of age, United States, 2002. *Advance Data From Vital and Health Statistics, 362,* 1–56.

Mustillo, S., Worthman, C., Erkanli, A., Keeler, G., Angold, A., & Costello, E. J. (2003). Obesity and psychiatric disorder: Developmental trajectories. *Pediatrics, 111,* 851–859.

National Center for Injury Prevention and Control. (2010). *Web-based injury statistics query and reporting system* [Interactive database]. Retrieved from http://www.cdc.gov/injury/wisqars/index.html

National Highway Traffic Safety Administration. (2009). *Seat belt use in 2008—Demographic results.* Retrieved from http://www-nrd.nhtsa.dot.gov/Pubs/811183.pdf

National Highway Traffic Safety Administration. (2011). *Young drivers: Traffic safety facts, 2009 data.* Retrieved from http://www-nrd.nhtsa.dot.gov/Pubs/811400.pdf

National Institute on Drug Abuse. (2005). *Prescription drugs: Abuse and addiction.* Retrieved from http://www.nida.nih.gov/PDF/RRPrescription.pdf

Neyens, D. M., & Boyle, L. N. (2008). The influence of driver distraction on the severity of injuries sustained by teenage drivers and their passengers. *Accident Analysis and Prevention, 40,* 254–259.

Ogden, C. L., & Carroll, M. D. (2010). *Prevalence of obesity among children and adolescents: United States, trends 1963–1965 through 2007–2008.* Retrieved from http://www.cdc.gov/nchs/data/hestat/obesity_child_07_08/obesity_child_07_08.pdf

Ogden, C. L., Carroll, M. D., Curtin, L. R., Lamb, M. M., & Flegal, K. M. (2010). Prevalence of high body mass index for age among U.S. children and adolescents 2007–2008. *Journal of the American Medical Association, 303,* 242–249.

O'Toole, T. P., Anderson, S., Miller, C., & Guthrie, J. (2007). Nutrition services and foods and beverages available at school: Results from the School Health Policies and Programs Study 2006. *Journal of School Health, 77*(8), 500–521.

Resnick, M. D., Ireland, M., & Borowsky, I. (2004). Youth violence perpetration: What protects? What predicts? Findings from the National Longitudinal Study of Adolescent Health. *Journal of Adolescent Health, 35,* 424e1–424e10.

Rideout, V. J., Foehr, U. G., & Roberts, D. F. (2010). *Generation M²: Media in the lives of 8 to 18 year olds.* Washington, DC: Kaiser Family Foundation.

Rolls, B. J. (2003). The supersizing of America: Portion size and the obesity epidemic. *Nutrition Today, 38,* 42–53.

Rounds, K. A. (2004). Preventing sexually transmitted infections among adolescents. In M. W. Fraser (Ed.), *Risk and resilience in childhood: An ecological perspective* (2nd ed., pp. 251–280). Washington, DC: NASW Press.

Santelli, J. S., Lindberg, L. D., Finer, L. B., & Singh, S. (2007). Explaining recent declines in adolescent pregnancy in the United States: The contribution of abstinence and improved contraceptive use. *American Journal of Public Health, 97,* 150–156.

Savin-Williams, R. C. (2006). *The new gay teenager.* Cambridge, MA: Harvard University Press.

Singh, G. K., Siahpush, M., & Kogan, M. D. (2010). Neighborhood socioeconomic conditions, built environments, and childhood obesity. *Health Affairs, 29,* 503–512.

Soni, A. (2009). *The five most costly children's conditions, 2006: Estimates for the U.S. civilian noninstitutionalized children, ages 0–17.* Retrieved from http://www. meps.ahrq.gov/mepsweb/data_files/publications/st242/stat242.pdf

Substance Abuse and Mental Health Services Administration. (1999). *The relationship between mental health and substance abuse among adolescents.* Rockville, MD: Author.

Substance Abuse and Mental Health Services Administration. (2007). *A day in the life of American adolescents: Substance use facts.* Rockville, MD: Author.

Substance Abuse and Mental Health Services Administration. (2008). *Results from the 2007 National Survey on Drug Use and Health: National findings.* Rockville, MD: Author.

Taylor, J., & Seltzer, M. (2011). Employment and post-secondary educational activities for young adults with autism spectrum disorders during the transition to adulthood. *Journal of Autism & Developmental Disorders, 41*(5), 566–574.

U.S. Census Bureau. (2008). *An older and more diverse nation by midcentury.* Retrieved from http://www.census.gov/newsroom/releases/archives/population/cb08-123.html

U.S. Department of Health and Human Services. (2000a). *Mental health: A report of the Surgeon General's conference on children's mental health: A national action agenda.* Washington, DC: Author.

U.S. Department of Health and Human Services. (2000b). *Reducing tobacco use: A report of the Surgeon General.* Washington, DC: Author.

U.S. Department of Health and Human Services. (2001). *Youth violence: A report of the Surgeon General.* Washington, DC: Author.

U.S. Department of Health and Human Services. (2004). *The health consequences of smoking: A report of the Surgeon General.* Washington, DC: Author.

U.S. Department of Health and Human Services. (2011). *Healthy People 2020: Summary of objectives.* Retrieved from http://www.healthypeople.gov/2020/topicsobjec tives2020/default.aspx

Weinstock, H., Berman, S., & Cates, W. (2004). Sexually transmitted diseases among American youth: Incidence and prevalence estimates, 2000. *Perspectives on Sexual and Reproductive Health, 36,* 6–10.

Wolraich, M. L., Wibbelsman, C. J., Brown, T. E., Evans, S. W., Gotlieb, E. M., Knight, J. R., et al. (2005). Attention-deficit/hyperactivity disorder among adolescents: A review of the diagnosis, treatment, and clinical implications. *Pediatrics, 115,* 1734–1746.

Xu, J., Kochanek, K. D., Murphy, S. L., & Teiada-Vera, B. (2010). Deaths: Final data for 2007. *National Vital Statistics Reports, 58,* 1–135.

CHAPTER 5

Aging and Caregiving

Elaine T. Jurkowski

INTRODUCTION

*E*very 8 minutes, a baby boomer turns 60 (U.S. Bureau of the Census, 2012). Currently worldwide, there are more centenarians, or people over the age of 100, than ever before. Our "longevity explosion" has also led to a rise in caregivers as well. At the current time, more than 5 million people (20% of the U.S. population), provide care for a chronically ill, disabled, or aged family member or friend during any given year (National Alliance for Caregiving, 2012). In 2010, according to the U.S. Census, nearly 38 million people (13% of the population) were 65 years of age or older in the United States. Estimates from various expert sources suggest that by 2030, this same age group will grow to about 72 million people and will represent about 20% of the population. In like manner, these same trends will be seen globally, and we will witness a growth in older adults living within our communities. As people live longer, we will see trends toward better educated and healthier older adults, who will remain in their home communities. This demographic shift will call for changes in our communities and in the preparation of a workforce to address the many and varied needs that this population shift will bring to communities. This chapter will provide an overview of some of the major issues that will affect the health of older adults and provide a response to address these needs for public health social workers.

CURRENT HEALTH STATUS OF OLDER ADULTS

Census data suggest that our population is graying, and we can expect greater longevity as time moves onward. Despite people living longer, questions remain: Will people continue living in relatively good health, and what can we expect in terms of life expectancy and of health status?

Life expectancy is a summary measure of the overall health of a population (FEDSTATS, 2010). According to a consensus group representing the aging consortium, the term *life expectancy* refers to the average number of years of life remaining for a person at a given age if death rates were to remain constant. In the United States, improvements in health have led to an increase in life expectancy during the past century and have also been a contributing factor to the expansion of our population over 60 years of age (Centers for Disease Control and Prevention [CDC], 2010; FEDSTATS, 2010).

Demographic data from the U.S. Bureau of the Census reveal that life expectancies at both age 65 and age 85 have risen (U.S. Bureau of the Census, 2010). Under current mortality conditions in 2010, people who survive to age 65 can expect to live an average of 18.5 more years, about 4 years longer than people aged 65 expected to live in 1960 (CDC, 2010). The life expectancy of people who survive to age 85 was documented in 2010 to be 6.8 years for women and 5.7 years for men (U.S. Bureau of the Census, 2010).

One cannot examine life expectancy without looking at racial variation or differences. Life expectancy varies by race, but the differences seem to decrease with age, according to vital statistics records (CDC, 2010). In 2006, life expectancy at birth was 5 years higher for White people than for African Americans. At age 65, White people can expect to live an average of 1.5 years longer than African Americans. Among those who survive to age 85, however, the life expectancy among African Americans is slightly higher (6.7 years) than White people (6.3 years; FEDSTATS, 2010).

Ironically, one would expect that with the wealth and living conditions available to people in the United States, that life expectancy for Americans would surpass that of other industrialized nations. However, life expectancy at age 65 in the United States is lower than that of many other industrialized nations. In 2005, women aged 65 in Japan could expect to live on average 3.7 years longer than women in the United States (CDC, 2010; FEDSTATS, 2010). Among men, the difference was 1.3 years (CDC, 2010; FEDSTATS, 2010).

Advancing age results in health limitations and chronic health conditions. As we have seen elsewhere in this book, chronic health conditions include heart disease, arthritis, hypertension, and respiratory diseases (Saleeby & Jurkowski, 2013). The prevalence of these chronic conditions, however, differs by sex and is not consistent across racial groups. For example, in 2008, women reported higher levels of arthritis (55% versus 42%) than men (BFRSS, 2010; FEDSTATS, 2010). Men reported higher levels of heart disease (38% versus 27%) and cancer (24% versus 21%; FEDSTATS, 2010). Between 1992 and 2007, the age-adjusted proportion of people aged 65 and over with a functional limitation declined from 49% to 42% (FEDSTATS, 2010). These functional limitations include feeding, bathing, toileting, transferring from bed to chair and vice versa, and dressing. Thus, it is no surprise that there was no significant change in the percentage of people aged 65 and over reporting physical activity between 1997 and 2008 (Federal Interagency Forum on Aging-Related Statistics, 2010).

Evidence in the literature suggests that social support can modify risk factors for isolation and depression among older adults. Despite these facts, the reality is that as people grow older, they tend not be as social as people in their early years of "growing older." In 2008, The Behavioral Risk Factor Surveillance system reported that some types of communicating, such as visiting friends or attending or hosting social events, declined with age. For Americans age 55 to 64, 13% of leisure time was spent socializing and communicating, compared with 8% for those aged 75 and over (BFRSS, 2010). Studies also suggest that increased isolation leaves one vulnerable for elder abuse and exploitation (Gallo, Jimenez, & Shivpuri, 2010; McGuire, Strine, Vachirasudlekha, Anderson, Berry, & Mokdad, 2009; Defries, McGuire, Andresen, & Brumback, 2009).

In addition to issues for older adults, such as isolation and elder abuse, the decline of one's cognitive health is also a major area of concern. The increase of incidence and prevalence of Alzheimer's disease worldwide, and more specifically in the United States, led the Centers for Disease Control and Prevention to embark on a "Healthy Brain Initiative, 2006–2011" (CDC, 2011). This initiative set out to assess the public health burden of cognitive impairment through surveillance, build an evidence base for public policy, and translate public policy into action through public health practice. The end result of this initiative was a renewed approach to addressing the issue of cognitive health through public health prevention, surveillances, and policy development (CDC, 2011).

CAREGIVER SUPPORT SERVICES

A recent study by the National Alliance for Caregiving (2009) and the AARP found that 65 million Americans (29% of the U.S. population) aged 18 or older are providing unpaid care for a chronically ill, disabled, or aged family member or friend. The typical caregiver is a 46-year-old woman with some college education who is employed. In all, 66% of family caregivers are women, and more than 37% have children or grandchildren under 18 years old living with them. On average, family caregivers spend 20 hr/wk caring for their loved ones, while 13% of family caregivers are providing 40 hr of care a week or more (National Alliance for Caregiving, 2009).

Female caregivers provide more hours of care and provide a higher level of care than male caregivers. However, 66% of male caregivers are working full or part time while only 55% of female caregivers are working full or part time. Many caregivers fulfill multiple roles. For example, 62% of caregivers are married or living with a partner, and 74% of caregivers work and manage caregiving responsibilities at the same time (Giovanetti & Wolff, 2010; Kusano et al., 2011; National Alliance for Family Caregiving, 2009).

Also, 36% of caregivers care for a disabled parent, while 14% of caregivers care for a special needs child, with an estimated 16.8 million of those children being under the age of 18 while the average length of caregiving is 4.3 years (Giovantti & Wolff, 2010).

The physical stress of caregiving, especially in relation to providing care for someone who is bedridden or wheelchair bound, can affect the physical health of the caregiver. One in 10 primary caregivers has reported that they are physically strained (Buyck et al., 2011). Similarly, about one in 10 caregivers report that caregiving has caused their physical health to worsen. A decline in a caregiver's physical ability to care for a loved one affects one's ability to continue providing care and increases the risk of one's own frailty later in life (Buyck et al., 2011; Hastrup, Van Den Berg, & Gyrd-Hansen, 2011).

Caregivers also experience emotional strain. A total of 16% of caregivers feel emotionally strained, and 26% say taking care of the care recipient is hard on them emotionally. Caregivers often report feeling frustrated, angry, drained, guilty, or helpless as a result of providing care. Caregiving can also result in feeling a loss of self-identity, lower levels of self-esteem, depression, constant worry, or feelings of uncertainty (McPherson, Wilson, Chyurlia, & Leclerc, 2011).

Consistent with the worry, strain, and depression related to caregiving is the constant stress of how to deal with the changes in one's loved one and one's own grief or loss. These issues, when considered as an aggregate, rather than by individual (Arai & Zarit, 2011) unique case, leads to building a rationale for community-based interventions to address caregiving needs (Rao, Abraham, & Anderson, 2009; White-Cooper, Dawkins, Kamin & Anderson, 2009).

Caregiving challenges call for the need for health literacy, or education about caregiving, and what to expect in the process. Similarly, public health approaches to community-based interventions are also necessary in efforts to build and provide resources to caregivers (Johansson, Long, & Parker, 2011). Consequently, public health social workers will move beyond the individual adaptation and coping needs to working with other professional stakeholders to address the issue from a mezzo and macro perspective (Stafinski, Menon, Marshall & Caufield, 2011). This perspective will include the assessment of community needs, building of resources, assurance of services, and policy development.

Healthy People 2020 Objectives Related to Aging and Caregiving

The seminal *Healthy People 2020* (U.S. Department of Health and Human Services [DHHS], 2010) document identifies 22 objectives related to aging and caregiving. These objectives basically fall into four specific areas; benefits, prevention, workforce issues, and caregivers. In terms of benefits, The Central Management System issued a document titled "Welcome to Medicare Benefits." *Healthy People 2020* strives to increase the proportion of older adults who will utilize this resource.

Prevention services include clinical preventative services, diabetes self-management, functional capacity, and falls. In 2008, only approximately 7% of the population was up to date on a core set of clinical preventative services; thus, *Healthy People 2020* strives to increase this amount by 10% (DHHS, 2010). *Healthy People 2020* also strives to increase these targets equally between male and female individuals. In 2008, the Behavioral Risk Factor Surveillance System indicated that only about 47% of the older adult population 60 years of age and older were comfortable with managing one or more chronic health conditions. *Healthy People 2020* strives to increase this target by 10% by the year 2020. Other prevention targets include reducing the proportion of older adults who have moderate-to-severe functional limitations and to reduce the rate of emergency department visits due to falls among older adults.

The workforce-related goals identified in *Healthy People 2020* call for an increase in the proportion of individuals in the health care workforce with geriatric certifications. This workforce specifically includes physicians, geriatric psychiatrists, registered nurses, dentists, physical therapists, and registered dietitians. According to workforce surveys identified in *Healthy People 2020*, it appears that anywhere from .3% to 4.0% of the workforce received training on issues related to older adults within their repertoire of training. This is a very narrow window, considering that soon one in four of our population will be an older adult.

Caregivers are an often-neglected group of unsung heroes whose unpaid affections and attention to loved ones help maintain the health, well-being, and longevity of those receiving care. *Healthy People 2020* strives to reduce the proportion of unpaid caregivers of older adults who report an unmet need for caregivers. In addition, another goal seeks to reduce the proportion of noninstitutionalized older adults with disabilities who have an unmet need for services and supports that will extend into the long-term nature of care needs.

Lastly, the notion of elder abuse seems foreign among a concerned group, the so-called care providers. However, it may be foreign simply because several states do not have the mechanism or the manpower to provide detection and intervention services. In addition, systems of care are often not provided. *Healthy People 2020* strives to increase the number of states, the District of Columbia, and tribes that collect and make publicly available information on the characteristics of victims, perpetrators, and statistics on cases of elder abuse, neglect, and exploitation.

According to the Administration on Aging, in 2004, only three states carried this out (DHHS, 2010). At the current time, many states have the mechanism to report the incidence and prevalence of elder abuse, neglect, and exploitation, but the data are not publicly available. Advocacy efforts to release these data to the general public are necessary.

THE CORE FUNCTIONS OF PUBLIC HEALTH IN RELATIONSHIP TO AGING AND CAREGIVING

The essential public health services functions of assessment, policy development, and assurance cannot be divorced from the field of aging and caregiving, if public health social workers expect to assure that the needs of an older adult population and the needs of caregivers are met. This section will address each of the core functions and showcase various strategies that public health social workers can meet the needs of older adult populations through effective intervention, action, and advocacy within each of these three core functions, and via the 10 essential health services.

The core function of "assessment" seeks to assure three essential public health services, which include (1) to monitor the health status to identify community health problems; (2) to diagnose and investigate health problems and health hazards in the community; and (3) to evaluate the effectiveness, accessibility, and quality of personal and population-based health services. Public health social workers carry out each of these essential functions within communities through needs assessment; the use of vital statistics and epidemiological data for planning; and the development of community-based interventions and immunizations, such as flu vaccines. Screening techniques for high-risk health behaviors such as diabetes and depression also take place through community health initiatives led by public health social workers. Evaluations of ongoing efforts are constantly at play and are important tools used to decide what impact activities and interventions have on the target population, and to justify resources. Public health social workers often take the lead in these initiatives. Epidemiological data are often used to help assess the need for public health and home health interventions and serve as the basis of needs assessments in community planning efforts.

Policy development activities identified through the core function includes three essential services. These include: (1) the development of policies and plans that support individual and community health efforts, (2) the enforcement of laws and regulations that protect health and ensure safety, and (3) the research for new insights and innovative solutions to health problems. Public health social workers are often at the helm of legislative efforts to build or amend current county, state, or federal legislation to expand programs and services for older adults and their caregivers. The Older Americans

Act, over 50 years old, is amended continually, and testimony for new programs and services often begins with public health social workers. Programs to demonstrate how individual management of health care resources rather than case management via home health agencies is another example of how policies and programs are developed to support community health efforts.

Caregiver support groups and caregiver educational materials, borne out of the Caregiver Support Act (2006), is another example of an intervention developed through public health social workers attempting to build policies and plans to support and protect health. New initiatives are followed up with evaluative strategies to help ascertain the efficacy of program efforts. Research into the effectiveness and efficacy of programs helps to build evidence-based interventions and provide interventions that impact change. This too is another venue for public health social workers to provide input or assume leadership (Centers for Disease Control and Prevention, 2012).

Lastly, the assurance function includes four essential public health services. These services include: (1) the linkage of people to needed personal health services and the assurance of the provision of health care when otherwise unavailable; (2) the assurance of a competent public health and personal health care workforce; (3) the practice of informing, educating, and empowering people about health issues; and, finally, (4) the mobilization of community-based partnerships to identify and solve health problems. Public health social workers working within home health agencies or aging-related services will broker services for older adults and their families. Oftentimes, these services will target some aspect of one's functional limitations, but will also enable older adults to remain in the least restrictive environment, and often their own homes. Services brokered for caregivers also help caregivers receive the needed respite so that they can maintain their caregiving role as effectively as possible.

The assurance of a competent public health workforce will be an essential goal for public health social workers to pursue as the population ages. Public health social workers can spearhead training sessions and continuing education units for a range of interdisciplinary professionals, including physicians, nurses, geriatric psychiatrists, dentists, and physical therapists. Often, the training that professionals receive on geriatrics and aging is severely limited, and professionals lack the necessary skills to engage older adults in a therapeutic relationship. Public health social workers target interventions at micro, mezzo, and macro levels for older adults and their caregivers, and in return educate and inform other members of the multidisciplinary team. Public health social workers can also exercise leadership within the professional arena to serve on advisory boards as an associate member, and provide insight on professional competencies required for effective practice with older adults and their caregivers. Public health social workers can also participate in building professional competencies related to aging and older adults within their individual state through partnerships with the state-based Department of Professional Regulation.

Public health social workers also work in a variety of settings to provide educational materials to the public on topics related to healthy aging, or on disease-specific topics for caregivers. These educational sessions can occur within the faith-based communities, at senior centers, through health fairs, through local AARP chapters, or in venues such as the public library or local educational institution. This type of educational effort helps raise the level of health literacy older adults and their caregivers may possess.

Lastly, within the assurance function, public health social workers also will play a pivotal role in mobilizing community partnerships to address issues that may impact older adults and their caregivers. Healthy Communities coalitions and Mental Health and Aging coalition groups are two strident examples, led by public health social workers, of how coalitions have been used to mobilize and leverage resources.

This section has articulated how the core functions and essential services associated with these core functions can be implemented by public health social workers in the course of their day-to-day activities. In an effort to carry out these responsibilities, a specific set of competencies are required, which have been articulated by a working group assembled through the National Association of Social Workers and the Social Work section of the American Public Health Association. The next segment of this chapter will articulate some of the specific competencies that public health social workers will need in an effort to serve older adults and their caregivers.

PUBLIC HEALTH SOCIAL WORK STANDARDS AND COMPETENCIES RELATED TO AGING AND CAREGIVING

In efforts to effectively meet the needs of older adults and their caregivers, public health social workers will need to utilize a range of competencies that embrace a theoretical base, methodological skills, and analytical processes; leadership and communication; public policy advocacy; and values and ethics.

When practicing with adults who are aging and their caregivers, a range of skills will be necessary for public health social workers within a specific theoretical base. These skills include understanding principles of social epidemiology; understanding patterns of growth and development from an intergenerational and life span perspective; and understanding the characteristics of health systems, including the dimensions of, use of, and access to health care. Skills in the areas of implementing the application of primary, secondary, and tertiary strategies to address the heath, social, and economic issues of individuals, families, and communities, and utilizing practice and epidemiologic theories to substantiate interventions and programming designed to promote health and behavioral change will also be essential for public health social workers. These skills will serve the community well in advancing needs assessments and the interpretation of secondary data/vital statistics. Building interventions that cut across the life span and utilize intergenerational approaches have been proven to be efficacious in the literature and will continue to build ties across generational lines. It will be necessary for public health social workers to facilitate interventions at primary, secondary, and tertiary levels within the public health system to advance the provision of care for people who are growing older.

A range of competencies within the methodological and analytical process are also essential for public health social workers to be effective in addressing the needs of people growing older and their caregivers. These skills will be essential in building evidence-based interventions and critiquing new initiatives that may come forward from state-based departments of aging, health promotion, or health. Such skills will also play a key role in devising community-wide intervention trials dedicated to meeting the needs of an older adult population. Some of the methodological competencies and skills that would be an asset for public health social workers include a knowledge base and understanding of areas such as research design, sampling, basic descriptive and inferential statistics, and validity/reliability assessment of measures; epidemiological/socio epidemiological concepts and community needs assessment; and program design, implementation, and evaluation. These competencies may be transformed by skills in data collection and interpretation from a variety of secondary data sources from vital statistics or National Center for Health Statistics databases. These skills can then lead to the formulation of hypotheses or research questions in collaboration with internal or external stakeholders, which in turn can then be used in the process of building an analytical strategy to influence the health of older adults and their caregivers, and facilitating planned social change efforts.

Public health social workers interested in older adult and caregiving issues exercise leadership and communication skills in their process to promote networking across professional disciplines. This networking, multidisciplinary team building, and group processing are essential ingredients in the building of relationships that will foster collaborative strategies to assure that consumers and other constituencies participate in the process of building partnerships. Leadership skills for public health social workers, which will also be effective in building community resources for older adults and their families, will include management and organizational theories and practices to the development, planning, budgeting, staffing, administering, and evaluating of public health programs, including the implementation of strategies promoting integrated service systems, especially for vulnerable populations.

Policy and advocacy skills will play a central role for public health social workers interested in mobilizing resources and programs through policy development. In order to facilitate policy development, the public health social worker will need to be knowledgeable of the federal and state mandates that guide the funding and implementation of health and social services programs for older adults and caregivers. Some background in the historical development and scientific basis of public health and social policies and practices for federal, state, and local agencies working with older adults and their caregivers will also be exceedingly useful and necessary. In efforts to impact change at a legislative level, one must apply critical thinking to every stage of policy development and practice. Other skills that will be paramount for public health social workers who want to be effective policy advocates will include the ability to clearly write concise policy statements, position papers, and/or testimonies to educate and inform various stakeholders.

In terms of the values and ethics that public health social workers should espouse when working with older adults and their caregivers, one must be consistent with the values and ethics prescribed by both the social work profession and by public health entities. These values and ethics have been detailed earlier within this textbook. This being said, one's knowledge base also should embody philosophical concepts and the rationale that undergirds the delivery of services that are family centered, comprehensive, community based, and culturally competent, as well as recognize individual, group, and community strengths/assets. In addition, public health social workers will utilize skills to include the development of cultural competence within public health settings and "partnerships with public health and social services communities and constituencies to foster community empowerment, reciprocal learning and involvement in design, implementation, and research aspects of public health and social systems" (Practice Standards Development Committee, 2005).

This chapter thus far has explored some of the demographics of older adults and their caregivers and some of the current issues impacting these target groups, explored *Healthy People 2020* objectives within the arena of aging and caregiving, and articulated how the core functions and essential services (Institute of Medicine, 1988) need to be practiced in efforts to reach the *Healthy People 2020* goals and objectives by the year 2020. This chapter has also explored which public health social worker skills and competencies are necessary in efforts to be effective in practice with older adults and their caregivers. Although this exploration may be sufficient to understand current practice, one must also keep an eye out for issues that the future will bring. The next section will discuss some of these issues.

ISSUES FOR THE FUTURE

A number of issues emerge as we consider the future needs of people growing older and their caregivers. These issues include meeting the community needs of a growing elderly population, addressing the health and cognitive health issues of older adults and their caregivers, developing a workforce to take care of people with aging minds and bodies, addressing and preventing elder abuse, encouraging healthy lifestyles and chronic disease management and encouraging strategies to promote functional living skills.

Health and Cognitive Health Issues of Older Adults and Their Caregivers

Alzheimer's disease is currently the 5th leading cause of death among Americans who are 65 years of age and older (CDC, 2011). This disease knows no boundaries, and will increasingly become a concern as baby boomers age. The need for preventative and curative strategies and interventions for the older adult will become increasingly important. In like manner, the need to arrive with programming to meet this target population will also be a challenge. In like manner, the need for cognitively stimulating activities to promote brain health will also be important to develop, test, and disseminate among the young-old, in an effort to provide some protective factors against acquiring Alzheimer's disease or cognitive decline.

Developing a Workforce to Address the Needs of an Aging Population

Building a competent workforce, prepared to deal with the science of aging, will be another challenge for the future. Many professional curricula lack the necessary training, background, and rigor in training with older adults. Incentives will also need to be a consideration as a strategy to attract professionals to work within the realm of the aging arena. Managed care environments may want to consider incorporating a geriatric practice case manager into the practice to address screening needs of older adult patients or their caregivers, prior to visits with the primary care physicians. Geriatric education competencies could be adopted across professions in an effort to begin to prepare medical, dental, and associated health professionals to adequately meet the health care needs of people growing older and/or their caregivers.

Prevention of Elder Abuse

The incidence and prevalence of elder abuse in communities that is being reported may actually just be a snapshot of the extent of the real problem. Reporting, tracking, and surveillance systems, if in existence within state public health or aging departments, are not transparent in their reporting. Adult Protective Services personnel are also largely underfunded or under-staffed to adequately fulfill their state mandates. Efforts to meet the goal of preventing elder abuse will require efforts from multiple stakeholders. As the availability of fiscal resources to family members begins to deteriorate, financial abuse may be on the rise. Specific efforts and strategies to under-stand the dynamics of elder abuse will be vital to address the privative needs associated with elder abuse. Public education efforts toward the recog-nition of signs that elder abuse may be occurring will also be needed in the future.

Chronic Disease Management

The advent of new medical technologies and new home health devices will lead older adults to remain in their home communities. Increasingly, individ-uals with chronic health care needs will be capable of treating themselves within their home-based community settings. Preventing chronic diseases will also be an important focus to help people manage their conditions and keep treatment expenditures controlled. Preventative screenings (cardi-ovascular, diabetes, colorectal cancer, and depression) and funding for these screenings will be on the rise in the future. The need for fiscal resources (insurance coverage) will be an issue in the process of building strong chronic disease-management systems within local communities (AARP, 2012; American Medical Association, CDC, 2011; Smith et al., 2010).

Promotion of Functional Living Skills

The baby boomer generation will demand more of the health care system, as well as themselves, as they attempt to pursue active aging principles in their care and rehabilitation. As part of this expectation, boomers will expect to maintain or regain functional living skills posthospitalization or rehabilitation stay. The shrinking availability of home health aides or rehabilitation aides may also force older adults to be more resilient and independent within a rehabilitation process that addresses functional living skills. Functional living skills, also referred to as "activities of daily living," include feeding, bathing, dressing, toileting, and transferring oneself from the bed to chair/ wheelchair (Katz, 1976).

Public Policy

A major issue to be addressed in the future will be legislation that impacts the health of older adults and their caregivers. Current discussions within the political arena have centered on reducing or containing the costs of Medicare and costs for long-term care and health care through the Patient Protection and Affordable Care Act (2010). Within the Elder Justice Act (2009), provision for the development of state wide tracking systems for the detection and surveillance of elder abuse was passed into law. The implementation of these laws is essential if state governments hope to adequately provide services to their older adult target groups. In a climate where fiscal resources are tight, and the need to balance budgets takes priority, public health social workers will need to carry the torch for older adults and lobby efforts from colleagues in other arenas to assist in efforts to help maintain or expand resources, rather than risk losing the current legislative and programming efforts.

CLASSROOM EXERCISES

Case Study 1

Julia is a 58-year-old woman who, like most people of her age, has a lot to look forward to. Julia is excited about the opportunity for a big promotion at her job, where she has been working for 35 years, and for the birth of her first grandchild. However, Julia has a barrier to all of her hopes and dreams. Julia's mother, Mary, was recently diagnosed with Alzheimer's and can no longer care for herself like she has in the past. The doctors thought it would be best if Mary moved in with Julia and her family so that they could take better care of Mary. In order to take care of her mother effectively, Julia had to quit her job and will not be able to spend as much time with her new grandchild.

Since her mother moved into her home, Julia describes her typical day as a challenge. She often complains of sleeping poorly at night and dreads getting up in the morning because she has to take care of Mary. Also, Julia lacks motivation to do the activities that she once loved. She has difficulty concentrating when it comes to preparing medications for her mother and in basic daily activities. Julia feels burdened daily since she has to care for her mother and feels as if she is isolated from society and over loaded. She has become withdrawn and irritable from other people in her family and sulks when she does not get her way. Julia has also become impatient with all aspects of life.

Discussion Questions

1. List some of the resources that could assist this family.
2. What resources are available within your community to address these needs?
3. As a public health social worker, how can you develop resources to address the family needs, using the core functions of assessment, policy development, and assurance?
4. What public health social work competencies would you utilize in building community resources to respond to the issues presented?

Case Study 2

Martin and Margie have been married for almost 60 years. They have four loving, grown children. Martin has always been a carefree, easy going man and a loving, doting husband. In addition, he has had a calm demeanor for most of his married life, and his children characterized him as the voice of reason between their two parents. He was also viewed as a model husband among the couple's circle of friends through their local church.

Recently, Margie was found, distraught and in tears, with bruises from Martin's cane after he erupted because he could not find his watch. He accused his wife of some conspiracy to harm him. After much family discussion, Martin was admitted to a locked unit, while the local Adult Protective Services division discussed the case and tried to determine whether charges of spousal abuse should be brought against Martin.

Discussion Questions

1. What happened in this scenario?
2. Why did Martin's behavior change so radically?
3. Was there a reason for this behavior change?
4. How can a caregiver survive behavioral issues?
5. List some of the resources that could assist this family.
6. What resources are available within your community to address these needs?
7. As a public health social worker, how can you develop resources to address the family needs, using the core functions of assessment, policy development, and assurance?
8. What public health social work competencies would you utilize in building community resources to respond to the issues presented?

INTERNET RESOURCES

FastStats: Older Persons, Health

(www.cdc.gov/nchs/fastats/older_americans.htm)

> This resource provides a number of important indicators and links related to risk factors and the health status of people who are growing older. Data from key repositories funded through the Centers for Disease Control and Prevention can be located within this site.

AgeStats.Gov

(www.agingstats.gov/Main_Site/Contacts/Resource_Links.aspx)

> This page provides web links to all federal government agencies working in areas related to older adults. It also provides links to all National Center for Health Statistics partners that have some interest in or provide data on issues that relate to older adults. Links are also available for practice-oriented agencies such as Veterans Affairs, Social Security, and Centers for Medicaid/Medicare.

Older Americans, Wellbeing: Key Indicators of Health in Older Adults, 2010

(www.agingstats.gov/Main_Site/Data/2010_Documents/docs/)

> This site provides a publication that details the leading 33 health indicators for older adults, with trend data from 1986 to 2010, aggregated by the Federal Interagency Forum on Aging-Related Statistics (Forum). The Forum was founded in 1986 to foster collaboration among federal agencies that produce or use statistical data on the older population.

Administration on Aging (AoA)

(www.aoa.gov)

> This federally funded website provides information about federally mandated programs and services for older adults. The site also provides information directed at elders and their families (Medicare benefits, long-term planning, and local programs), information on emergency preparedness, aging statistics, AoA programs, grant opportunities and AoA-funded resource centers. The segment on AoA programs addresses the Older Adults Act and the Aging Network; home- and community-based long-term care, elder rights protection, health prevention, wellness programs, and user-friendly resources.

Family Caregiver Alliance: National Center on Caregiving

(www.caregiver.org/caregiver/jsp/home.jsp)

This site provides a wealth of information for caregivers and their family members. The site provides up-to-date information on public policy and research, caregiving information and advice, fact sheets and publications, newsletters, and support groups. The press room provides caregiving releases and information about caregiving that is up to date.

National Alliance for Caregivers

(www.caregiving.org/)

This website has publications for caregivers that include brochures designed for family caregivers and reports on alliance programs and research. Also, there are resources such as a beginner's caregiver booklet for family members who have just started their journey in the caregiving world. Lastly, the website has a list of worldwide events that are presented by the National Alliance for Caregivers and coalitions for anyone who is interested.

AARP

(www.aarp.org/relationships/caregiving/)

This website has a section dedicated just to caregivers. It has a resource center for caregivers who are new to the profession, how the caregiver can provide care, housing options for caregivers, legal and financial matters, and end-of-life care. The website also has a section for caregivers to offer personal advice and tips from their own experiences.

REFERENCES

AARP. (2012). Retrieved from http://www.aarp.org/relationships/caregiving/

Administration on Aging (AoA). (2012). Retrieved from http://www.aoa.gov

AgeStats.Gov. (2012). Retrieved from http://www.agingstats.gov/Main_Site/Contacts/Resource_Links.aspx

Anderson, L. A., Day, K. L., Beard, R. L., Reed, P. S., & Wu, B. (2009). The public's perceptions about cognitive health and Alzheimer's disease among the US population: A national review. *The Gerontologist, 49*(s1), 3–11.

Arai, Y., & Zarit, S. H. (2011). Exploring strategies to alleviate caregiver burden: Effects of the National Long-Term Care insurance scheme in Japan. *Psychogeriatrics, 11*(3), 183–189. doi:10.1111/j.1479-8301.2011.00367.x

Behavioral Risk Factor Surveillance System (BFRSS). (2010). *Data system portal.* Retrieved from: http://www.cdc.gov/brfss/smart/2010.htm

Buyck, J., Bonnaud, S., Bourmendil, A., Andrieu, S., Bonenfant, S., Goldberg, M., et al. (2011). Informal caregiving and self-reported mental and physical health: Results from the Gazel Cohort Study. *American Journal of Public Health, 101*(10), 1971–1979.

Centers for Disease Control. Executive Summary Progress Report on The CDC Healthy Brain Initiative: 2006–2011. Atlanta, GA: CDC Office of Communications; 2011.

Centers for Disease Control and Prevention. (2012). *Resources for older Americans.* Retrieved from http://www.cdc.gov.nchs_for_you/older_americans.htm

DeFries, E. L., McGuire, L. C., Andresen, E. M., Brumback, B. A., & Anderson, L. A. (2009). Caregivers of older adults with cognitive impairment. *Preventative Chronic Disease, 6*(2), A46.

Family Caregiver Alliance: National Center on Caregiving. (2010). Retrieved from http://www.caregiver.org/caregiver/jsp/home.jsp

FastStats—Older Persons, Health. (2010). Retrieved from http://www.cdc.gov/nchs/fastats/older_americans.htm

Federal Interagency Forum on Aging Related Statistics. (2010). *Older Americans well-being: Key indicators of health in older adults, 2010.* Retrieved from http://www.agingstats.gov/Main_Site/Data/2010_Documents/docs/

Gallo, L. C., Jimenez, J. A., & Shivpuri, S. (2010). Domains of chronic stress, lifestyle factors, and allostatic load in middle-aged Mexican-American women. *Annals of Behavioral Medicine, 41*(1), 21–31.

Giovanetti, E. R., & Wolff, J. L. (2010). Cross-survey differences in national estimates of numbers of caregivers of disabled older adults. *Milbank Quarterly, 88*(3), 310–349.

Hastrup, L. H., Van Den Berg, B., & Gyrd-Hansen, D. (2011). Do informal caregivers in mental illness feel more burdened? A comparative study of mental versus somatic illnesses. *Scandinavian Journal of Public Health, 39*(6), 598–607. doi: 10.1177/1403494811414247

Institute of Medicine. (1988). *The future of public health.* Washington, DC: National Academies Press.

Johansson, L., Long, H., & Parker, M. G. (2011). Informal caregiving for elders in Sweden: An analysis of current policy developments. *Journal of Aging & Social Policy, 23*(4), 335–353. doi:10.1080/08959420.2011605630

Katz, S. (1976). Assessing self-maintenance: Activities of daily living, mobility, and instrumental activities of daily living. *Journal of the American Geriatrics Society 31*(12), 721–727.

Kusano, C. T., Bouldin, E. D., Anderson, L. A., McGuire, L. C., Salvail, F. R., Simmons, K. W., et al. (2011). Adult informal caregivers reporting financial burden in Hawaii, Kansas, and Washington: Results from the 2007 Behavioral Risk Factor Surveillance System. *Disability and Health Journal, 4*(4), 229–237.

McGuire, L. C., Strine, T., Vachirasudlekha, S., Anderson, L. A., Berry, J. T., & Mokdad, A. H. (2009). Modifiable characteristics of healthy lifestyle in US older adults with or without serious psychological distress, 2007 Behavioral Risk Factor Surveillance System. *International Journal of Public Health, 54*, 84–93.

McPherson, C. J., Wilson, K. G., Chyurlia, L., & Leclerc, C. (2011). The caregiving relationship and quality of life among partners of stroke survivors: A cross-sectional study. *Health and Quality of Life Outcomes, 9*(1), 29.

National Alliance for Caregiving. (2009). *Caregiving in the U.S. - Executive summary.* Bethesda, MD: The Author.

National Alliance for Caregivers. (2012). Retrieved from http://www.caregiving.org/

National Center for Chronic Disease Prevention and Health Promotion. (2011). *The CDC Healthy Brain Initiative: 2006-2011*. Atlanta, GA: Centers for Disease Control and Prevention.

Practice Standards Development Committee, Beyond Year 2010: Public health social work practice project at the UNC School of Social Work. (2005). *Public health social work standards and competencies*. Columbus, OH: Ohio Department of Health. Available at http://oce.sph.unc.edu/cetac/phswcompetencies_May05.pdf. Retrieved March 5, 2012.

Rao, J. K., Abraham, L., & Anderson, L. A. (2009). Novel approach, using end-of-life issues, for identifying times for public health surveillance. *Preventing Chronic Disease, 6*(2), A57.

Saleeby, P., & Jurkowski, E. T. (2013). Chronic diseases, appearing in the Handbook for Social Work in Public Health, In R. Keefe & E. T. Jurkowski, (Eds.), New York, NY: Springer Publishing Company.

Smith, C. E., Piamjariyakul, U., Yadrich, D. M., Ross, V. M., Gajewski, B., & Williams, A. R. (2010). Complex home care: Part III—Economic impact on family caregiver quality of life and patients' clinical outcomes. *Nursing Ecomomics, 28*(6), 393-414.

Stafinski, T., Menon, D., Marshall, D., & Caufield, T. (2011). Societal values in the allocation of healthcare resources: Is it all about the health gain? *The Patient, 4*(4), 207-225.

U.S. Department of Health and Human Services. (2010). *Healthy People 2020: Health objectives for the nation*. Baltimore, MD: US Government Printing Office.

White-Cooper, S., Dawkins, N. U., Kamin, S. L., & Anderson, L. A. (2009). Community-institutional partnerships: Understanding trust among partners. *Health Education Behavior, 36*, 334-347.

PART III

Medical Topics

*T*he needs of various populations throughout the United States and the world are as varied as the people themselves. Public health social workers must be skilled in providing skills in all health care settings where their clients seek services. The chapters in this section help students pursuing a career in public health social work prepare to become familiar with some of the most pressing medical topics and the people dealing with medical issues addressed in these topics.

Chapter 6 addresses immigrant health care. The author of this chapter draws upon her rich history as a practitioner and professor living in New York City, where she works with individuals who have immigrated to the United States from every continent. The author reminds readers that to be effective practitioners they must develop skills to become culturally humble, self-aware of their own cultural biases, and forward thinking in how to bring a client's cultural value system into the helping process. In order to achieve these skills, a public health social worker must have a sound grasp of social work ethics, be sensitive to the issues surrounding why immigrants relocate to the United States, understand what "health" means to them, and understand how the various health and social policies often discriminate against immigrants.

Chapter 7 focuses on the devastating effects of HIV/AIDS. The authors highlight how few illnesses have had as massive an effect on global populations such as HIV/AIDS. The authors ask students that, while reading the chapter, to pay attention to issues surrounding the disparate rates of health care access and outcomes for various groups affected and infected by HIV. Chapter 8 investigates the involvement of social work in the field of genetics. Many public health social workers find this topic to be somewhat foreign to them and lack the knowledge of how to work with families dealing with such issues surrounding biomedical technology and the ethical, legal, and psychosocial impacts of genetics testing.

Chapter 9 considers the rapidly growing field of disabilities and secondary conditions. The authors emphasize that as our population ages, so too will the population living with disabling conditions. Public health social workers will need to develop skills that help integrate people living with disabilities into existing community services and develop additional services as current services become overwhelmed with the unmet needs of the service-seeking public.

This chapter provides an excellent foundation for Chapter 10, which is devoted to chronic health conditions. As the authors point out, the number of people living with disabilities grows, so too do the number of people living with chronic health conditions. Consequently, public health social workers will need to know not only how to work with individuals living with chronic conditions and their families, but also how to work with individuals at risk for developing chronic conditions. This work will require that we have not only good direct-practice skills but also skills in policy development and advocacy.

Perhaps no other health problem has affected so many people as has substance abuse, the focus of Chapter 11. The authors point out that substance abuse is ubiquitous and affects every aspect of the abuser's life. Although much progress has been made in the treatment of substance abuse disorders, many individuals receive no or inadequate treatment. Furthermore, the cost of treatment poses a significant burden to society as people develop addictions to more than one substance, thus complicating treatment. New and synthetic drugs are being developed that have unknown effects, and populations that had not had a significant history of abuse—such as the elderly—now require our ability to help them with this ever-developing health problem.

Throughout the text, the chapters focus largely on health care in the United States. Chapter 12 takes a look at global health. The chapter authors consider the impact of economic burden on prevalence and incidence rates of various illnesses around the world. They highlight efforts put forward by various nations to contain rates of malaria, tuberculosis, and HIV. In each case, social determinants play a significant role in perpetuating the illness. The authors encourage the readers to think about which skills are needed to practice public health social work in foreign countries and how these skills need to be altered to fit the new environments in which the social worker practices.

The final chapter in this section addresses the broad topic of mental health. As the authors quote, there is no health without mental health. The mental health concerns throughout the nation are vast and include suicide, depression, severe and persistent mental illnesses, eating disorders, and dementia. Public health social workers who wish to focus only on major medical/health issues will find that they require additional skills that allow them to work effectively with people living with mental health issues as well. Mental health concerns present a significant financial burden to society. As public health social workers, we must be able to not only treat the person living with the mental illness but also to advocate for policy changes in service provision, fiscal allocation, and the development of evidence-based practices that have been shown to be effective in treating mental health disorders.

This section provides the reader with a number of topics to consider. As you read the chapters, think about other topics that are important to address that have not been covered. Begin researching these topics by looking at the federal initiatives in place to address them. What do you believe public health social workers should do to remedy the problems associated with these health issues? Bring these ideas to your instructor and have him/her discuss them with the class. Think about how you could use the information you collected to help your home communities address the health issues you identified.

CHAPTER 6

Immigrants and Health Care

Elaine Congress

INTRODUCTION

P ublic health social workers have long been committed to promoting improved health care to everyone. Yet the health of immigrants has frequently been compromised because of language barriers, cultural differences, access to health care, and poverty. This chapter will focus on five key areas: (1) ethical standards and competencies that provide a foundation for public health social work with immigrants, (2) theories on immigration that support public health social work, (3) prevention and practice in public health social work with immigrants, (4) dilemmas and challenges that emerge in public health social work with immigrants, and (5) guidelines for public health social work with immigrants and refugees.

ETHICAL STANDARDS FOR SOCIAL WORKERS AND PUBLIC HEALTH PROFESSIONALS

Both the National Association of Social Workers (NASW) and the American Public Health Association (APHA) have ethical codes to guide the professional practice of their members (Public Health Leadership Society, 2002; NASW, 2008). Although the NASW Code of Ethics does not specify health care, social workers are advised "to strive to ensure access to needed information, services, and resources ... for all people" (NASW, 2008, p. 5) and to provide service to clients without discrimination related to ethnicity, race, national origin, or immigration status. Consequently, social workers have an ethical responsibility to provide health care services to all immigrants, including immigrants who are undocumented. Similarly,

Thomas, Sage, Dillenberg, and Guillory (2002) stated that ethical practice requires public health programs to bring together various approaches that anticipate and respect a community's diverse values, beliefs, and cultures.

RELATIONSHIP TO PUBLIC HEALTH SOCIAL WORK CORE COMPETENCIES

A concern for health outcomes of various immigrants is consistent with public health social work core competencies. Public health social workers are advised to demonstrate the following skills: "(Conduct) critical analyses of inequities in health status based on race/ethnicity, socioeconomic position, and gender"; "recognize various strengths, needs, values and practices of diverse cultural, racial, ethnic, and socioeconomic groups to determine how these factors affect health status, health behaviors and program design"; and, finally, promote the "application of primary, secondary, and tertiary strategies to address the heath, social and economic issues of individuals, families, and communities" (Public Health Social Work Standards and Competencies, 2005, p. 2). To apply the core competencies to work with immigrants, this chapter will consider (1) inequities related to health status of immigrants, (2) the values and practices of diverse immigrant groups that may affect health behaviors and status, and (3) the strategies public health social workers use in promoting the health outcomes for immigrants.

For the last 20 years a major goal of the U.S. Department of Health and Human Services Healthy People initiative has been to reduce health disparities among all Americans. While *Healthy People 2010* addressed eliminating health disparities, *Healthy People 2020* expanded this goal to achieve health equity and improve the health of all people.

Health disparities adversely affect groups of people who have systematically experienced greater obstacles to health based on their racial or ethnic group; religion; socioeconomic status; gender; age; mental health; cognitive, sensory, or physical disability; sexual orientation or gender identity; geographic location; or other characteristics historically linked to discrimination or exclusion." *Health equity* is described as the "attainment of the highest level of health for all people. Achieving health equity requires valuing everyone equally, with focused and ongoing societal efforts to address avoidable inequalities, historical and contemporary injustices, and the elimination of health and health care disparities" (U.S. Department of Health and Human Services, 2010).

While the Healthy People documents have usually focused on reducing disease and illness and increasing health care services, there is now the recognition that the absence of disease does not necessarily mean the promotion of good health. Instead, primary prevention is a key ingredient to helping people live longer and healthier lives.

HEALTH ISSUES FOR IMMIGRANTS

Although *Healthy People 2010* and *2020* address health disparities among ethnic and racial minorities, neither specifically mentions immigrants. Prior to the Immigration and Nationality Act (1965), the federal government limited the number of immigrants who could enter the country. The act abolished quotas and eliminated race, national origin, and ethnicity as the basis for immigration status. Since 1965, an increasing number of immigrants from Asia, Africa, and Latin America have immigrated to the United States, with the majority of new immigrants being from racial and ethnic minorities (Congress, 2009).

Keefe (2010) considered the issues surrounding health outcomes and mortality for racial and ethnic minorities in seven major areas: heart disease and stroke, cancer, HIV/AIDS, respiratory diseases, diabetes, maternal and child health, and mental health. The top two causes of death in the United States are heart disease and cancer (Kochanek, Xu, Murphy, Minino, & Kung, 2011). The mortality rates for each of these diseases are much higher among ethnic and racial minority group members (Akresh, 2007).

Differences in cardiovascular care contribute to greater mortality among ethnic and racial minorities (Smedley, Stitch, & Nelson, 2003). While racial/ethnic differences in the diagnosis and treatment of cancer may be less well documented than with cardiovascular illness, there is some evidence that certain ethnic minorities have higher rates of cancer than Whites (Ward et al., 2004). Moreover, ethnic minorities are often diagnosed with cancer at a later stage, when the disease is less treatable. This may be particularly true for immigrants with limited health care access who do not receive secondary prevention in the form of early diagnosis.

People of color have higher rates of HIV/AIDS and subsequent death due to the disease than Whites. The likelihood of death within 3 years of receiving a diagnosis is much greater than for White populations (Hall, McDavid, Ling, &, 2006).

Mental health continues to be an area where ethnic minorities receive less treatment than Whites. Some of the reasons for the lack of treatment include the lack of health insurance to cover mental health care, reliance on cultural beliefs about mental health and its treatment, and distrust of formal mental health services and service providers. Hispanics are less likely to pursue mental health treatment than either Whites or African Americans (Wells, Klap, Koike, & Sherbourne, 2001). Many immigrants come from countries where mental health treatment does not exist and/or there is a stigma associated with mental illness (Congress, 2004).

APPROACH TO IMMIGRANT HEALTH ISSUES

To understand public health issues in work with immigrants, a longitudinal perspective that looks at the immigrant experience in the country of origin, in transition, and current situation is often helpful. Building upon Drachman's (1992) three-stage approach, a cultural health assessment tool can be used to understand more fully health issues for immigrants (Congress, 2010). This model looks at the physical and mental health challenges that immigrants face in their home country before immigrating, then at immigrants' experiences in transition from their home countries to the United States, and finally at threats to their physical and mental health since migrating.

The Push Pull theory of migration (Lee, 1966; Misra & Ganda, 2007) focuses on the macro-level factors, including the political, economic, geographic, and social factors that affect immigrants in their countries of origin and countries of destination; the mezzo-level factors including the social and community relationships of those who immigrate and those who stay behind; and the micro-level factors, including the characteristics of individuals who immigrate from those who do not.

Important questions include the following: What health problems did immigrants experience in their country of origin, and how much did these contribute to the decision to immigrate? Were there food shortages, economic hardships, malnutrition, hunger, disease, torture, or fear for their personal and family safety and loss of family members because of war or disease? Were their transit experiences traumatizing? For many, especially refugees, long airplane rides followed by years spent in refugee camps posed traumas that were not easily resolved. For others, especially those who entered the United States from southern areas and who did not have adequate documents, the dangers of crossing deserts with limited water and food compromise health and affect the physical and mental health of immigrants once they arrive.

Is the health of immigrants better in the United States? Immigrants may have survived food shortages or physical abuse before immigrating that has detrimentally affected their health. Mental health issues may emerge related to the stress of relocating and memories of past traumatic events. In the United States many immigrants must deal with poverty as well as fears about deportation, detention, and violence.

Some immigrants hold low-wage jobs in farming, fishing, forestry, maintenance, meat and poultry industries, landscaping, services, and garment sweatshops that do not provide health insurance. A large number of immigrants are employed as migrant and seasonal farm workers (MFSW). This group has greater morbidity and mortality rates than the majority of Americans (Hansen & Donohoe, 2003). Life expectancy of MFSW is 49 as compared to 75 in the general population (Sandhuaus, 1998). Some of the health risks these farm workers encounter are extreme hot weather conditions, infectious disease (tuberculosis, parasites, HIV, urinary tract infections), chemical and pestilence-related illness that affect the respiratory system, musculoskeletal and traumatic injuries, maternal exposure to poisonous sprays, and child labor. Given that these jobs are often hazardous, immigrants are disproportionately involved in serious and fatal work-related injuries.

IMMIGRANT ACCESS FOR HEALTH CARE

A major reason for health care inequities is the disparate access to health care. A primary reason for the inequities in health care access is the limited health care insurance. Immigrants, even those with "green cards," are much less likely to have health care than nonimmigrants. Undocumented immigrants are especially disadvantaged in accessing health care. In many families there often are U.S. citizens and undocumented immigrants. While special government programs may provide health care to documented and undocumented children, their undocumented parents are often denied health care except for emergency treatment. Thus, health care access within immigrant families is often limited because of immigrant status.

The long-awaited Health Care Reform Act, passed in April 2010, did little to expand health care coverage to immigrants. Legal immigrants (i.e., "green card holders") still have limited Medicaid coverage, because the current federal restrictions require a 5-year waiting period of "lawful residing" before Medicaid coverage will be granted. Since 2009, some states have chosen to provide Medicaid and State Children's Health Insurance Program (SCHIP) benefits to children and pregnant women. However, not all states provide coverage.

On a more positive note, all immigrants, legal and undocumented, have access to public health programs providing immunizations and/or treatment of communicable diseases.

Many states have developed special programs for immigrants, but these programs may vary depending on state budgets. These programs are primarily for children (Health Care Plus) or pregnant women.

Having access to primary health care is seen as essential in providing preventive and other important health services. In lieu of a regular health provider, many uninsured immigrants receive only emergency health care. A recent government study indicated that 30% of Hispanics (the fastest growing immigrant group) lack a usual source of health care as compared to less than 15% of Whites (Livingston, Minushkin, & Cohn 2008). Hispanic children are especially at risk as they are three times less likely to have access to regular health care, despite the availability of special state and federal health care programs (Akresh, 2009). A study in Los Angeles found that one fourth of foreign-born individuals never had medical checkups, and one in nine have never visited a doctor (Goldman, 2006).

Disparities in health care access is seen as a contributing factor to poorer health care outcomes for immigrants (Institute of Medicine, 2002). Lower life expectancies related to cardiac conditions and breast cancer have also been linked to disparities in access to preventive and therapeutic care. Although the increase in childhood asthma among Hispanic children is well documented, only 2% of Hispanic children are prescribed routine medications to prevent further asthma attacks (US Department of Health and Human Services, Agency for Health Care Research and Quality, 2000).

Even if immigrants are able to access health care, facilities and transportation are often lacking, especially in rural areas, where many immigrants live. This problem is compounded for immigrants in small towns and rural areas, where health care providers and facilities, especially those who are culturally and linguistically sensitive to immigrant health needs, may not be available.

HEALTHY IMMIGRANT PHENOMENON

On the basis of the research findings indicating that many immigrants have limited access to health care, should one conclude that immigrants always have negative health outcomes and lower life expectancies? The "healthy immigrant phenomenon" or "immigrant paradox" suggests that although immigrants have higher poverty rates and less access to health care than U.S.-born Whites, they may have similar or better health outcomes (Fennelly, 2006; McDonald & Kennedy, 2004). In 2008, the Centers for Disease Control and Prevention supported this theory by reporting that Hispanics have a higher life expectancy than Whites (Center for Disease Control and Prevention, 2007). Life expectancy at birth for Hispanics is 80.6 years, whereas for Whites it is 78.1 years and for Blacks 72.9 years. In 2006, life expectancy for all Americans at birth was estimated to be 77.7 years. These results are consistent with others that show a Hispanic mortality advantage despite this population's lower socioeconomic status (Institute of Medicine, 2002).

How is this outcome possible? Do immigrants arrive in a healthier state than native-born Americans? Strict health policies and eligibility criteria for entry into the United States may lead to healthier people immigrating (Misra & Ganda, 2007). Applying the Push Pull theory, perhaps the healthier people are more able to immigrate, while the disabled and elderly have health conditions that prevent them from immigrating (push). Also, the healthier may be more likely to want to start over in new country (pull). Others have proposed that immigrant health may deteriorate the longer the immigrants stay in the United States and become acculturated to less healthy habits. Change of diet and less exercise (Cho et al., 2004; Goel, McCarthy, Phillips, & Wee, 2004) may lead to serious health conditions such as obesity, diabetes, and cardiovascular disease (Himmelgreen et al., 2003; Koya & Egede, 2007; Mizra & Ganda, 2007) that may not have been prominent in the home countries.

Much of the research on the Healthy Immigrant Phenomenon has been on maternal and child health outcomes (Mendoza, 2009). Higher rates of low birth weight and infant mortality have been found among U.S.-born Hispanic women, rather than among recent Hispanic immigrants. The research on older children, however, has been less conclusive. There is some evidence suggesting that children of immigrants may develop less healthy eating and other behaviors (e.g., overeating of fried foods, getting little exercise) as they become more acculturated to life in the United States that contributes to negative health outcomes (Hernandez & Charney, 1998).

Lara et al. (2005) found that acculturation of children and adults had both positive and negative outcomes. While acculturated non-U.S. born immigrants may have developed poor health behaviors such as smoking, drinking, using recreational drugs, and developing poor eating habits, they have also benefited from greater access to health care.

CULTURAL ISSUES AND IMMIGRANTS

One explanation for disparate health outcomes has been attributed to cultural differences among various racial and ethnic groups, including differences in language abilities, knowledge about prevention, and fear and distrust of health care providers. Social workers must be aware of these differences so that they can empower members of immigrant groups to become involved in health care decisions.

LANGUAGE BARRIERS

Immigrants' ability to acquire knowledge about relevant treatment options may be compromised by language barriers. Language differences may decrease access to primary and preventive care, impair patient comprehension, decrease patient adherence, and diminish patient satisfaction (Wilson, Chen, Grumbach, Wang, & Fernandez, 2005). Having a language-concurrent physician or access to professional interpretation services is important to good health care. One problem that often arises in immigrant families is when children are used as interpreters. This practice often creates inappropriate boundaries for children, who are assuming too great a role in helping to address their parent's health care needs and missing school for their parent's medical appointments (Congress, 2004).

DISTRUST/FEAR OF HEALTH CARE PROVIDERS

Many immigrants (particularly undocumented immigrants) have had negative experiences while seeking health care services. Providers who focus only on proper documentation, especially when patients and their families are in crisis, often contribute to negative experiences. Many immigrants perceive health care professionals as part of government immigration enforcement who may work to separate undocumented immigrants from their families for deportation. Some states have passed profiling laws that make many immigrants particularly anxious about contacting health care providers except for emergencies. In other cases, some cities and states have passed laws and regulations to protect immigrants who seek health care (Congress, 2010). A social worker's job is to inform immigrants of these laws and regulations that may protect them.

KNOWLEDGE ABOUT AVAILABLE HEALTH CARE

Many immigrants come to the United States from countries that have very limited health care services. Newly arrived immigrants may not know about the extensive and very complex health care services available in the United States. The following example illustrates how a lack of knowledge of primary prevention can detrimentally affect utilization and may have unexpected negative consequences. An immigrant woman brought her 2-year-old child to the emergency room with a very high fever. When the examining doctor asked about the child's immunization record, the mother replied that she had not brought her child to a doctor in the past because he had never been sick. The doctor then asked the emergency room social worker to report the mother to Child Protective Services (Congress, 2004).

In the previous case scenario, the mother, an undocumented immigrant, came from a country that had no preventive care: The only available medical treatment was for emergencies. The mother did not know she could have brought her child to the local well-baby clinic and receive free health care under the SCHIP program. Although she would have been able to receive immunizations for her child in all states, in some states she would not have been able to receive ongoing health care for her child after immunizations were completed.

CHALLENGES IN PUBLIC HEALTH SOCIAL WORK WITH IMMIGRANTS

Primary and Secondary Prevention

The previous case example illustrates a major challenge in public health work with immigrants, especially immigrants from developing countries. Many immigrants come from countries in which primary and secondary prevention services do not exist and only limited tertiary prevention services are available. *Healthy People 2020* focuses on primary prevention as a way to prevent the development of disease for which treatment is needed. As part of the health acculturation process, public health social workers seek to educate immigrants about the value of prevention and consistency in following through on medical treatment. For example, the immigrant who feels better after an initial visit to the doctor may not complete a prescribed course of antibiotics or return for a follow-up appointment. While maintaining respect for immigrants and their beliefs, public health social workers seek to educate immigrant clients about public health issues and available medical treatment.

Cultural Beliefs About Health and Illness

An understanding about immigrants' beliefs about health, illness, and health care is essential for public health social workers to be effective working with immigrants. In Western, developed countries, illnesses are perceived to be related to a physical cause, such as bacteria, viruses, or a poor diet, while some immigrants, especially those from rural developing countries, attribute illness to a spiritual or supernatural cause or to being out of balance with nature (Smith, 2009). As a result, many immigrants are likely to use herbal remedies, acupuncture, and spiritual folk healers to cure both physical and mental diseases. Many immigrants see the mind and body as one, while Western health providers separate physical and mental symptoms and treatment. As public health social workers it is important that we respect the values and beliefs of immigrant clients. Yet because of professional education and employment, public health social workers promote a Western approach to diagnosis and treatment.

Many immigrants use a combination of Western medicine and folk remedies. A dilemma may arise when immigrant clients decide to pursue only a folk remedy without using primary, secondary, or tertiary prevention health methods. Although social workers are respectful of differing health beliefs, there can be a conflict, especially if the practice is potentially life threatening. For example, a parent may choose to seek help from a faith healer rather than a surgeon for a child with a brain tumor. Goldberg (2000) identified a challenge for social workers who strive to respect the beliefs of all cultures but also support basic human rights.

Conflicts Within Health Care Facilities

Social workers may face a dilemma in advocating for their patients' right to choose alternative health care with the health practices of their employing institutions.

The NASW Code of Ethics states that social workers have an ethical responsibility to their employer (NASW, 2008). What if the immigrant's behavior seems contrary to accepted medical practice or hospital procedures? What should the social worker do if the relative of a hospitalized patient continues to bring in food that is antithetical to a prescribed diet? Research suggests that many minorities are particularly wary of making end-of-life decisions (Gutheil & Heyman, 2005). What if the hospital policy proscribes a clear discussion about end-of-life decisions and a client refuses to participate in these discussions, stating that doing so will bring bad luck?

Individual Versus Family Approach

Health care in the United States is very individualistic. Public health social workers are committed to improving the health of all people. The relationship between the public health professional (e.g., doctor, nurse, social worker) and the patient is considered very private and confidential. HIPAA (the Health Insurance Portability and Accountability Act) laws continually reinforce the importance of confidentiality between provider and patient. Yet many immigrant patients continue to view themselves as members of a family and community. For example, the family rather than the "identified patient" may show up for an initial intake in a behavioral health care clinic. An immigrant client on a restricted calorie diet may plan to eat a special dessert prepared by relatives. When an immigrant is hospitalized in intensive care, "family members' who are part of the community may want to remain by the bedside."

Informed Consent

An important concern for public health social workers is helping clients to make informed decisions regarding their health care. Immigrants may face certain risks in being able to make informed-consent decisions. Informed consent includes presumption of competence, voluntary action, and disclosure before consent. Presumption of competency implies that a client can gather diverse information, exercise judgment, and make a decision that may differ from that of the practitioner (Palmer & Kaufmann, 2003). There may be an erroneous perception that immigrants who do not understand English have limited education and understanding of medical terms and may not be competent to make their own decisions. The use of professional interpreters and explanation of medical conditions and procedures in simple vocabulary helps immigrants to make competent health care decisions. In order for patients to be ruled incompetent to make their own decisions, a court decision must be made that is not based on language or cultural differences between the patient and health provider.

Another important aspect of informed consent involves voluntary action without duress or coercion. Voluntary action may be hampered when there are institutional pressures that prevent clients from making independent decisions. Immigrants may be overly influenced by the health care provider's authority and not able to exercise their own independent judgment.

A final condition for informed consent is that consent must be preceded by the disclosure of adequate information. All possible risks and side effects must be reviewed and understood before clients can be expected to operate informed consent, even when the information may lead clients to refuse treatment. In working with immigrants, public health social workers must ensure that their clients have a complete understanding of possible consequences of different types of treatment. Having the option to exercise informed consent may be a new experience for many immigrants. Consequently, a thorough explanation of possible consequences of treatment in terms that immigrants can understand is essential.

PRIMARY, SECONDARY, AND TERTIARY PREVENTION

Primary Prevention

A primary strategy to promote positive health care outcomes among immigrants is education about primary prevention. Immigrants who come from countries in which the diet was limited may not know about the importance of a well-balanced diet that promotes lifelong health. Many immigrants who come from countries in which food was scarce may see obesity as a sign of health rather than cause for concern. Public health social workers can engage in education campaigns within schools and communities to promote healthy diet habits.

A continuing challenge is that often access to healthy foods may be limited in poor minority neighborhoods. A primary prevention strategy for a public health social worker may be to promote accessibility to fresh food. In accordance with the healthy immigrant phenomenon, the children of immigrants may be less healthy than their parents. An example is the increase of obesity among young people linked not only to poor diet but also to limited recreational facilities. On a primary prevention level, the public health social worker can work with community leaders to ensure that immigrant children and their families have access to recreational facilities.

Secondary Prevention

Early detection of illness has been important in preventing the onset of illness or minimizing its consequences. For example, immigrants at high risk for diabetes because of obesity can receive early screening and counseling about diet. Offering free screening tests can help in early disease detection among immigrants. Advertising in ethnic newspapers and at community events may serve to inform immigrants about existing free health care programs.

Tertiary Prevention

Public health social workers can develop culturally competent programs for working with immigrants. Hire bilingual staff who, in addition to speaking the languages of various immigrants, understand different cultures and can facilitate the treatment of ill immigrants. Within health care institutions social workers can help other health care professionals understand the needs of immigrant patients and their families. Public health social workers often assume the roles of cultural broker to educate other health care providers about the cultural and social backgrounds of immigrant patients (Congress, 2004).

GUIDELINES

The following guidelines may be helpful to public health social workers in their work with immigrants

(1) Communication

The public health social worker should strive to improve communication between all participants in health care. The "need to contour public health according to the cultural ways of different groups" has been well documented in public health literature (Gibbie, Rosenstock, & Hernandez, 2003, p. 80). Health care providers must work to ensure that immigrant voices are heard in health care settings and seek to improve communication and understanding between immigrants and health care providers.

(2) Education

Many immigrants do not fully understand medical conditions and available treatments. Public health social workers can take responsibility in educating their immigrant clients about illness, treatment, and prevention. Although immigrants, especially undocumented immigrants, may have limited access to services, social workers have a role in educating clients as to what health benefits they can receive. Education, however, does not apply only to immigrants. Social workers also can serve as culture brokers educating doctors and other medical personnel about cultural beliefs and practices of their immigrant patients.

(3) Empowerment

Building on clients' strengths, public health social workers can also help empower immigrant clients to take responsibility for their own health care. Often immigrants, especially women, neglect taking care of their own health to be sure that their family's needs are taken care of. Public health social workers can work with immigrants in empowering them to articulate what their health needs are and to seek adequate health care.

(4) Advocacy

Advocacy is an important component of public health social work with immigrant populations. This activity is fundamental to both the social work field as the NASW Code of Ethics (2008) advises social workers to engage in "social and political action to insure that all people have equal access to the resources, employment, services and opportunities they require to meet their basic human needs" (p. 27), while the APHA code proposes that "public health should advocate for, or work for the empowerment of disenfranchised community members ensuring that the basic resources and conditions necessary for heath are accessible for all people in the community" (Thomas, Sage, Dillenberg, & Guillory, 2002, p. 1958). Public health social workers need to advocate within each prevention stage to ensure that the goals of *Healthy People 2020* are within the reach of immigrants. For primary and secondary prevention, education, and community development, education about early detection and preventive treatment, as well as increased free screening services, are needed.

Tertiary prevention involves greater access for both documented and undocumented immigrants for health care, as well as the provision of culturally competent treatment for immigrants within institution settings. Advocacy needs to take place not only within health care settings, but also in the larger community. On a local level, social workers can advocate for immigrants to live in a healthy and safe environment. On state and national levels, public health social workers must advocate for laws and policies to be adopted that provide immigrants with access to affordable and available health care. In accordance with *Healthy People 2020* initiatives, the goal for public health social work is not only to improve health outcomes and access, but also to ensure good health and long life expectancy for all immigrants.

CASE EXAMPLE: IMMIGRANT FAMILY

Carmen Perez is a 35-year-old Latina woman who saw the hospital social worker to discuss discharge plans for her 60-year-old mother, Rosa, who had been hospitalized for the last 2 days following a trip to the emergency room. The emergency room physician diagnosed Rosa's condition as chronic kidney disease, which may lead to the possibility that Rosa will have to go on dialysis. Additional tests have been ordered so as to ascertain the seriousness of her condition. Rosa does not want to return to the hospital and says that the spiritualist can provide the care that she needs.

The social worker learned that Carmen was having increasing conflicts with her 16-year-old son, Juan Jr., who had begun to cut school and stay out late at night. Her 14-year-old daughter, Lucia, had gained 50 pounds over the past 2 years and now weighs 200 pounds. Lucia had become very depressed, tearful, and did not want to go to school. Last week, Carmen found that Lucia had hidden two bottles of aspirin in her room. In contrast to her two older children, who presented many problems, Carmen described her 10-year-old daughter, Maria, as "an angel." Maria is very quiet and very helpful with household chores and accompanying her to appointments. She goes to school regularly without any complaints, and earns passing grades, but does not socialize with other children.

Carmen also has some health problems of her own. Because of excessive bleeding, she had recently gone to the emergency room. Carmen had brought Maria to interpret and learned that she (Carmen) needed more tests and possible surgery. Carmen is not eligible for Medicaid and does not have funds for follow-up treatment.

Carmen indicated Juan Jr. was the source of much family conflict as he believed he did not have to respect Pablo, Carmen's boyfriend, who is not Juan's father. Juan complained that his mother and stepfather were "dumb" because they did not speak English. He felt that his parents did not understand how difficult his school experiences were and believed that teachers favor lighter skin Latinos. Juan has much darker skin than anyone in his family.

At age 20, Mrs. Perez moved to the United States from Mexico with her first husband, Juan Sr. She states they were very poor in Mexico and had heard there were better job opportunities in the United States. At the time, Juan Jr. was 2 and Maria was pregnant with Lucia. One year later Juan Sr. died in an automobile accident on a visit back to Mexico. Shortly afterward, Carmen met Pablo, who had come to New York from Guatemala to visit a terminally ill relative. After she became pregnant with Maria, Pablo and Carmen began to live together. Pablo indicated that he was very fearful of returning to Guatemala, stating that several people in his village had been killed in political conflicts. Because Pablo and Carmen were undocumented immigrants, they had been able to find only occasional "off the books" work. Carmen, however, was able to work more regularly as a home care worker and babysitter, and Pablo was embarrassed that Carmen was the primary breadwinner.

Carmen is very close to her mother, Rosa, who had come to live with the family 9 years ago. Rosa has not been able to help recently because of her health problems. Rosa, who does not have health insurance, first consulted a spiritualist to help her with her health concerns before she came to the emergency room with a severe backache and fatigue. Pablo has no relatives in New York, but has several friends at the social club in his neighborhood. Recently, he has started to stay out late with his friends and often arrives home after excessive drinking.

Discussion

This Latino family has numerous physical and mental health problems. In terms of health issues, the grandmother, Rosa, has serious kidney problems and may need dialysis, while Carmen has gynecological problems that require further investigation and possible surgery. Lucia is extremely overweight and is at risk for diabetes and has expressed some suicidal thoughts. Suicide among Latina adolescents is rising and a suicide assessment risk is indicated. Pablo needs treatment for alcohol abuse, even though he is still in denial about his alcohol problems. There also are family issues in that Juan Jr. does not respect the man who is not his father.

Rosa, Carmen, and Pablo are all undocumented immigrants and unemployed. Consequently, they are able to access only emergency treatment. Moreover, Juan Jr. can receive medical treatment only if he lives in a state that provides health care services to children and adolescents regardless of immigration status. Lucia and Maria are United States citizens because of their birthplace, and Carmen might be able to apply for health care benefits for them.

In the current immigration climate the parents may be fearful that if their undocumented immigrant status is discovered they will be deported and the two youngest children will have to go into Child Protective Services care.

Cultural issues are very relevant in understanding the needs of this family. The grandmother consulted a spiritualist before seeking medical treatment and then only on an emergency basis. With a possible life-threatening disease how much should the public health social worker insist that Rosa follow up with Western medical assessment and treatment rather than pursuing care from a spiritualist?

Discrimination, racism, and sexism are also evident in this case example. Juan Jr. feels discriminated against because he is the darkest in his family, as well as at school. Also, neither parent is able to work regularly because they are undocumented immigrants. It has been easier for Carmen to work as a domestic or child care worker. The fact that she is the one who has brought income into the family, rather than Pablo, has led to increased relationship conflict.

Questions

1. What areas of strength do you see in this family?
2. From a micro-practice perspective, how would the public health social worker assess and develop appropriate interventions for individual family members as well as the family as a whole?
3. From a mezzo-practice perspective, how would a public health social worker assess and develop appropriate interventions?
4. From a macro-practice perspective, how would a public health social worker assess and develop appropriate interventions?
5. What primary, secondary, and tertiary prevention methods would be helpful for this family and other similar families?

INTERNET RESOURCES

Henry Kaiser Family Foundation

(www.kaiseredu.org/Issue-Modules/Immigrants-Coverage-and-Access-to-Health-Care/Policy-Research.aspx)

The Kaiser Family Foundation has compiled a database of resources regarding insurance coverage and access to health care, including costs and coverage, health indicators, linguistic competency, issues facing specific immigrant populations, and the effects of health and welfare reform.

National Alliance on Mental Illness (NAMI): Cultural Competence

(www.nami.org/Content/NavigationMenu/Find_Support/Multicultural_Support/Cultural_Competence/Cultural_Competence.htm)

NAMI provides information and resources for practitioners and organizations on culturally appropriate mental health services. The website also includes a "Toolkit for Assessing Cultural Competence in Peer-Run Mental Health Organizations."

National Council of La Raza (NCLR): Health and Nutrition

(www.nclr.org/index.php/issues_and_programs/health_and_nutrition/)

The NCLR Institute for Hispanic Health works to reduce the prevalence of health disparities and various negative health outcomes common to Latinos in the United States.

Southeast Asia Resource Action Center

(www.searac.org/content/health-policy-resource-hub)

Provides policy briefs, reports, fact sheets, and resources on health policies specific to Southeast Asian immigrants and other immigrant populations as well.

U.S. Department of Health and Human Services (DHHS): Health Resources and Service Administration

(www.hrsa.gov/culturalcompetence/index.html)

The DHHS website includes information and links for health care professionals on cultural and linguistic competence in the areas of health communication.

REFERENCES

Addressing Racial and Ethnic Disparities in Health Care" Fact Sheet. AHRQ Publication No. 00-PO41, February 2000. Agency for Healthcare Research and Quality, Rockville, MD. http://www.ahrq.gov/research/disparit.htm

Akresh, I. R. (2007). Dietary assimilation and health among Hispanic immigrants to the United States. *Journal of Health and Social Behavior, 48*, 404–417.

Akresh, I. R. (2009). Health service utilization among immigrants to the United States. *Population Research and Policy Rev, 28*, 795–815.

Centers for Disease Control and Prevention. (2007). *Leading causes of death.* Retrieved from http://www.cdc.gov/nchs/FASTATS/lcod.htm

Cho, Y., Frisbie, W. P., Hummer, R. A., & Rogers, R. G. (2004). Nativity, duration of residence, and the health of Hispanic adults in the United States. *The International Migration Review, 38*(1), 184–211.

Congress, E. (2004). Cultural and ethnic issues in working with culturally diverse patients and their families: Use of the culturagram to promote cultural competency in health care settings. *Social Work in Health Care, 39*(3/4), 249–262.

Congress, E. (2009). Introduction: Legal and social work issues with immigrants. In F. Chang-Muy & E. Congress (Eds.), *Social work with immigrants and refugees: Legal issues, clinical skills, and advocacy* (pp. 3–37). New York: Springer Publishing Company.

Congress, E. (2010). Developing a cultural health assessment tool (CHAT). Paper presented at the 138th annual meeting of the American Public Health Association, Denver, CO.

Drachman, D. (1992). A stage of migration framework for service to immigrant populations. *Social Work, 37*, 68-72.

Fennelly, C. (2006). *The healthy migrant effect. Minnesota Medicine.* Retrieved November 1, 2010. http://www.minnesotamedicine.com/PastIssues/PastIssues2007/March2007/FennellyClinicalMarch2007/tabid/1641/Default.asp

Gibbie, K., Rosenstock, L., & Hernandez, L. (Eds.). (2003). *Who will keep the public healthy in the 21st century?* Washington, DC: National Academy Press.

Goel, M. S., McCarthy, E. P., Phillips, R. S., & Wee, C. C. (2004). Obesity among immigrant subgroups by duration of residence. *Journal of the American Medical Association, 292*(23), 2860-2867.

Goldberg, M. (2000). Conflicting principles in multicultural social work. *Families in Society 81*(1), 12-33.

Goldman, N., Kimbro, R., Turra, C., & Pebley, R. (2006). Socioeconomic gradients in health for white and Mexican-origin populations. *American Journal of Public Health, 96*(12), 2186-2193.

Gutheil, I., & Heyman, J. (2005). Working with culturally diverse older adults. In E. Congress & M. Gonzalez (Eds.), *Multicultural perspectives in working with families* (2nd ed., pp. 11-127). New York: Springer Publishing Company.

Hall, H. I., McDavid, H., Ling, K., & Sloggett, A. (2005). Survival after diagnosis of AIDS, United State. Annals of Epidemiology, *15*(8), 630-665.

Hansen, E., & Donohoe, M. (2003). Health issues of migrant and seasonal farmworkers. *Journal of Health Care for the Poor and Underserved, 14*(2), 153-163.

Hernandez, D. J., & Charney, E. (1998). *From generation to generation: The health and well-being of children in immigrant families.* Washington, DC: National Academies Press.

Himmelgreen, D. A., Perez, E., Martinez, D., Bretnall, A., Eells, B., & Peng, Y. (2003). The longer you stay, the bigger you get: Length of time and language use in the U.S. are associated with obesity in Puerto Rican women. *American Journal of Physical Anthropology, 125*(1), 90-96.

Institute of Medicine. (2002). *Unequal treatment: Confronting racial and ethnic disparities in health care.* Washington, DC: National Academies Press.

Keefe, R. H. (2010). Health Disparities: A primer for public health social workers. *American Journal of Public Health, 25*, 237-257.

Kochanek, K., Xu, J., Murphy, S., Minino, A., & Kung, H. (2011). Preliminary data for 2009. *Vital Statistics Report, 59*(4). Retrieved from http://www.cdc.gov/nchs/data/nvsr/nvsr59/nvsr59_04.pdf

Koya, D. L., & Egede, L. (2007). Association between length of residence and cardiovascular disease risk factors among an ethnically diverse group of United States immigrants. *Society of General Internal Medicine, 22*, 841-846.

Lara, M., Gamboa, C., Kahramanian, M., Morales, L., Hayes, D., & Bautista, D. (2005). Acculturation and Latino health in the United States: A review of the literature and its sociopolitical context. *Annual Review Public Health, 26*, 367-397.

Livingston, G., Minushkin, S., & Cohn, D. (2008). *Hispanics and health care in the United States: Access, information and knowledge.* Retrieved July 28, 2011, from http://pewhispanic.org/reports/report.php?ReportID=91

Lee, E. (1966). A theory of migration. *Demography, 3*, 47–57.

McDonald, J. T., & Kennedy, S. (2004). Insights into the "Healthy Immigrant Effect": Health status and health service use of immigrants to Canada. *Social Science & Medicine, 59*(8), 1613–1637.

Mendoza, F. (2009). Health disparities and children in immigrant families: A research agenda. *Pediatrics, 124*(3), 187–195.

Misra, A., & Ganda, O. (2007). Migration and its impact on adiposity and type 2 diabetes. *Nutrition, 23*, 696–708.

National Association of Social Workers. (2008). *Code of ethics.* Washington, DC: Author.

Palmer, N., & Kaufmann, M. (2003). The ethics of informed consent: Implications for multicultural practice. *Journal of Ethnic and Cultural Diversity in Social Work, 12*(1), 1–26.

Public Health Leadership Society. (2002). Principles of ethical practice of public health, version 2.2. Washington DC: Public Health Leadership Society.

Public Health Social Work Standards and Competencies. (2005). Retrieved July 29, 2011, from www.oce.sph.unc.edu/cetac/phswcompetencies_may05.pdf

Sandhuaus, S. (1998). Migrant health: A harvest of poverty. *American Journal of Nursing, 98*(9), 52–54.

Smedley, B. D., Stitch, A. Y., & Nelson, A. R. (2003). *Unequal treatment: Confronting racial and ethnic disparities in health care.* Washington, DC: National Academies Press.

Smith, S. (2009). Social work and physical health issues of immigrants. In F. Chang-Muy & E. Congress (Eds.), *Social work with immigrants and refugees* (pp. 103–133). New York: Springer Publishing.

Thomas, J. C., Sage, M., Dillenberg, J., & Guillory, V. J. (2002). A code of ethics for public health. *American Journal of Public Health, 92*(7), 1957–1059.

US Department of Health and Human Services, Agency for Health care Research and Quality. (2000). *Addressing racial and ethnic disparities in health care fact sheet AHR.* Retrieved from September 17, 2012. http://www.ahrq.gov/research/disparit. htm

U.S. Department of Health and Human Services. (2010). *The Secretary's Advisory Committee on National Health Promotion and Disease Prevention Objectives for 2020. Phase I report: Recommendations for the framework and format of Healthy People 2020. Section IV. Advisory Committee findings and recommendations.* Aceessed September 17, 2012 from http://www.healthypeople.gov/hp2020/advisory/PhaseI/ sec4.htm#_Toc211942917.

Ward, E., Jemal, A., Cokkinides, V., Gopal, K., Singh, G., Cardinez, C., et al. (2004). Cancer disparities by race/ethnicity and socioeconomic status. *CA Cancer Journal for Clinicians, 54*, 78–93.

Wells, K., Klap, R., Koike, K., & Sherbourne, C. (2001). Ethnic disparities in unmet need for alcoholism, drug abuse and mental health care. *American Journal of Psychiatry, 57*(1), 36–54.

Wilson, E., Chen, A., Grumbach, K., Wang, F., & Fernandez, A. (2005). Effects of limited English proficiency and physician language on health care comprehension. *Journal of General Internal Medicine, 20*, 800–806.

CHAPTER 7

HIV/AIDS and Public Health Social Work

Julie Cederbaum and Robert H. Keefe

INTRODUCTION

*T*he year 2013 marks the 32nd year since the discovery of the human immunodeficiency virus (HIV). During this short period of time, HIV/AIDS has become the leading cause of death and lost years of productivity for adults aged 15 to 59 worldwide (Lee, 2004). Virtually no country exists that is unaffected by HIV (UNAIDS, 2010). Once thought to be a problem among certain "high-risk" populations, such as men who have sex with men (MSM), injection drug users (IDUs), and sex workers, HIV/AIDS spares no group and affects members of every race, ethnicity, sex, religion, socioeconomic class, and age.

Public health social workers play a pivotal role in the prevention of HIV through their work in health education and health promotion, counseling, and services to HIV-infected and noninfected individuals. The services provided include risk-reduction strategies, primary (to those who are HIV negative) and secondary prevention (to those who are already infected with HIV), help with medication adherence and compliance, care coordination and management, and counseling. Some of the primary issues that HIV-infected persons and persons at high risk for HIV infection face include substance use, stigma, discrimination, incarceration, and problems accessing care. This chapter highlights the disparities and inequities many people with HIV in the United States face with the goal of learning how public health social workers can effectively provide health education and health promotion, HIV-risk reduction strategies, and other services to persons infected and affected by HIV.

CORE FUNCTIONS OF PUBLIC HEALTH

In 1998, the National Institutes of Health established three core functions of the practice of public health: assessment, assurance, and policy development. This section highlights the ways in which these three core functions are carried out in working with people infected and affected by HIV/AIDS.

Assessment

Assessment involves monitoring the health status of an individual, family, group, or community in order to identify and diagnose health issues and evaluate the effectiveness, accessibility, and quality of available health services. It promotes health education, prioritizes funding for services, increases public awareness, and decreases stigma related to HIV.

One area in which public health social workers practice their assessment skills is in jails and prisons, where a disproportionate number of individuals are living with or are at risk for contracting HIV. Available research has concluded that because of consensual and forced sex acts while incarcerated, many men in prison are exposed to HIV (Rapposelli et al., 2002). These men may not know their HIV status. Consequently, they can unintentionally spread the virus to other prisoners who themselves spread the virus to sexual partners in jails and, later, in their home communities. In response to this assessment, a public health policy change may be to offer HIV testing to inmates upon entry to and exit from incarceration facilities.

Adimora et al. (2002) provided an excellent example of public health assessment related to HIV. They interviewed mothers who tested HIV positive after childbirth. Many states encourage testing pregnant women and require testing of newborn infants for HIV. Because many of the mothers had not received prenatal care they were unaware of their HIV status until their newborn babies were tested. During interviews the researchers discovered that all of the fathers of the babies born to these mothers had been incarcerated within a 24-month period. The fathers denied being members of any high-risk groups; however, they did report that they had been tattooed while in prison and shared tattooing paraphernalia such as aluminum foil and metal guitar strings. Because of the disproportionate rates of incarceration in these fathers' home communities, there were many fewer available men than women. The mothers reported that there was much "man-sharing" in which one male individual would have concurrent sexual relationships with several different women, who, due to the disproportionate sex ratios resulting from incarceration, lacked the bargaining power in their relationships to require the men to be monogamous.

This example illustrates how an individual event (tattooing), when practiced without adhering to low-risk practices (using "clean" metal guitar strings or aluminum foil), led to infecting families (the mothers and their unborn children) and a community (fellow prison/jail inmates and members of the home community). Due to the lack of access to "clean" needles for tattooing or bleach to clean used guitar strings and aluminum foil, the men lacked self-protective methods that could have prevented the spread of HIV.

Assurance

Assurance is the guarantee from a community to its citizens that they will have a competent health care workforce to remedy problems discovered during community assessments. The health force works to develop additional health services that may not otherwise be available. For example, the services may be public health clinics for prenatal care and sexually transmitted infections, and other ad hoc services, including free annual flu shots.

Consider our example above. Most state and federal prisons do not allow for condom distribution and "clean" needle exchange. In order to assure that inmates can be self-protective, several states have begun to allow jails to distribute condoms (Harawa, Sweat, George, & Sylla, 2010; Sylla, Harawa, & Reznick, 2010; Tucker, Chang, & Tulsky, 2007). Despite this more open stance on inmate sexual practices, some states will allow inmates to have condoms in the jails and prisons but will not distribute them. Although condoms have become available in some major city jails (such as New York City; Philadelphia; Los Angeles; San Francisco; and Washington, DC) since the late 1990s, ongoing work is needed to expand both HIV testing and condom access in other correctional facilities (Tucker, Chang, & Tulsky, 2007). As a result, the communities (in this case a county jail) have not used evidence-based research on best practices that would help eliminate the spread of an infectious disease (i.e., HIV).

Policy Development

Policy development involves putting into place plans that support health efforts on both individual and community levels. These policies are meant to enforce laws and regulations that protect health and ensure its safety. In all states, it is illegal for individuals to knowingly spread the HIV virus (Burris, Beletsky, Burleson, Case, & Lazzarini, 2007; Gostin, 2000; Tucker, Chang, & Tulsky, 2007). This policy extends to individuals who may not have been tested for HIV but have reason to suspect that they may be HIV infected.

Once again, consider our example from above. The mothers interviewed in the Adimora et al. (2002) study who did not know they were HIV positive and consequently spread the virus to their unborn children would not be considered blameworthy for infecting their child, but what about the fathers? A quick review of HIV-screening instruments will point out that "partner incarceration" was not listed as a high-risk category. The men who had become HIV positive could safely say that they were not members of high-risk groups as per the screening-instrument criteria. If, as they stated, they had not engaged in unsafe sex practices or used "dirty" needles, they were not blameworthy. Still, the men did exchange aluminum foil and metal guitar strings while administering tattoos. By using these paraphernalia, the men exchanged body fluids (i.e., blood gathered on the metal guitar strings and aluminum foil). The former inmate who is perhaps somewhat concrete in his thinking and lacks abstract thinking skills may not be able to make the connection between the foil and strings with "dirty" needles used by intravenous drug users. Interestingly, the men indicated they knew intravenous drug use is a high-risk activity that could transmit the HIV virus, but not the guitar strings and foil.

This distinction brings into question the effectiveness of the policy. Should the federal government consider altering HIV-screening instruments to add a question of partner incarceration? If this question is added, it is possible that culpability shifts from the individual to the correctional facilities. For instance, consider an individual who is sentenced to jail. This individual enters jail HIV negative and while there is infected with the HIV virus. In the event this individual is in a jail that does not allow condom distribution or needle exchange and infects a sexual partner once released from jail, who would be held culpable? In this jail, the inmate is not allowed the opportunity to practice self-protection if he is engaging in consensual or nonconsensual sexual activity with another inmate who has HIV, particularly if the inmate is not aware of his own HIV-positive status. In such a case might the state be held culpable? These and other questions concerning HIV policy need to be addressed and further evaluated and offer public health social workers, who wish to pursue jobs in health policy, with interesting career opportunities.

Healthy People 2020

The U.S. Department of Health and Human Services (DHHS, 2011) sets specific benchmarks for various health conditions as published in its Healthy People report. There are 11 objectives with respect to HIV/AIDS: (1) reduce the number of cases of AIDS among adults and adolescents; (2) reduce the number of new AIDS cases among adolescent and adult MSM;

(3) reduce the number of new AIDS cases among adolescents and adults who inject drugs; (4) reduce the number of new cases of HIV/AIDS diagnosed among adults and adolescents; (5) increase the proportion of substance abuse treatment facilities and other HIV/AIDS education, counseling, and support services; (6) increase the proportion of adults with tuberculosis who have been tested for HIV; (7) reduce the number of deaths from HIV infection; (8) increase the proportion of new HIV infections diagnosed before progression to AIDS; (9) increase the proportion of persons surviving more than 3 years after being diagnosed with AIDS; (10) reduce the number of new cases of perinatally acquired HIV and AIDS diagnosed each year; and (11) increase the proportion of sexually active persons who use condoms.

Some objectives, such as "reducing the number of deaths due to HIV infection," are familiar and have been a focus of the HIV service delivery system for many years, while others, such as "increase the proportion of adults with tuberculosis who have been tested for HIV," reflect the changing trends in HIV infection. The DHHS has been effective in achieving many of these benchmarks: the number of cases of HIV among adolescent and adult MSM had declined for many years such that the DHHS would consider this objective to be on the verge of being met. In recent years, however, the rates have increased and may reflect the increase in numbers of men and adolescent males who do not self-identify as gay or homosexual but engage in high-risk sexual behaviors with other male partners. Many of these men may also be married or in relationships with women who are unaware of the men's sexual relations occurring outside the heterosexual relationships.

Other social issues, including disproportionate rates of incarceration among people of color—particularly men—have led to increases in tuberculosis (an AIDS-defining condition), which some have indicated is running rampant in jails and prisons (Bick, 2007; MacNeil et al., 2007). Incarceration has also led to an increase in the number of women diagnosed with HIV whose infected male partners return home after release from corrections facilities and reengage in the romantic relationships they left behind. The men in turn transmit HIV to their female partners. Many of the women do not learn of their status until they are tested during pregnancy. Because of this problem, the DHHS maintains the goal of increasing HIV testing during the prenatal period with the goal of decreasing the rates of perinatally transmitted cases of HIV. Further, lack of needle-exchange programs in the United States perpetuates the use of "dirty needles," which in turn increase HIV transmission among IDUs. Despite clear and convincing evidence that needle-exchange programs reduce the rates of HIV infections while not increasing the numbers of individuals who inject recreational drugs (DesJarlais & Semaan, 2008; Wodak & Cooney, 2006), many communities refuse to allow such programs to operate in their communities.

Cultural determinants impact other methods that have been known to curtail HIV transmission, including condom use and HIV testing. Clear and convincing evidence exists that condoms reduce the spread of HIV. In some communities, however, condom use is heavily frowned upon. For instance, in the African American and Latino communities men have been found to limit condom use, believing it to be unmanly (Lane et al., 2004). Many African American and Latina women report that they have limited bargaining power in their relationships due to fewer available men and therefore cannot mandate that their male partners use condoms for fear of losing their man to another woman (Guttentag & Secord, 1983). Beyond condom use, early testing has been shown to increase the longevity of individuals diagnosed with HIV (Beckwith et al., 2005). Stigma and cultural beliefs about HIV transmission influence HIV testing in many communities. Therefore, despite recommendations from the Centers for Disease Control and Prevention (CDC) that all sexually active individuals be tested yearly (CDC, 2007), many individuals do not get tested. Yearly screening has major public health implications as HIV-positive individuals who are tested early in their illness will likely live longer than HIV-positive individuals who are tested later.

For the *Healthy People 2020* objectives to be attained, treatment facilities that offer HIV education, counseling, and testing need to be continually enhanced to meet the existing and emerging community needs. Various organizations nationwide continue to operate on shoestring budgets that do not allow them to reach out to communities impacted by HIV.

Disparities and Inequities in HIV/AIDS in the United States

The CDC estimates that there are more than 1,000,000 individuals residing in the United States who are infected with HIV (CDC, 2010e). Of the estimated 56,300 new annual cases, 53% are among gay/bisexual men, 27% are among women, 45% are among African Americans (CDC, 2010a), and 34% are among individuals aged between 13 and 29 (Hall et al., 2008). Since the introduction of Highly Active Antiretroviral Therapy (HAART) in 1995, there have been significant changes in illness course, life expectancy, and quality of life for people with HIV in the United States. Although the incidence of new infections has not decreased, deaths from AIDS-related complications have declined, thereby increasing the number of people living with HIV.

Despite the increased longevity, HIV is a major contributor to excess loss of life. In 2007, HIV was the sixth leading cause of death for all persons aged between 25 and 44 and the fourth leading cause for individuals aged between 35 and 44 (Minino, Xu, & Kochanek, 2010). Furthermore, HIV was the fourth leading cause of death among African American men and women (aged 25–54) and the fourth leading cause of death among Hispanics (aged 35–44). Reported cases of AIDS in the United States have been primarily concentrated in large metropolitan areas (85%), with 10 of those accounting for 42% of all reported cases (Kaiser Family Foundation, 2007). The Northeastern U.S. has the highest AIDS rate (21.1 per 100,000) (CDC, 2007).

HIV/AIDS Among Women

Worldwide, sexually transmitted diseases (STDs), including HIV, affect women more than men (Aral, Hawkes, Biddlecom, & Padian, 2004; Kates & Leggoe, 2005). Women are at risk for STDs due to their own risky behavior and increased biological risk for infection. They may also be at risk due to the behaviors of their partners, who may have multiple sexual partners (including sex workers), engage in gender roles that harm women (power, negation, and coercion by male partners over female partners), and enforce financial dependence (Aral et al., 2004; Myer, Kuhn, Stein, Wright, & Denny, 2005). In the United States, women account for an increasing number of newly diagnosed AIDS cases and deaths (CDC, 2004a; Kates & Leggoe, 2005). Although deaths from 2002 to 2006 dropped by 19.2% among men, they dropped only by 11.7% among women (CDC, 2007). This drop may be related to access to care, not making or being unable to make health care a priority, or a later stage of illness at time of diagnosis.

HIV/AIDS Among MSM

Although many groups once deemed at highest risk (i.e., sex workers and IDUs) have shown a decline in rates of new HIV infections (which is likely due to aggressive and effective campaigns, including needle exchange and condom distribution and negotiation training), this trend has not been the case among MSM, which is the group most severely affected by HIV and the only risk group where rates of new infections have steadily increased since the 1990s (CDC, 2010b). As a group, MSM are 44 to 86 times more likely to be diagnosed with HIV as compared to other men and 40 to 77 times more likely than women (CDC, 2010b). Almost one-half of all new HIV infections are found among MSM, particularly White male individuals (46% of new infections) who are more likely to be older (30–49 years) when infected (CDC, 2010b). More than half of all new infections among Black MSM occurred among 13- to 29-year-olds, making infections among young Black MSM twice that of Whites. Young Hispanic MSM are also at increased risk (43% of HIV infections occurred in the youngest age group, 13 to 29 years [CDC, 2010b]).

HIV/AIDS Among African Americans and Hispanics

Race and ethnicity correlate with other determinants of health, such as poverty, access to quality health care, health care-seeking behaviors, illicit drug use, and living in communities with a high prevalence of STDs (CDC, 2002). African Americans and Hispanics are at increased risk of sexually acquired HIV infection due to lower socioeconomic status, urbanicity, and the impact of these factors on risky behaviors such as drug and alcohol use, violence, and imprisonment (UNAIDS, 2004). Male and female African Americans account for 46% of HIV/AIDS cases in the United States (CDC, 2010c). Black men accounted for two-thirds of all new infections; Black women are 15 times more likely to be HIV infected than White women. Among all women, African American female individuals account for 64% of all HIV/AIDS cases (CDC, 2008). Estimates of AIDS prevalence among African Americans increased by 12% between 2005 and 2008. If these rates continue, 1 in 16 Black men, and 1 in 30 Black women, will be diagnosed with HIV at some point in their lives (CDC, 2010c). Significant racial and ethnic disparities among adolescents exist as well (CDC, 2008).

Like African Americans, Hispanic/Latinos account for a growing number of HIV infections in the United States. Recent reports show 17% of all new infections were among this group, making them 2.5 times more likely than Whites to become infected (CDC, 2010d). Among Hispanic/Latinos, men account for the majority of new infections (76%). Rates of HIV infection among Hispanic/Latina women are 4 times that of White women. Similar to African Americans, rates of new infections among Hispanic/Latinos rose 5% between 2005 and 2008, which may reflect the growing migration trends in the United States (CDC, 2010a). Among Hispanic/Latino teens, 13- to 19-year-olds account for 19%, and 20- to 24-year-olds account for 24%, of all AIDS cases in the United States (KKF, 2010).

HIV/AIDS and Drug Use

Substance use/abuse has a bifold link to HIV infection: (1) needle sharing among IDUs exposes individuals to bodily fluids that carry the virus and (2) individuals are more likely to engage in risky sexual behavior while under the influence of alcohol or other drugs (Ehrenstein, Horton, & Samet, 2004; Logan & Leukefeld, 2000; Nadeau, Truchon, & Biron, 2000; Rees, Saitz, Horton, & Samet, 2001; Stein et al., 2005; Tortu et al., 2000). Drug and alcohol use can impair safe-sex related judgment and increase impulsivity (Semaan, Des Jarlais, & Malow, 2007; Semple et al., 2009). Use is also connected with unprotected sexual intercourse, trading sex for drugs, and engaging in sex with multiple partners (Cooper, 2006; Leigh, Ames, & Stacy, 2008; Raj et al., 2009; Raj, Saitz, Cheng, Winter, & Samet, 2007; Semaan, Des Jarlais, & Malow, 2007). Substance use remains significantly associated with HIV among other sexually transmitted infections (Bachmann et al., 2000; Heimer, Grau, Curtin, Khoshnood, & Singer, 2007; Plitt et al., 2005; Semple, Amaro, Strathdee, Zians, & Patterson, 2009). IDU is thought to account directly or indirectly to 36% of infections (CDC, 2002). IDUs account for 12% of new infections and 19% of all HIV-infected persons (CDC, 2010a).

Summary

Since 1981, HIV has progressed from an illness affecting small, specific, socially segregated populations. However, today no group is completely risk free. Although the illness has been somewhat "managed" in the Western industrialized world, there remain significant disparities. There is clear epidemiological evidence of the disproportionate number of AIDS cases and new HIV infections among MSM, IDUs, and African Americans and Latinos in the United States. Beyond race/ethnicity, being female also increases one's risk of contracting HIV due to increased biological suscepti-bility (Myer, Kuhn, Stein, Wright, & Denny, 2005). The introduction of HAART has led to a dramatic shift in the HIV epidemic. HIV is now considered a chronic auto-immune disorder. Public health social workers must focus both on primary and secondary prevention strategies, services to persons infected and affected by HIV/AIDS, and continued advocacy for access to ser-vices for this highly vulnerable population.

Public Health Social Work Practice in HIV

As part of our core competencies, public health social workers seek to promote optimal health; inform and educate individuals, families, and com-munities; and mobilize communities to make normative changes to promote better health outcomes. When working with individuals and com-munities with HIV or at risk for HIV, public health social workers must be aware of the history of the disease and the differing beliefs and stigma associ-ated with it. This section will discuss these ongoing issues as well as barriers to HIV testing, and ways in which public health social workers can effectively intervene.

Public Health Social Work Standards and Competencies

Public health social work is characterized by its use of an epidemiologic approach to the prevention and treatment of social health issues (Ruth, Wyatt, Chiasson, Geron, & Bachman, 2006) and the psychosocial support provided to individuals and families coping with chronic illnesses like HIV. Among the core practice standards and competencies in public health social work are health education and health promotion.

Most of our work is accomplished within interdisciplinary and transdisciplinary teams in hospitals, clinics, and other community-based settings. Public health social workers may work directly with individuals and families, create community- or policy-level changes, and use evidence-based strategies to enhance health promotion that strengthen social support systems to reduce social stressors that worsen health outcomes. Here we describe how three important public health social worker standards and competencies can be employed to make individual and structural changes for persons infected, affected, and at risk for HIV/AIDS.

Standard: Identify, Measure, Assess, and Monitor Social Problems Affecting Health Status

We alleviate social problems such as HIV by using our social epidemiology, program evaluation, and research skills to document the impact of HIV on communities. To start, public health social workers can help people understand the dynamics of HIV in their communities. Much of this information is already collected at the county, state, and federal levels but is not always translated for use in all communities, particularly rural or nonurban areas. Once we understand what the epidemic looks like in a community, we seek funding for services that help reduce the spread of HIV. We can then disseminate information on the impact of the services in a number of ways, including working with schools, public health departments, health clinics, and local community-based organizations in tracking the effectiveness of HIV-prevention programs; providing medical services for people who are HIV infected; and linking HIV-infected and affected individuals and their families to various social services. Knowing which groups are using services allows public health social workers to create targeted awareness campaigns that are regionally and culturally appropriate. The campaigns provide opportunities for local governments to evaluate and allocate funds in ways that are most effective for their communities and to maximize the potential for bringing about change in the neediest communities.

Standard: Develop Primary Prevention Strategies That Promote Health and Well-Being

Public health social workers are poised not only to assist their communities to identify HIV prevention needs, but also to make use of HIV-prevention strategies. By using our knowledge and accessing evidence-based prevention projects funded at the state and federal levels (e.g., the CDC provides opportunities for community-based organizations to receive the supplies, training, and technical assistance to help implement evidence-based interventions through their Diffusion of Effective Behavioral Interventions project), public health social workers can bridge the gap between research and practice that is essential to building effective prevention strategies.

Standard: Provide Quality Services Within a Cultural, Community, and Family Context

Our efforts, of course, must be carried out in a context that accounts for differences in age, race/ethnicity, culture, language, and gender. Understanding the community beliefs concerning a sensitive and stigmatized chronic condition like HIV helps us to promote the inclusion of people with HIV in planning efforts, and increase our knowledge of how best to intervene by way of tailored promotion and prevention messages.

HIV-related stigma is generally viewed as more negative than other conditions, such as mental illness and physical disability (Corrigan et al., 2000). Among persons living with AIDS, self-stigma has been linked to lower self-esteem, depression, and anxiety (Lee et al., 2002; Treisman & Angelino, 2004). Persons living with HIV/AIDS struggle with their own internalized negative attitudes about the illness and often have prejudicial attitudes and may discriminate against others living with HIV before knowing they are infected themselves (Bogart et al., 2008). Because of this internal and external stigma, individuals are often reluctant to disclose their HIV status or request that their status remain a family secret. There are varied beliefs about how HIV began, who is at risk for HIV, how it is transmitted, and the reasons why specific groups are at greater risk. We must be aware of cultural nuances concerning HIV so that we can respectfully work within these belief systems, as well as work to make normative changes.

Where Public Health Social Workers Make a Difference in HIV/AIDS

There are many ways in which public health social workers can impact primary and secondary HIV prevention. In this section, we will highlight health promotion and health education.

Health Promotion/Health Education

Larger scale health promotion is a method of action firmly grounded in public health social work that includes efforts at the local, regional, or national levels to promote HIV testing, abstinence, condom use, and clean needle exchange. We encourage and link people to resources that support good nutrition, exercise, and mental health to promote healthy lifestyles.

Health education related to primary and secondary HIV prevention is a vital part of our healthy community dialogues. These conversations must include discussions about community attitudes and beliefs related to HIV (i.e., how "real" is HIV to people in the community, what are their beliefs about transmission and are these beliefs accurate, do they believe condoms are effective in preventing HIV), community norms related to sexual health practices (i.e., do individuals believe abstinence is realistic, do most people use condoms), and their ability and intention to avoid behaviors that put them at risk for HIV. We know that individuals are deeply impacted by the norms of their referent groups (Azjen, 2002) and therefore we need to inform and educate individuals and communities by using a comprehensive framework; we need to change knowledge, attitudes, and beliefs not just for the individual, but the community as well.

Unprotected Sex

Changing risky sexual behaviors is the primary intervention target for HIV prevention. These risks include early sexual initiation, number of sexual partners, concurrent sexual partnering, and condom use. With young people (under the age of 12 years), abstinence promotion has been shown to effectively delay the onset of sexual activity (Kirby, 2008; Jemmott, Jemmott, & Fong, 2010). With adolescents, a more effective approach is the combination of abstinence and safe-sex promotion (most often condom use) during sexual intercourse (Kohler, Manhart, & Lafferty, 2008; Isley et al., 2010). With adults, condom use promotion is the most common approach.

There are many factors that shape how people view the importance of condom use during intercourse. Marston and King (2006) found that the primary motives for using condoms fell into seven categories: (1) the assessment of sex partners as being "clean" or "unclean"; (2) the important influence sex partners had on behavior (i.e., promoting of safe behaviors); (3) the beliefs that condoms were stigmatizing and were associated with lack of trust; (4) the gender stereotypes, which determined expectations and behavior; (5) the penalties and rewards from society for engaging in sex; (6) the reputation and social displays of sexual activity or inactivity; and (7) the effect of social expectations that hamper communication about sex. As such, interventions may be focused on how persons perceived their partners, and increasing partner communication and negotiation.

Alcohol and Drug Use

Given the well-documented link between engaging in unsafe sex and substance use with HIV (Ehrenstein, Horton, & Samet, 2004; Heimer et al., 2007; Plitt et al., 2005; Semple et al., 2009; Stein et al., 2005), it is vital to highlight substance use/misuse information and HIV education. To do so, we would include the ways alcohol and other drug use can influence engaging in sex without using condoms, having sex with multiple partners, and in engaging in transactional sex (i.e., exchanging sex for money). It is through promoting HIV knowledge and healthy sex and substance use behaviors that public health social workers can promote HIV-risk reduction within communities.

The intervention for IDUs that is found to be the most effective is reducing "needle sharing" (i.e., two or more people using the same needle without proper "cleaning" between injections) by making available needle exchange and bleach kits where IDUs can safely (and without judgment) exchange "used" needles for new needles. Both methods use the Harm Reduction model, which is guided by a set of strategies to reduce negative consequences of drug use. Harm Reduction includes meeting people "where they are," addressing conditions of use, and helping individuals employ strategies for safer use, which can lead to abstinence (as opposed to targeting abstinence first [Marlatt, 1996]). Grounded in public health social worker principles, harm reduction is a practical yet compassionate framework for reducing the damaging consequences of addictive behaviors (Marlatt, 1996).

Testing/Knowing Your Status

Testing may be the greatest and most important prevention campaign for HIV. HIV testing provides individuals with the opportunities to assess their risk, learn their status, gain new health-promotion skills, connect with service providers (if needed), and make a pledge to HIV-exposure harm reduction. There are other opportunities to promote HIV prevention, such as creating awareness events linked to World AIDS Day (December 1st); National HIV/AIDS Awareness days, including women, Native Americans, Asian and Pacific Islanders, Caribbean Americans, the elderly, gay men, Latinos, African Americans (www.aids.gov/awareness-days/); and National HIV Testing Day (June 27th). There are also creative ways to raise awareness, such as having people participate in poster contests (i.e., www.whatifitwereyou.org/) that may appeal to younger demographics. All of these approaches provide an opportunity to promote prevention and testing while reducing stigma through knowledge acquisition.

Stigma

Stigma is present in all communities and cultures; however, stigma affects each community differently. For example, in the African American community, stigma has been linked to increased psychological distress (Black & Miles, 2002; Lichtenstein et al., 2002). Rao et al. (2008) found that Blacks were more likely to report greater stigmatization, in which others discriminated against them, compared to Whites, who reported higher stigma related to keeping their status a secret and fear of interpersonal rejection. Reluctance to disclose to children is related to fear that the children would disclose the information to others who in turn would discriminate against them (Bogart et al., 2008). Most often children heed this advice, which places them at increased risk for anxiety and depression. For example, children of HIV-positive parents have reported being discriminated against by teachers, friends, and community members, which can lead to angry expressions of internalized stigma (Witte & deRidder, 1999). Children who hide HIV from others report stress and loneliness while relying on support from their immediate family only (Bogart et al., 2008). They express fears of abandonment upon parental death and blame their parent, perceiving one to be "reckless" and "loose" and see contracting HIV as a result of lack of good judgment and self-discipline (Witte & deRidder, 1999).

For both adults and adolescents, fears of disclosure are linked to social support. Perceived social support from family is inversely related to perceived HIV-related stigma (Galvan et al., 2008). Lower levels of HIV-related stigma are also positively correlated with better mental, physical, and social functioning (Galvan et al., 2008; Murphy et al., 2006).

SUMMARY

There are many ways in which pubic health social workers can influence knowledge, attitudes, beliefs, and behaviors related to primary and secondary prevention of HIV. In this section, we have detailed approaches that can be employed to increase awareness, reduce stigma, and promote health. As we have repeatedly stated, knowledge is a key component in reducing HIV risk. Although hard to imagine, there are still subgroups that have limited or incorrect knowledge of HIV transmission and risk. These misunderstandings may be normed by culture, faith systems, and personal experiences. Health literacy around HIV is also important. Based on the Health Belief Model (Janz & Becker, 1984), for individuals to think HIV testing is important, they must believe that they (1) are at risk for contracting HIV; (2) will face serious consequences if infected; (3) can do things to reduce their susceptibility to HIV; and (4) can address the anticipated barriers to taking action, which are outweighed by the benefits. For individuals to reduce their risk for HIV, they need to be clear about who is affected by HIV and how HIV is transmitted. They need to know about HIV testing, including how and where testing is done, and how they can access these services.

CLASSROOM EXERCISES

Case Scenario 1: Michael O'Brian

Michael O'Brian is an 18-year-old, gay, White male freshman at the state university who has recently "come out" to his friends and family. He states the "coming out" process was positive and that he is ready to start dating. Michael informs you that he is seeking services to learn more about self-protective measures so that he does not contract HIV or another STD. In your role as a social work intern at the student counseling center, you are to provide individual services to help students make the transition to college life and to link students to campus and other community resources that promote a healthy and positive college experience.

Exercises and Questions

It is likely that Michael is only one of many students who have recently "come out" and need services to protect them against HIV and other STDs. How would you gather information to formulate a needs assessment to assure adequate services are provided? Focus your thoughts on:

1. Gathering information of the number of students who may be in the "coming out" process and are at risk for contracting HIV or other STDs. Pay attention to differences you may find based on students' race, ethnicity, gender, spiritual/religious ideas, class, and other demographic variables.
2. Developing services for new students who need to develop self-protection skills against contracting HIV and other STDs. How would you go about evaluating the effectiveness of these services?
3. Reflecting on the services provided to sexual minorities, you discover there is little service coordination to help prevent HIV and other STDs. Discuss how you would develop a community assessment, network with university campus allies, and develop a strategic plan that you would present to your own college/university administration to help prevent HIV and other STDs among sexual minorities.
4. Researching the policies on services for students at the university, you discover there is a gap in the policy on HIV and other STD prevention. Write a concise policy statement and discuss how you would implement the policy.
5. Reviewing ethical issues, which ones do you see as potential challenges in your work with Michael? Think about the values of your own college/university, community, and cultural background.

Case Scenario 2: Re'shaun Lucas

Re'shaun Lucas is a pregnant 25-year-old, African American female who has recently been diagnosed with HIV. She does not know how long she has been HIV positive, but is certain that she contracted the virus from her husband, Jorell, age 27. Re'shaun decided to be tested after she heard a radio public-service announcement informing listeners that African Americans have been disproportionately infected with HIV. She told Jorell that they should both be tested but he refused to go, stating that there was no way he could be HIV positive. After Re'shaun's test came back positive Jorell agreed to be tested and found out that he too is HIV positive. Re'shaun states that Jorell has been sick off and on for the past 2 years, but he thought he was just run down. Upon further discussion, Jorell acknowledged that during his youth he engaged in high-risk behaviors that he was unaware could put him at risk for contracting HIV but has since given up those behaviors. They both report they are committed to each other and their family and that they are coming to the county department of health for information and guidance to help assure that Re'shaun does not transmit the virus to her unborn infant.

Exercises and Questions

Like many African Americans, Re'shaun and Jorell were unaware of their HIV status. At this time it is of utmost importance that they are provided with current information to help them plan for the healthy birth of their unborn child and to have a continued intimate relationship in which they do not reinfect each other. As a public health social worker employed at the county health department, your supervisor assigns you the task of reaching out to the African American community to find additional cases of pregnant women who may need services. To complete this assignment, discuss how you would

1. Use community organizing skills to reach out to African Americans in the community at risk for HIV.
2. Evaluate existing services to assure that they are providing culturally sensitive services.
3. Bring various community leaders together to address the rising rates of HIV in the African American community.
4. Build a coalition to advocate for the development of culturally sensitive services in existing agencies treating people living with HIV.

Case Scenario 3: Miguel Hernandez

Miguel Hernandez is a 52-year-old, Mexican American male who was recently diagnosed with HIV at the HIV/AIDS community agency in his county. Miguel reports that he has a long history of IDU but plans to start using clean needles offered by the agency's needle-exchange program. He states that he is worried that his friends who go to the same "shooting gallery" to shoot up may also be infected. Miguel believes these friends are unlikely to know their own HIV status and is concerned they may be spreading HIV. Furthermore, many of these friends do not speak English and are likely missing the harm-reduction messages the agency is putting out to the community. As the agency's outreach worker you are expected to provide services to all individuals in the county. Your supervisor has assigned you the task of reaching out to members of the IDU community who are not accessing the needle exchange program, particularly non-English-speaking residents. As you begin this project, think about:

1. Macro-level methods you can use to get the word out to various groups about the needle-exchange program, particularly non-English-speaking groups.
2. The data you will need to collect to assure everyone that you are reaching at-risk populations.
3. How to communicate effectively with diverse community members, including faith-based and other health organizations.
4. Identifying public health laws, regulations, and policies related to needle-exchange programs.
5. Community values that may impede reaching out to populations at risk of contracting HIV via intravenous drug use.

Key Issues

There are a number of key issues intimately intertwined with primary and secondary prevention. Racial/ethnic segregation, gender, poverty, and lack of access to health care remain predictors of HIV exposure. Further, factors such as legal status, acculturation, and cultural norms impact not only risk profiles, but the structural factors that place these groups in areas with greater concentrations of persons who are HIV infected. Attention has been given to structural factors that influence beliefs, norms, and behaviors, but to date there is little consensus on how best to influence these factors. In general, structural barriers can be viewed as fourfold: (1) the access to the product or item of interest, (2) the physical structures in the environment, (3) the community social structures, and (4) the messages derived from media and community culture (Cohen, Scribner, & Farley, 2000). Health behaviors are predicted by perception of neighborhood safety, housing, employment, and other opportunities. As such, engaging in HIV-risk behaviors cannot be viewed as just a product of group, race, and/or socioeconomic status, but rather also of social conditions (Cohen et al., 2000).

Neighborhoods that are saturated with violence and physical deterioration, among other stressors, reinforce high-risk community norms (Sampson et al., 1997). Other structural barriers can include local opportunity and community norms related to future orientation of an impaired community. We know that the more intimate the community, the more likely its members are to engage in it and have similar behaviors. Thus, the degree of social disintegration characterizing the community, socioeconomic status, and makeup all significantly contributes to determining sexual debut. By not accounting for neighborhood structure and safety, we overlook important factors that may influence engaging in HIV risk behaviors. As such, public health social workers must focus on how to most effectively intervene at various levels, moving beyond targeted individual-level change.

Comprehensive strategies are needed to meet the needs of those individuals most at risk for HIV infection. For example, individuals engaging in sex with multiple partners need to use condoms and decrease sexual concurrency to help reduce HIV exposure. For IDUs, comprehensive strategies, including harm-reduction techniques and access to substance use treatment, can help decrease HIV risk. For all groups, reducing the number of unprotected sex exposures, decreasing sexual activity while under the influence of alcohol and other drugs, increasing clean needle use among IDUs, reducing stigma, and promoting HIV testing are all efforts that will help to improve HIV prevention efforts.

INTERNET RESOURCES

Centers for Disease Control and Prevention (CDC)

(www.cdc.gov/hiv/topics/surveillance/basic.htm)
(www.cdc.gov/hiv/resources/factsheets/us.htm)
(www.cdc.gov/hiv/topics/surveillance/resources/reports/)

CDC National Prevention Information Network

(www.cdcnpin.org/)

Kaiser Family Foundation

(www.kff.org/hivaids/3029.cfm)

AIDS.gov

(http://aids.gov/)

World Health Organization

(www.who.int/hiv/en/)

United Joint Nations Programme on HIV/AIDS

(www.unaids.org/en/)

HIV/AIDS and Social Work Conference

(www.bc.edu/schools/gssw/academics/ce/conferences.html)

International Conference on AIDS

(www.aids2012.org/)

NASW HIV/AIDS Spectrum

(www.socialworkers.org/practice/hiv_aids/default.asp)

Professional Association of Social Workers in HIV and AIDS

(www.paswha.us/)

HIV Stops with me.org

(http://hivstopswithme.org/about-us)

POZ magazine

(www.poz.com/)

Division of HIV/AIDS Prevention at the CDC, Diffusion of Effective Intervention

(www.effectiveinterventions.org/en/home.aspx)

StopAIDS

(www.stopaids.org)

AIDS Education Global Information System

(www.aegis.com)

Project Inform

(www.projinf.org)

AIDSAction

(www.aidsaction.org)

Gay Men's Health Crisis

(www.gmhc.org)

The Body

(www.thebody.com)

Lifelong AIDS Alliance, Men's Program

(www.homohealth.org)

Be Greater than AIDS

(www.greaterthan.org/)

The Banyan Tree Project

(www.banyantreeproject.org/)

National Association of People Living with HIV/AIDS

(www.napwa.org/)

National Native American AIDS Prevention Center

(http://nnaapc.org/)

Me, Myself, & HIV

(http://hiv.staying-alive.org/)

REFERENCES

Adimora, A. A., Schoenbach, V. J., Bonas, D. M., Donaldson, K. H., Martinson, F. E. A., & Stancil, T. R. (2002). Concurrent sexual partnerships among women in the United States. *Epidemiology, 13,* 320–327.

Aral, S. O., Hawkes, S., Biddlecom, A., & Padian, N. (2004). *Disproportionate impact of sexually transmitted diseases on women.* Retrieved October 14, 2005, from http://www.cdc.gov/ncidod/EID/vol10no11/04-0623_02.htm

Azjen, I. (2002). Perceived behavioral control, self-efficacy, locus of control, and the theory of planned behavior. *Journal of Applied Social Psychology, 32,* 665–683.

Bachmann, L. H., Lewis, I., Allen, R., Schwebke, J. R., Leviton, L. C., Siegal, H. A., et al. (2000). Risk and prevalence of treatable sexually transmitted diseases at a Birmingham substance abuse treatment facility. *American Journal of Public Health, 90,* 1615–1618.

Beckwith, C. G., Flanigan, T. P., delRio, C., Simmons, E., Wing, E. J., Carpenter, C. C. J., et al. (2005). It is time to implement routine, not risk-based, HIV testing. *Clinical Infectious Disease, 40,* 1037–1040.

Bick, J. A. (2007). Infection control in jails and prisons. *Clinical Infectious Diseases, 45*(8), 1047–1055.

Black, B. P., & Miles, M. S. (2002). Calculating the risk and benefits of disclosure in African American women who have HIV. *Journal of Obstetric, Gynecologic, & Neonatal Nursing, 31,* 688–697.

Bogart, L. M., Cowgill, B. O., Kennedy, D., Ryan, G., Murphy, D. A., Elijah, J., et al. (2008). HIV-related stigma among people with HIV and their families: A qualitative analysis. *AIDS & Behavior, 12,* 244–254.

Burris, S., Beletsky, L., Burleson, J., Case, P., & Lazzarini, Z. (2007). Do criminal laws influence HIV risk behavior? An empirical trial. *Arizona State Law Journal, 39,* 467–519.

Centers for Disease Control and Prevention (CDC). (2002). Youth Risk Behavior Survey—United States, 2001. *Morbidity and Mortality Weekly Report, 51,* 13–15.

CDC. (2004). *HIV/AIDS surveillance in adolescents: L265 slide series.* Retrieved October 9, 2005, from http://www.cdc.gov/hiv/graphics/adolesnt.htm

CDC. (2007). *HIV/AIDS surveillance report.* Retrieved November 19, 2008, from http://www.cdc.gov/hiv/topics/surveillance/resources/reports/2005report/pdf/2005surveillancereport.pdf

CDC. (2008). *HIV/AIDS among African Americans.* Retrieved November 19, 2008, from http://www.cdc.gov/hiv/topics/aa/resources/factsheets/aa.htm

CDC. (2010a). *HIV/AIDS surveillance.* Retrieved February 26, 2011 from http://www.cdc.gov/hiv/topics/surveillance/resources/factsheets/pdf/surveillance.pdf

CDC. (2010b). *HIV among gay, bisexual and other men who have sex with men (MSM).* Retrieved February 26, 2011 from http://www.cdc.gov/hiv/topics/msm/pdf/msm.pdf

CDC. (2010c). *HIV/AIDS among African Americans.* Retrieved February 26, 2011 from http://www.cdc.gov/hiv/topics/aa/pdf/aa.pdf

CDC. (2010d). *HIV/AIDS among Hispanic/Latinos.* Retrieved February 26, 2011 from http://www.cdc.gov/hiv/hispanics/resources/factsheets/pdf/hispanic.pdf

CDC. (2010e). *HIV in the United States.* Retrieved February 26, 2011 from http://www.cdc.gov/hiv/resources/factsheets/PDF/us.pdf

Cohen, D. A., Scribner, R. A., & Farley, T. A. (2000). A structural model of health behavior: A pragmatic approach to explain and influence health behaviors at the population level. *Preventive Medicine, 30,* 146–154.

Cooper, M. L. (2006). Does drinking promote risky sexual behavior? A complex answer to a simple question. *Current Directions in Psychological Science, 15*(1), 19–23.

Corrigan, P. W., River, L. P., Lundin, R. K., Wasowski, K. V., Campion, J., Mathisen, J., et al. (2000). Stigmatizing attributions about mental illness. *Journal of Community Psychology, 28*(1), 91–102.

DesJarlais, D. C., & Semaan, S. (2008). HIV prevention for injecting drug users: The first 25 years and counting, *Psychosomatic Medicine, 70,* 606–611.

Ehrenstein, V., Horton, N. J., & Samet, J. H. (2004). Inconsistent condom use among HIV-infected patients with alcohol problems. *Drug and Alcohol Dependence, 73,* 159–166.

Galvan, F. H., Davis, E. M., Banks, D., & Bing, E. G. (2008). HIV stigma and social support among African Americans. *AIDS Patient Care and STDs, 22,* 423–436.

Gostin, L. O. (2000). *Public health law: Power, duty and restraint.* Los Angeles: University of California Press.

Guttentag, M., & Secord, P. (1983). *Too many women? The sex ratio question.* Newbury Park, CA: Sage Publications.

Hall, H. I., Song, R., Rhodes, P., Prejean, J., An, Q., Lee, L. M., et al. (2008). Estimation of HIV incidence in the United States. *Journal of the American Medical Association, 300,* 520-529.

Harawa, N. T., Sweat, J., George, S., & Sylla, M. (2010). Sex and condom use in a large jail unit for men who have sex with men and male-to-female transgenders. *Journal of Healthcare for Poor and Underserved, 21*(3), 1071-1087.

Heimer, R., Grau, L. E., Curtin, E., Khoshnood, K., & Singer, M. (2007). Assessment of HIV testing of urban injecting drug users: Implications for expansion of HIV testing and prevention efforts. *American Journal of Public Health, 97,* 110-116.

Isley, M. M., Edelman, A., Kaneshiro, B., Peters, D., Nichols, M. D., & Jensen, J. T. (2010). Sex education and contraceptive use at coital debut in the U.S.: Results from Cycle 6 of the National Survey of Family Growth. *Contraception, 82*(3), 236-242.

Janz, N. K., & Becker, M. H. (1984). The health belief model: A decade later. *Health Education & Health Behavior, 11,* 1-47.

Jemmot, J. B., Jemmott, L. S., & Fong, G. T. (2010). Efficacy of theory-based abstinence-only intervention over 24 months. *Archives of Pediatrics and Adolescent Medicine, 164*(2), 152-159.

Kaiser Family Foundation. (2007). *HIV/AIDS policy fact sheet: The HIV/AIDS epidemic in the United States.* Retrieved November 19, 2008, from http://www.kff.org/hivaids/upload/3029-071.pdf

Kaiser Family Foundation. (2010). *HIV/AIDS policy fact sheet: Latinos and HIV/AIDS.* Retrieved January 22, 2011 from http://www.kff.org/hivaids/upload/6007-08.pdf

Kates, J., & Leggoe, A. W. (2005). *HIV/AIDS policy fact sheet: The HIV/AIDS epidemic in the United States.* Retrieved September 25, 2005, from http://www.kff.org/hivaids/upload/Fact-Sheet-The-HIV-AIDS-Epidemic-in-the-United-States-2005-Update.pdf

Kirby, D. B. (2008). The impact of abstinence and comprehensive sex and STD/HIV education programs on adolescent sexual behavior. *Sexuality Research and Social Policy, 5*(3), 18-27.

Kohler, P. K., Manhart, L. E., & Lafferty, W. E. (2008). Abstinence-only and comprehensive sex education on the initiation of sexual activity and teen pregnancy. *Journal of Adolescent Health, 42,* 344-351.

Lane, S. D., Rubinstein, R. A., Keefe, R. H., Webster, N., Cibula, D., Rosenthal, A., & Dowdell, J. (2004). Structural violence and racial disparity in HIV transmission. *Journal of Health Care for the Poor and Underserved, 15*(3), 319-335.

Lee, J. W. (2004). *The World Health Report, 2004: Changing history.* Geneva, Switzerland: World Health Organization.

Lee, M. B., & Rotheram-Borus, M. J. (2002). Parents' disclosure of HIV to their children. *AIDS, 16,* 2201-2207.

Leigh, B. C., Ames, S. L., & Stacy, A. W. (2008). Alcohol, drugs, and condom use among drug offenders: An event-based analysis. *Drug and Alcohol Dependence, 93,* 32-38.

Lichtenstein, B., Laska, M. K., & Clair, J. M. (2002). Chronic sorrow in the HIV-positive patient: Issues of race, gender, and social support. *AIDS Patient Care and STDs, 16*(1), 27-38.

Logan, T. K., & Leukefeld, C. (2000). Sexual and drug use behaviors among female crack users: A multi-site sample. *Drug and Alcohol Dependence, 58,* 237-245.

MacNeil, J. R., McRill, C., Steinhauser, G., Weisbuch, J. B., Williams, E., & Wilson, M. L. (2007). Jails, a neglected opportunity for tuberculosis prevention. *American Journal of Preventive Medicine, 28*(2), 225–228.

Marlatt, G. A. (1996). Harm reduction: Come as you are. *Addictive Behaviors, 21,* 779–788.

Marston, C., & King, E. (2006). Factors that shape young people's sexual behaviour: A systematic review. *The Lancet, 368,* 1581–1586.

Minino, A. M., Xu, J., & Kochanek, K. (2010). Deaths: Preliminary data for 2008. *National Vital Statistics Reports, 59*(2). Retrieved February 2, 2011 from http://www.cdc.gov/nchs/data/nvsr/nvsr59/nvsr59_02.pdf

Murphy, D. A., Austin, E. L., & Greenwell, L. (2006). Correlates of HIV-related stigma among HIV-positive mothers and their uninfected adolescent children. *Women & Health, 44*(3), 19–42.

Myer, L., Kuhn, L., Stein, Z. A., Wright, T. C., & Denny, L. (2005). Intravaginal practices, bacterial vaginosis, and women's susceptibility to HIV infection: Epidemiological evidence and biological mechanisms. *The Lancet Infectious Disease, 5,* 786–794.

Nadeau, L., Truchon, M., & Biron, C. (2000). High-risk sexual behaviors in a context of substance abuse: A focus group approach. *Journal of Substance Abuse Treatment, 19,* 319–328.

Plitt, S. S., Garfein, R. S., Gaydos, C. A., Strathdee, S. A., Sherman, S. G., & Taha, T. E. (2005). Prevalence and correlates of *Chlamydia trachomatis, Neisseria gonorrhoeae, Trichomonas vaginalis* infections, and bacterial vaginosis among a cohort of young injection drug users in Baltimore, Maryland. *Sexually Transmitted Diseases, 32,* 446–453.

Raj, A., Reed, E., Santana, M. C., Walley, A. Y., Welles, S. L., Horsburgh, R., et al. (2009). The associations of binge alcohol use with HIV/STI risk and diagnosis among heterosexual African American men. *Drug and Alcohol Dependence, 101,* 101–106.

Raj, A., Saitz, R., Cheng, D. M., Winter, M., & Samet, J. H. (2007). Associations between alcohol, heroin, and cocaine use and high risk sexual behavior among detoxification patients. *The American Journal of Drug and Alcohol Abuse, 33,* 169–178.

Rao, D., Pryor, J. B., Gaddist, B. W., & Mayer, R. (2008). Stigma, secrecy, and discrimination: Ethnic/racial differences in the concerns of people living with HIV/AIDS. *AIDS and Behavior, 12,* 265–271.

Rapposelli, K. K., Kenney, M. G., Miles, J. R., Tinsley, M. J., Rauch, K. J., Austin, L., Dooley, S., Aranda-Naranjo, B., & Moore, R. A. (2002). HIV/AIDS in correctional settings: A salient priority for the CDC and HRSA. *AIDS Education and Prevention, 14*(5, Suppl. B), 103–113.

Rees, V., Saitz, R., Horton, N. J., & Samet, J. (2001). Association of alcohol consumption with HIV sex- and drug-risk behaviors among drug users. *Journal of Substance Abuse Treatment, 21,* 129–134.

Ruth, B. J., Wyatt, J. W., Chiasson, E., Geron, S., & Bachman, S. (2006). Social work and public health: Comparing graduates from a dual-degree program. *Journal of Social Work Education, 42,* 429–439.

Sampson, R. J., Raudenbush, S. W., & Earls, F. (1997). Neighborhood and violent crime: A multilevel study of collective efficacy. *Science, 277,* 918–924.

Semaan, S., Des Jarlais, D. C., & Malow, R. M. (2007). STDs among illicit drug users in the United States: The need for intervention. In S. O. Aral & J. M. Douglas (Eds.), *Behavioral intervention for prevention and control of sexually transmitted diseases.* New York: Springer Publishing.

Semple, S. J., Amaro, H., Strathdee, S., Zians, J., & Patterson, T. (2009). Ethnic differences in substance use, sexual risk behaviors, and psychosocial factors in a sample of heterosexual methamphetamine users. *Substance Use and Misuse, 44,* 1101-1120.

Stein, M. D., Herman, D., Trisvan, E., Pirraglia, P., Engler, P., & Anderson, B. (2005). Alcohol use and sexual risk behavior among human immunodeficiency virus-positive persons. *Alcoholism: Clinical and Experimental Research, 29,* 837-843.

Sylla, M., Harawa, N., & Reznick, O. G. (2010). The first condom machine in U.S. jail: The challenge of harm reduction in a law and order environment. *American Journal of Public Health, 100,* 982-985.

Talbot, C. (2000, December, 4). *United Nations AIDS report confirms worst epidemic in history.* Retrieved from http://www.wsws.org/articles/2000/dec2000/aids-d04.shtml

Tortu, S., Beardsley, M., Deren, S., Williams, M., McCoy, H. V., Stark, M., et al. (2000). HIV infection and patterns of risk among women drug injectors and crack users in low and high sero-prevalence sites. *AIDS Care, 12*(1), 65-76.

Treisman, G. J., & Angelino, A. F., (Eds.). (2004). *The psychiatry of AIDS: A guide to diagnosis and treatment.* Baltimore: John's Hopkins University Press.

Tucker, J. D., Chang, S. W., & Tulsky, J. P. (2007). The catch 22 of condoms in U.S. correctional facilities. *BMC Public Health, 7,* 296.

UNAIDS. (2004). *AIDS epidemic update.* Retrieved April 10, 2005, from http://www.unaids.org/wad2004/EPI_1204_pdf_en/EpiUpdate04_en.pdf

UNAIDS. (2010). *Report on the global AIDS epidemic.* Retrieved February 26, 2011 from www.unaids.org/globalreport/Global_report.htm

U.S. Department of Health and Human Services. (2011). *Healthy People 2020.* Retrieved March 1, 2011 from http://www.healthypeople.gov/2020/about/default.aspx

Witte, S. S., & deRidder, N. F. (1999). "Positive feelings": Group support for children of HIV-infected mothers. *Child and Adolescent Social Work Journal, 16*(1), 5-12.

Wodak, A., & Cooney, A. (2006). Do needle syringe programs reduce HIV infection among IDUs? A comprehensive review of the international evidence. *Substance Use and Misuse, 41,* 777-813.

CHAPTER 8

Public Health Social Work and Genetic Health Services Delivery

Joseph Telfair

INTRODUCTION

*T*he health and well-being of Americans are far better today than at any time in our past. Many of the serious infectious diseases that threatened our citizens in the earlier part of the last century have all but disappeared. At present, Americans face new challenges, and thanks to advances in the bio-medical, technological, and public health sciences there are new opportunities to advance health promotion and disease prevention. Although national progress toward improved health is notable, significant disparities in the receipt of individual and population-based specialized services that result from modifiable social, economic, and cultural factors remain, leading to disparate rates in morbidity and mortality. Consequently, it is clear that not all groups have benefited equally from this progress. In their role as genetic services workers, public health social workers play a critical role in assisting clients with inherited and metabolic disorders and in assisting providers with addressing these disparities.

As pointed out elsewhere and in this text, since the early days of the profession, social workers have been engaged in the delivery of services to persons at risk for and having diverse health conditions (Combs-Orme, 1990; Gitterman, Black, & Stein, 1985; Watkins, 1985). In 1935, Congress enacted Title V of the Social Security Act, authorizing the Maternal and Child Health Services Programs. This legislation, which is administered through funded "block" grants to states and territories, has provided a foundation and structure for assuring the health of mothers and children for more than 65 years. Title V was designed to improve health and assure access to high-quality health services for the maternal and child health (MCH) population, comprising those individuals with disabilities and chronic illnesses, both inherited and acquired. Public health social workers have had prominent service and leadership roles within Title V programs at the local, state, and national levels (Black 1985).

The National Association of Social Workers (NASW) Genetics & Social Work Practice Standards Working Group (NASW, 2003) stated,

> Current and emerging advances in the science of genetics provide significant promise for enhanced health and well-being and an opportunity for social workers to make a major contribution. As rapid discoveries in genetics (the study of single genes and their effects) and genomics (the study of the functions and interaction of all the genes in the genome) continue to identify genetic components of common diseases... A social worker is often the first to provide psychosocial services to individuals and families with genetic disorders. Therefore, it is imperative that social workers become more aware of the ethical, legal, and psychosocial implications of a genetic diagnosis, genetic testing, and genetic research in order to empower individuals and families to speak out for their rights as public citizens. In addition, the profession must continue to be active in shaping public policy as well as organizational policy as it relates to genetics and service delivery. Without specialized training, it is inappropriate for social workers to assume the role of genetic counselors, but they have important contributions to make within the social work scope of practice." (pp. 1, 2)

Khoury, Gwinn, Burke, Bowen, and Zimmern (2007) expressed concern that without a more integrated approach between primary health care delivery and public health, genomics could easily widen the schism that has long existed between medicine and public health. As pointed out in the Secretary's Advisory Committee on Genetics, Health and Society (SACGHS) recent report "Genetics, Education and Training" (2011), the challenges to achieving a more genomics-informed public health workforce are multifaceted. First, the public health workforce is diverse and follows many educational and training paths, including a variety of professionals with formal training and certifications, volunteers, and community (lay) health workers. Thus, a "one-size-fits-all" approach is not feasible. Second, many providers in the field today received their formal education before genomics became a critical aspect of medicine and health. This includes most social workers who provide genetic health services at the local and state levels who were often assigned these roles with no formal introduction or training (Guttmacher et al., 2001). Third, attitudes, perceptions, and beliefs shape the acceptance and adoption of genomics by the public health community (text adopted from SACGHS, 2011, p. 31). The latter challenge of prioritization for many public health providers' acceptance of genetic services, especially in the context of limited public health funding, include skepticism about genomics and genomics research being seen as a low-yield investment and a low priority because of other, more important local issues, national and international preventative or modifiable environmental causes of morbidity and mortality (Khoury et al., 2007), and the SACGHS report makes it clear that public health providers perceive neither public health genomics to be part of their job, nor a professional priority (SACGHS, 2011).

The purpose of this chapter is twofold: (1) to succinctly discuss the role of the public health social worker as part of the genetic services professional workforce and (2) to provide information that will allow the reader to have a better understanding of requirements and practices of public health social workers as members of the genetic services workforce.

WHY SOCIAL WORKERS AS MEMBERS OF THE GENETIC HEALTH WORKFORCE?

The literature makes it clear that there have been changes in genetics over the past 30 years that include (a) mapping of the human genome, providing insights into basic biological processes and into genetic contributions to common diseases; (b) expanding roles in clinical settings where there is a growing availability of genetic tests, starting with the test for cystic fibrosis, increase of electronic medical records, and greater emphasis on family history; (c) growing interest in personalized medicine and increased importance of the Internet; and (d) educating and training where there is an increased recognition for genetics in medical and public health classroom and continuing education (Holtzman, 2006; Jenkins et al., 2001). However, what has not changed is that there remain: (a) a limited ability to identify variants of complex diseases, develop tests for common diseases, and understand the environmental variables and epigenetic phenomena for disease onset; (b) a limited ability to convince practitioners that genetics matter, a tendency of clinicians and others to define diseases as "genetic" and "nongenetic," an uncertainty about what components belong to nongeneticists, little ability to convince nongeneticists to provide services and to know what issues need to be referred on to other professionals, a limited time to collect family history, and a failure to recognize its importance; and (c) limited education for health practitioners on genetics content, a lack of consensus on what genetics content should be included, a disconnect between classroom instruction and tasks that occur in the clinical setting, segregated support for genetics content from other subjects, as well as a lack of financial support for educational programs in genetics, and an inability to tie genetics education programs directly to changes in practitioner behavior (Guttmacher, Porteous, & McInerney, 2007; McInerney, 2008).

Lapham, Kozma, Weiss, Benkendorf, and Wilson (1999) stated, "Emerging genetic advances mandate that all health professionals have basic knowledge of genetics in order to provide adequate services to their clients"

(p. 57). In 2003, the Human Genome Project (HGP) was completed, resulting in a delineation of the complete sequence of the human genome. The sequence data helped advance research into the genetic basis of diseases, including common, multifactorial diseases. Expanded genetic knowledge and technologies are now leading to new approaches for diagnosing some common chronic diseases and conditions (SACGHS, 2011). These developments are moving genetics beyond a clinical specialty focused on rare, inherited diseases. As a result of these advances, clients will be using the results of genetic technologies increasingly in their own health care decision making. Yet many health and public health professionals lack sufficient knowledge about the application and interpretation of genetics in the clinic or in the community.

Clients and health care providers are challenged to keep pace with this dynamic and rapidly evolving field. The emerging understanding of the role of genetics in common diseases is increasing the need for knowledge of risk assessment, genetic diagnoses, appropriate treatment approaches, and communication in professional and public education, as well as the synergistic interaction with social, economic, and cultural factors that influence a client's ability to understand and appropriately access medical and public health systems.

Public health social workers bring a wealth of knowledge about system negotiation and "wrap-around" support services at the local, national, and global levels. Adaptation to the unique environments of the population they serve is one of their professional competencies—especially having an understanding of assets and needs to address intervention, prevention, and wellness gaps. For example, in the specialty area of MCH, one of the most common entry points for public health social workers and other public health professionals into the genetic services area (Wang & Watts, 2009), the expansion of screening and early-detection technologies for many common chronic diseases means that public health social workers will become increasingly integral to both community education and service provision. Moreover, expanded newborn screening increases the need for primary care providers to be educated about the critical nature of a positive result and emphasizes the need for just-in-time resources for referral and client management (especially with pediatric cancers and diabetes). Parents and families also have educational needs related to newborn screening (for rare diseases like Tay-Sachs and sickle cell disease), not only if their child has a positive screen and requires follow-up, but also as new issues emerge. These issues include (a) the increasing rates of false positives, (b) the interpretation of results from over-the-counter and direct-to-consumer mail order tests, and (c) the clarity of policy and clinical implications for practice as more tests are added to the newborn screening genomic panels (Etchegary et al., 2010; Wilde, Meiser, Mitchell, & Schofield, 2010).

The need for social workers to play a role in assuring that clients have access to and participate in counseling and testing is reflected in the *Healthy People 2020* (HP2020) genomic objectives: (a) genetic counseling for women with a family history of breast and/or ovarian cancer and (b) genetic testing for persons with colorectal cancer to detect Lynch syndrome (U.S. Department of Health and Human Services, 2011).

In addition to the HP2020 objectives, public health social workers employed as genetic services workers are trained and expected to carry out their duties and responsibilities in line with the three core public health functions linked to essential services: assessment, policy development, and assurance. Tasks carried out by these social workers are covered in the following discussion.

(a) **Assessment**—involves monitoring health status to identify community health problems; diagnosing and investigating health problems and health hazards in the community; and evaluating effectiveness, accessibility, and quality of personal and population-based health services. Public health social workers carry out their assessments through participation in data gathering on the epidemiological, medical, and social needs of their clients; conducting needs, assets, and risk assessments of clients to determine eligibility of services; solving problems to address social, cultural, family, and community concerns; and assisting primary care and specialist (e.g., genetic counselors) providers in medical and wellness assessments.

(b) **Policy development**—involves developing policies and plans that support individual and community health efforts, enforcing laws and regulations that protect health and ensure safety, and conducting research aimed at gaining new insights and innovative solutions to health problems. Public health social workers bring their skills to work with diverse stakeholders who help to broaden their influence, which in turn leads to effectively carrying out the functions of developing policies and plans that support individual and community health efforts.

(c) **Assurance**—involves linking people with genetic disorders to needed personal health services and assuring access to, provision of, and use of health care when otherwise unavailable; assuring a competent public health and personal health care workforce; informing, educating, and empowering people about health issues; and mobilizing community partnerships to identify and solve health problems. This work is carried by implementing the functions of delivery of MCH services; assuring availability of competent providers; conducting health needs assessments; and assessing type, quality, and extent of services delivered (see the section "Genetics and Public Social Work Standards and Competencies in Practice").

There are additional client needs that public health social workers must attend to if they are to be effective in their assurance role. For example, McInerney (2008) concluded that 32% of the consumers of genetics services surveyed indicated that their health care providers' genetics knowledge was poor, and 78% said they received no genetics information from the provider most important to their family in either primary or specialty care. The study suggests that there are fundamental gaps in competencies that need to be addressed. Lapham, Kozma, Weiss, Benkendorf, and Wilson (2000), reporting on the results of the Human Genome Education Model (HuGEM) research survey, made it clear that public health social workers and other genetic health professionals must work together to assure a competent workforce that can identify, anticipate, and assist both health care professionals and consumers to address the arising legal, ethical, policy, and social issues, as genetic knowledge and technologies are developed and this information is made available to individuals and groups. More recently, Rogowski, Grosse, and Khoury (2009), citing national public health workforce data, highlighted the cooperation across disciplines (primary and clinical health care and genetics), as well as the nature and lack of genetics education of health care professionals as factors limiting the integration of genetics into health care. Finally, the SACGHS report makes this point very clear by stating:

> Cooperation and collaboration in processing, applying, and interpreting genetic information will be essential. Without educated health care professionals and consumers, society will not benefit from genetic advances. Without an educated public health workforce, opportunities will be lost for deploying prevention and early detection programs for a wide variety of chronic diseases. And, without an informed public, patients and consumers may make poorly informed choices, or fail to seek needed professional health services. (p. 7)

The knowledge, skills, competencies, and standards for social workers in public health and genetics serve as a guide to address these gaps in practice at the micro (individual), mezzo (group), and macro (community, organization, state) levels. The narrative to follow will provide a discussion of the work done to assure that public health social workers are competent and contributing members of the genetic services workforce.

GENETICS AND PUBLIC SOCIAL WORK STANDARDS AND COMPETENCIES IN PRACTICE

Educators and practitioners in the genetics health workforce point out that it is important to teach the underlying concepts and appreciation of the future clinical importance of genetics so that professionals in the fields of medicine and public health will be motivated to learn about it (Guttmacher et al., 2007; Lin Fu & Puryear, 2000). It is vital to educate health professionals about the basic concepts of genomics so that they can understand and use genetics-based probability and risk assessment and communicate effectively about them to clients. This is imperative on the micro, mezzo, and macro practice levels so that practitioners approach each client as a biological individual, target appropriate courses of prevention, provide diagnostic and treatment services (micro) to engage practitioners at all levels in the development of genetic health services (mezzo), and work within systems to provide necessary quality services (macro).

Social workers who work in genetic health services settings must have a basic understanding of medical genetics. At a minimum, the following must be well understood. The current edition of McKusick's *Mendelian Inheritance in Man* lists more than 14,000 entries, of which more than 13,000 are autosomal, 788 are X-linked, 43 are Y-linked, and 60 are in the mitochondrial genome (Jorde, Carey, Bamshad, & White, 2003). Each human is estimated to have approximately 30,000–40,000 different genes. The genes are classified into the following four major groups: (1) chromosome disorders—the entire chromosome is missing, duplicated, or otherwise altered (Down and Turner syndromes); (2) single gene disorders—also known as "Mendelian" conditions, in which single genes are altered (sickle cell, cystic fibrosis, and hemophilia); (3) multifactorial disorders—result from a combination of multiple genetic and environmental causes (cleft lip, cleft palate, heart disease, diabetes); and (4) mitochondrial disorders—include a relatively small number of diseases, caused by alterations in the small cytoplasmic mitochondrial chromosome. Of all disease classifications, single-gene disorders have probably received the greatest amount of attention (Guttmacher & Collins, 2002; Jenkins et al., 2001; Jorde et al., 2003).

Given the rapid proliferation of genetic technologies and the shift toward personalized health care, the education and training needs of social work and other genetic health professionals on the front lines of public health and health care delivery is a high priority, as is the need for a supported and informed public (Reichert, 1980; Wilkinson, Rounds, & Copeland, 2002).

Genetics service specialists and public health social workers know that issues facing practitioners and clients specific to the delivery of genetic health services are complex and multifactorial. Practitioners recognize that ongoing education and training are needed to enhance their strengths (knowledge, skills) and address limitations of their work. These enhanced strengths include:

1. Recognition that public health risk-prevention recommendations are typically community or population wide, with limited ability to tailor the intervention or message to the high-risk individual or family.

2. Recognition that health-risk appraisals will benefit from a knowledge of genetics by helping to identify individuals with inherited suscepti- bilities to major diseases, such as heart disease and cancer—at-risk individuals in presymptomatic stages may be offered preventive interventions earlier.

3. Recognition of the extraordinary impact that common chronic dis- eases will have on the world's aging population, making it critical for genetic health specialists to apply an understanding of genetic mechanisms to reduce risk and disability and develop successful interventions.

4. Recognition that fundamental to a public health-based genetics curri- culum is a course that focuses on ethical, legal, and social issues (especially disparities) arising from the application of the advances of genetics and molecular biology into public health research, edu- cation, and practice.

5. Recognition that issues of privacy and confidentiality are important in light of genetic information about health risk and their potential effects on discrimination in employment and health insurability.

6. Recognition that, in addition to being available and affordable, genetic services must be culturally appropriate and acceptable, particularly to racial and ethnic minorities.

7. Recognition that access cannot be discussed without considering the genetic literacy of the American public, which is a prerequisite if clients are to make truly informed decisions and preserve their autonomy.

8. Recognition that providers should serve as a link between patients and genetic specialists.

9. Recognition that since there is a genetic basis for virtually every disease, formal linkages should also be established between the gen- etics community and subspecialty care providers, including social workers, psychologists, and consumer support groups.

10. Recognition that because genetics services are being provided without any systematic approach, oversight, or assessment of what will be needed, services in the future should address essential public health functions.

11. Until the Patient Protection and Affordable Care Act of 2010 preexist- ing-condition provision is in full effect, solutions addressing barriers to access appropriate genetic health services, such as low genetic lit- eracy of the U.S. public, lack of insurance coverage, and ethnocultural issues, remains a challenge (Greendale & Pyeritz, 2001; Lin Fu & Puryear, 2000; Wang & Watts, 2007, 2009).

Recognizing the growing influence of a changing and challenging field, as well as the need for "social workers to establish the social work profession as a leader in the field of genetics, to support the development of programs, training, and information that provide social workers with current genetic information for use with clients, and to support policies that provide protection for clients..." (NASW, 2003, p. 4), NASW published a Social Work Practice Update in 1998 that defined the role of social workers in genetics, emphasizing practice, policy, and ethical issues (as cited in Taylor-Brown & Johnson, 1998). The NASW policy statement on genetics provided a framework all social workers could use to understand ethical and practical issues in genetic testing and research (NASW, 2003). Chaired by Joan O. Weiss, ACSW, a pioneer and leader of over 40 years in the field of genetics and social work, the NASW Genetics & Social Work Practice Standards Working Group published its nine standards in 2003 (NASW, 2003).

The impetus for the workgroup was to add specificity to the 1998 update and make clear the competencies needed for execution of the social worker's role in encouraging clients to become their own advocates in bringing genetic issues to the forefront of quality health care that had been defined in part by the completion of the HGP (NASW, p. 2). The workgroup recognized that

> a social worker is often the first to provide psychosocial services to individuals and families with genetic disorders. Therefore, it is imperative that social workers become more aware of the ethical, legal and psychosocial implications of a genetic diagnosis, genetic testing and genetic research in order to empower individuals and families to speak out for their rights as public citizens... Without specialized training, it is inappropriate for social workers to assume the role of genetic counselors, but they have important contributions to make within the social work scope of practice. Social workers can take an active part in ensuring that their clients are protected against genetic discrimination in areas such as health and life insurance, employment, and adoption. (p. 2)

The workgroup further pointed out that critical issues in the field of genetics of importance to social workers include: (a) the benefits and risks of gene therapy, stem cell research, reproductive technology, and tissue cloning; (b) the need for social workers to become more informed and sensitive to related ethical, legal, and psychosocial considerations to be helpful to their clients; (c) the importance of becoming knowledgeable about genetic resources in the community; and (d) the ethical and practical issues involved with genetic testing, such as informed consent, confidentiality, self-determination, equal access, and the implications of knowing one's genetic makeup (modified from pp. 3, 4). The workgroup believed the NASW standards (a) allow the social worker to address genetics as an expanding field of knowledge, emphasizing the need for clarification of, understanding of, and education about this specialized area and (b) are designed to enhance social workers' awareness of the skills, knowledge, values, methods, and sensitivity needed to work effectively with clients, families, health care providers, and the community and to increase their understanding of the impact that the field of genetics has, and will have, on them (pp. 4, 5). The workgroup indicated that six specific objectives of the standards are as follows (p. 5): (1) to inform social workers about genetics as an expanding field of social work knowledge; (2) to improve the quality of social work services provided to clients with genetic disorders; (3) to provide a basis for the development of continuing education materials and programs in genetics;

TABLE 8.1   National Association of Social Workers Standards for Integrating Genetics into Social Work Practice

STANDARD	EXPLANATION/PURPOSE
Standard 1: Ethics and Values	When integrating genetics and social work practice, social workers shall function in accordance with ethical principles and standards of the profession as articulated in the NASW Code of Ethics (NASW, 1999)
Standard 2: Genetics Knowledge	Social workers shall acquire a basic understanding about genetics as a science and a field of study, including its biological, psychosocial, ethical, and legal aspects
Standard 3: Practice Skills in Working with Individuals, Families, Groups, and Communities	Social workers shall use appropriate practice theories, skills, and interventions that reflect their understanding of genetic factors in their work with individuals, families, groups, and communities
Standard 4: Client/Practitioner Collaborative Practice Model	Social workers shall be able to work with their clients with genetic concerns in a partnership that includes mutual respect, shared information, and effective communication
Standard 5: Interdisciplinary Practice	Social workers shall participate in multidisciplinary teams that deliver comprehensive genetics services
Standard 6: Self-Awareness	Social workers shall have and continue to develop an understanding of their own personal, cultural, and spiritual values and beliefs pertaining to genetics and genetic therapies
Standard 7: Genetics and Cross-Cultural Knowledge	Social workers shall have and continue to develop specialized knowledge and understanding about the history, traditions, values, and family systems of client groups as they relate to genetics
Standard 8: Research	Social workers shall contribute to, support, and be cognizant of the development of research-based and practice-relevant knowledge of the psychosocial, cultural, economic, and ethical implications of genetics on individuals, families, and society
Standard 9: Advocacy	Social workers shall safeguard the privacy and confidentiality of genetic information of their clients and advocate for and with clients when appropriate to ensure fair social policies and access to quality genetic services

Source: NASW (2003).

(4) to ensure that social work services to clients with genetic disorders are guided by the NASW Code of Ethics; (5) to advocate for clients' right to self-determination, confidentiality, access to genetic services, and nondiscrimination; and (6) to encourage social workers to participate in the formulation and refinement of public policy (at the state and federal levels) relevant to genetic research, services, and treatment of populations with genetically identified predispositions or conditions. These standards are listed in Table 8.1.

In practice, these standards are consistent with a number of public health social work standards (Practice Standards Committee, 2005; Wilkinson et al., 2002). The standards relevant to the focus of this chapter are listed in Table 8.2.

Collectively, both sets of standards and the list of essential services provide structured guidance for the public health social worker's role of identifying, planning, developing, implementing, and/or evaluating programs designed to address the social and interpersonal needs of populations in

TABLE 8.2   Practice-Linked Public Health Social Work Standards

STANDARD	EXPLANATION/PURPOSE
Professional Standard #8	Public Health Social Work uses social planning, community organizational development, and social marketing to assure public accountability for the well-being of all, with emphasis on vulnerable and underserved populations
Professional Standard #9	Public Health Social Work uses social planning, community organizational development, and social marketing to develop primary prevention strategies that promote the health and well-being of individuals, families, and communities
Professional Standard #10	Public Health Social Work uses social planning, community organizational development, and social marketing to develop secondary and tertiary prevention strategies to alleviate health and related social and economic concerns
Professional Standard #11	Public Health Social Work provides leadership and advocacy to assure the elimination of health and social disparities wherever they exist such as, but not limited to, those based on community, race, age, gender, ethnicity, culture, or disability
Professional Standard #12	Public Health Social Work provides leadership and advocacy to assure and promote policy development for providing quality and comprehensive public health services within a cultural, community, and family context
Professional Standard #13	Public Health Social Work supports and conducts data collection, research, and evaluation
Professional Standard #14	Public Health Social Work assures the competency of its practice to address the issues of public health effectively through a core body of social work knowledge, philosophy, code of ethics, and standards

Source: Practice Standards Committee (2005).

order to improve the health of a community and pre- and postgenetic services, decision making, and participation efforts that promote the health of individuals and families.

CONCLUSION

Public health genetics is a complex and challenging field. A knowledgeable and competent workforce can assure that those individuals who need to know of and benefit from genetics counseling can do so. Public health social workers continue to make significant contributions to the genetic health workforce by playing a significant role in assuring that this client population has access to and is able to appropriately utilize genetic health services at the micro level of delivering direct services (Caumartin, Baker, & Marrs, 2000; Gorin & Moniz, 1996). Advocacy and the provision of appropriate, competent, knowledgeable, targeted support services (at the micro, mezzo, and macro levels) are core values of social work. In practice, these efforts lead to increased capacity and empowerment of clients to make decisions for themselves, their families, and their communities.

The social worker's role is critical, one that faces many inherited challenges, particularly in (a) defining one's role; (b) working with others to overcome negative attitudes and beliefs about the importance of one's role; and (c) significantly contributing to the development and maintenance of a competent genetic health workforce that emphasizes continuous and up-to-date education and training—a reality faced by all genetic health professionals. Also, building and sustaining collaborative service networks is a crucial role played by public health social workers when working with health professionals and clients in assuring the delivery of genetic health services. Lastly, it is at the macro level that the public health social workers can have the greatest impact by policy and program development, program implementation, assessment (evaluation and research), and advocacy.

Based on assessment data from professionals and consumers, research carried out by the SACGHS (2011) made it clear that the following 12 competencies (skills and knowledge) are thought to be critical for providers of public health genetic services, whether at the local, state, or national level. Specific to the practice of genetics and public health social work, these competencies are listed as follows:

1. Maintain up-to-date knowledge on the development of genomic science and technologies within one's professional field and apply genomics as a tool for achieving public health goals.
2. Demonstrate basic knowledge of the role that genetics and genomics play in the development of disease and in the screening of and interventions for disease prevention and health promotion programs.

3. Describe the importance of family history in assessing clients' predisposition to disease.
4. Effectively identify opportunities and integrate genetic and genomic issues into public health practice, policies, or programs.
5. Maintain up-to-date knowledge of genetics and genomics-related policies, legislation, statutes, and regulations.
6. Describe the potential physical and psychological benefits, limitations, and risks of genetic and genomic information for individuals, family members, and communities.
7. Collaborate with existing and emerging health agencies and organizations; academic, research, private, and commercial enterprises; and community partnerships to apply genetics and genomics knowledge and tools to address public health problems.
8. Identify the resources available to assist clients seeking genetic and genomic information or services, including the types of genetics professionals available.
9. Conduct outcomes evaluation of available genetic and genomic programs and services to determine their effectiveness.
10. Identify the political, legal, social, ethical, and economic issues associated with integrating genomics into public health.
11. Use information technology (IT) to obtain credible, current information about genetics; utilize IT skills to share data and participate in research, program planning, evaluation, and policy development for health promotion and disease prevention.
12. Identify appropriate and relevant genetics research findings that can be translated into public health policies or practices.

CLASSROOM EXERCISE

Case Scenario—Antonio Lopes is the father of a newborn male with homozygous sickle cell disease who needs to find a culturally accessible medical home. Mr. Lopes and his wife are second-generation Latinos and have encountered challenges in getting primary and specialized care for their newborn due to the perception about what is and "who has" sickle cell disease, as well as eligibility for State Child Health Insurance Plan coverage.

Exercises and Questions

There are a number of misconceptions and myths about genetic diversity and inheritance due to limited education and understanding by the general public and practitioners, and in the health literature. How would you go about addressing the concerns and needs of the Lopes family as a public health social worker serving the individual in the context of the larger community? Focus your discussion on:

1. Deciphering what the myths about genetic inheritance held by public health stakeholders are.
2. Approaches to integrating NASW public health social work and genetic standards into a plan of action to assist families like the Lopeses.
3. Approaches to educating primary care, specialist, and other providers about the application and interpretation of genetics in the clinic and at the community and state service levels.

INTERNET RESOURCES

The following websites may be helpful to you as you move forward with your interests in genetics and genomics:

Secretary's Advisory Committee on Genetics, Health, and Society

(http://oba.od.nih.gov/SACGHS/sacghs_home.html)

National Human Genome Research Institute

(www.genome.gov/)

History of Social Work and Genetics

(www.socialworkers.org/practice/standards/geneticsstdfinal4112003.pdf)

Social Work's Role in Genetic Services

(www.socialworkers.org/practice/health/genetics.asp)

REFERENCES

Black, R. B. (1985). The state of the art in public health social work education: Public health and maternal child health content in graduate and continuing education programs. In A. Gitterman, R. B. Black, & F. Stein (Eds.), *Public health social work in maternal and child health: A forward plan*. Rockville. MD: Bureau of Health Care Delivery and Assistance, Health Resources and Services Administration, U.S. Department of Health and Human Services.

Caumartin, S. M., Baker, D. L., & Marrs, C. F. (2000). Training in public health genetics. In M. J. Khoury, W. Burke, & E. Thomson (Eds.), *Genetics and public health in the 21st century: Using genetic information to improve health and prevent disease* (pp. 569–578). Auckland, New Zealand: Oxford University Press.

Combs-Orme, T. (1990). Social work practice in maternal and child health: An orientation. In T. Combs-Orme (Ed.), *Social work practice in maternal and child health* (pp. 1–23). New York: Springer Publishing Company.

DHHS Title V—Maternal and Child Health Services Block Grant. Retrieved March 15, 2012, from http://www.ssa.gov/OP_Home/ssact/title05/0501.htm

Etchegary, H., Cappelli, M., Potter, B., Vloet, M., Graham, I., Walker, M., et al., (2010). Attitude and knowledge about genetics and genetic testing. *Public Health Genomics, 13,* 80–88.

Gitterman, A., Black, R. B., & Stein, F. (Eds.). (1985). *Public health social work in maternal and child health. A forward plan.* Rockville, MD: Bureau of Health Care Delivery and Assistance, Health Resources and Services Administration, U.S. Department of Health and Human Services.

Gorin, S., & Moniz, C. (1996). From health care to health: A look ahead to 2010. In P. R. Raffoul & C. A. McNeece (Eds.), *Future issues for social work practice.* Boston: Allyn & Bacon.

Greendale, K., & Pyeritz, R. E. (2001). Empowering primary care health professionals in medical genetics: How soon? How fast? How far? *American Journal of Medical Genetics, 106,* 223–232.

Guttmacher, A., & Collins, F. S. (2002). Genomic medicine: A primer. *New England Journal of Medicine, 347,* 1512–1513.

Guttmacher, A. E., Jenkins, J., & Uhlmann, W. R. (2001). Genomic medicine: Who will practice it? A call to open arms. *American Journal of Medical Genetics, 106*(3), 216–222.

Guttmacher, A. E., Porteous, M. E., & McInerney, J. D. (2007). Educating health-care professionals about genetics and genomics. *Genetics, 8,* 151–157.

Holtzman, N. A. (2006). What role for public health in genetics and vice versa. *Public Health Genomics, 9*(1), 8–20.

Jenkins, J., Blitzer, M., Boehm, K., Feetham, S., Gettig, S., Johnson, A., et al., (2001). Recommendations of core competencies in genetics essential for all health professionals. *Genetics in Medicine, 3,* 155–159.

Jorde, L. B., Carey, J. C., Bamshad, M. J., & White, R. J. (2003). *Medical genetics* (3rd ed.). St. Louis, MO: Mosby.

Khoury, M. J., Gwinn, M., Burke, W., Bowen, S., & Zimmern, R. (2007). Will genomics widen or help heal the schism between medicine and public health? *American Journal of Preventive Medicine, 33*(4), 310–317.

Lapham, V. E., Kozma, C., Weiss, J. O., Benkendorf, J. L., & Wilson, M. A. (1999). Genetics education of health professionals. *Genetics in Medicine, 1*(2), 57.

Lapham, V. E., Kozma, C., Weiss, J. O., Benkendorf, J. L., & Wilson, M. A. (2000). The gap between practice and genetics education of health professionals: HuGEM survey results. *Genetics in Medicine, 2*(4), 226–231.

Lin Fu, J., & Puryear, M. (2000). Access to genetic services in the United States: A challenge to genetics in public health. In M. J. Khoury, W. Burke, & E. Thomson (Eds.), *Genetics and public health in the 21st century: Using genetic information to improve health and prevent disease.* Auckland, New Zealand: Oxford University Press.

McInerney, J. D. (2008). Genetics education for health professionals: A context. *Journal of Genetic Counseling, 17*, 145–151.

National Association of Social Workers. (1999). *Code of ethics of the national association of social workers*. Washington, DC: Author.

National Association of Social Werkers Genetics & Social Work Practice Standards Working Group. (2003). *NASW Standards for Integrating Genetics into Social Work Practice*. Washington, DC: NASW.

Practice Standards Development Committee, Beyond Year 2010. (2005). *Public health social work standards and competencies*. Columbus, OH: Ohio Department of Health. Retrieved March 5, 2012, from http://oce.sph.unc.edu/cetac/phswcompeten cies_May05.pdf

Reichert, K. (1980). Essentials of social work practice in public health programs. In *Social work in a state-based system of child health care*. Based on Proceedings of The Tri-Regional Workshop for Social Workers in Maternal and Child Health Services. The Department of Maternal and Child Health, UNC-CH, and The Office for Maternal and Child Health Bureau of Community Health Services Department of Health and Human Services.

Rogowski, W. H., Grosse, S. D., & Khoury, M. J. (2009). Challenges of translating genetic tests into clinical and public health practice. *Nature Reviews Genetics, 10*(7), 489–495.

Secretary's Advisory Committee on Genetics, Health, and Society. (2011). *Genetics, education and training: Report of the Secretary's Advisory Committee on Genetics, Health, and Society*. Retrieved February 2011, from http://oba.od.nih.gov/oba/SACGHS/reports/SACGHS_education_report_2011.pdf

Taylor-Brown, S., & Johnson, A. (1998). Social work's role in genetic services. In *NASW practice update*. Washington, DC: National Association of Social Workers.

U.S. Department of Health and Human Services (2011). *Healthy People 2020*. Washington, DC. Retrieved March 15, 2012, from http://www.healthypeople.gov/2020/topicsobjectives2020/objectiveslist.aspx? topicId=15

Wang, G., & Watts, C. (2007). The role of genetics in the provision of essential public health services. *American Journal of Public Health, 97*(4), 620–625.

Wang, G., & Watts, C. (2009). *Genomics and public health practice: Lessons from state pilot projects*. Ann Arbor, MI: Center for Public Health and Community Genomics.

Watkins, E. (1985). The conceptual base for public health social work. Public health social work in maternal and child health: A forward plan. In A. Gitterman, R. Beck Black, & F. Stein (Eds.), *Proceedings of a conference conducted by the School of Social Work, Columbia University, 1985* (pp. 17–33). New York: School of Social Work, Columbia University.

Wilde, A., Meiser, B., Mitchell, P. B., & Schofield, P. R. (2010). Public interest in predictive genetic testing, including direct-to-consumer testing, for susceptibility to major depression: Preliminary findings. *European Journal of Human Genetics, 18*(1), 47–51.

Wilkinson, D. S., Rounds, K. A., & Copeland, K. C. (2002). Infusing public health content into foundation and advanced social work courses. *Journal of Teaching in Social Work, 22*(3/4), 139–154.

CHAPTER 9

Disabilities and Secondary Conditions

Patricia Welch Saleeby and Elaine T. Jurkowski

INTRODUCTION

*P*ublic health professionals who work with persons with disabilities will face numerous challenges. To address this critical workforce issue, this chapter explores the core functions of public health and disabilities and provides an overview of key issues in public health social work practice and with people living with disabilities. The ways in which health disparities and health inequities are related to disabilities is explained. Public health social work standards and competencies are discussed in relation to both disabilities and secondary conditions. *Healthy People 2020* objectives related to disabilities and secondary conditions are highlighted. Finally, strategies for public health social work practice with people who have disabilities and secondary conditions are presented for further capacity building.

OVERVIEW

Over the past several decades, new opportunities for public health social workers have emerged in relation to professional practice with persons with disabilities. First and foremost, there has been an increase in the community census of people with disabilities, and this growth is expected to continue as a result of two factors—the aging population in the United States and the likelihood of disability increasing with age. Advocacy efforts, including those led by social workers and public health professionals, have resulted in heightened attention to the experiences of people with disabilities and greater exertion on their behalf, including their integration into the community. With the growing number of persons with disabilities living and actively participating in the community, interaction with public health social workers across clinical settings, including the public health arenas, will continue to be significant.

Despite the progress and the growth in disability rights spearheaded by legislation like the Americans with Disabilities Act (1990), the Individuals with Disabilities Education Act (1975), and Section 504 of the Rehabilitation Act (1973), persons with disabilities continue to experience ongoing economic, financial, and social problems, such as stigma and discrimination (Fine & Asch, 1988; Gray & Hahn, 1997). While health disparities are prevalent among people with disabilities, only recently have public health agencies recognized disability as a significant population group and have included disabilities as a targeted population in public health initiatives such as *Healthy People 2010* and *2020* (Lollar, 2002).

As a result, public health social workers will be faced with numerous challenges in the coming years. However, most social workers and public health professionals have little or no experience working with persons with disabilities and consequently find themselves at a disadvantage dealing with them and their disability-specific issues. Both schools of social work and of public health continue to lack the necessary disability content in their curriculum, as well as relevant training opportunities to adequately prepare practitioners (Jurkowski & Welch, 1999; Tanenhaus, Meyers, & Harbison, 2000). Adequate exposure and preparation of public health social workers in working with the disability population is critical for facilitating effective and appropriate services (Jurkowski & Welch, 2002).

To address this critical workforce issue, this chapter provides an overview of key disability-related issues in public health social work. Specifically, health disparities and health inequities as experienced by persons with disabilities are described in conjunction with secondary conditions and *Healthy People 2020* objectives. The core functions of public health, as well as public health social work standards and competencies, are discussed in relation to disabilities. Finally, strategies for public health social work practice with people who have disabilities as well as future issues are presented for further capacity building.

KEY ISSUES IN PUBLIC HEALTH SOCIAL WORK AND DISABILITIES

According to the Institute of Medicine (IOM) landmark report, *Disability in America: Toward a National Agenda for Prevention*, disability is considered the nation's largest public health problem (Pope & Tarlov, 1991). Approximately 49.7 million, or 19.3% of Americans aged 5 years and above, have a disability or long-lasting condition (U.S. Census Bureau, 2000; Waldrop & Stern, 2003). *Disability* is defined as having difficulty in performing certain functional tasks (seeing or hearing) or activities of daily living (eating or dressing), or by meeting other criteria (having a developmental or learning disability; Pope & Tarlov, 1991). A disability can also be considered a permanent or long-term behavioral, cognitive, physical, psychological, or sensory impediment to be treated by working with individual recovery, adaptation, or both (Longmore, 1997).

Race and ethnicity are among the factors that have the strongest association with disability (Bradsher, 1995; Smart & Smart, 1997); consequently, race and ethnicity must be considered in addressing disability-related public health programs and policies. Regarding gender, women with disabilities face additional complications for having worse health outcomes due to their impairments and the greater likelihood of experiencing poverty—both of which put them at increased health risk (Parish & Ellison-Martin, 2007).

Persons with disabilities are frequently marginalized and discriminated against in the community, and consequently they represent a significantly underserved population in society. They frequently endure higher rates of environmental barriers, poverty, unemployment, and social isolation compared to the general population (Kaye, 1997). Limited access to health care services as a result of barriers such as negative attitudes and physical inaccessibility is common. Barriers to care are especially significant since persons with disabilities generally have a greater need for appropriate and accessible health care services (Iezzoni, McCarthy, Davis, & Siebens, 2000). All of these factors contribute to the health disparities that exist among persons with disabilities.

HEALTH DISPARITIES AND DISABILITIES

In most cases, persons with disabilities have not been identified as an underserved population for the purposes of screening, prevention, treatment, and intervention and so they are not specifically targeted in education and outreach efforts by public health policies, programs, and services. As indicated by Krahn and Campbell (2011), "Promoting health, quality of life, and participation of persons with disabilities is a relatively recent development in public health" (p. 12). Secondary conditions have been defined in a few different ways. Some views favor a narrow scope of identifying secondary conditions as primarily physiological in nature, such as pressure sores, urinary tract infections, and deconditioning (Rowland, 2011).

Broader views of secondary condition definitions include environmental factors, such as access to health services and structural barriers located within the environment that affect the health status of people with disabilities (Rowland, 2011). The *Healthy People 2010* Report (Chapter 6, "Disability and Secondary Conditions") identified secondary conditions as "medical, social, emotional, family, or community problems that a person with a primary disabling condition likely experiences." The lack of a universal definition of secondary conditions leads to the inability to compare the results of studies across states and population groups.

Historically, the focus has been on preventing disability in terms of birth defects, chronic illnesses, developmental disabilities, and injury; in fact, very few prevention efforts have addressed the unique needs of those persons already affected by disability (Lollar, 2002). However, health disparities may be considered persistent differences in health conditions across any demographic group (Keefe, 2010). A more contemporary approach recognizes disability as an actual minority group that experiences disparities compared to people without disabilities (Krahn & Campbell, 2011). According to DATA2010 (Centers for Disease Control and Prevention, 2010), the largest U.S. population-based health data set for people with disabilities, despite improvements in health over the previous decade, specific health disparities exist for people with disabilities.

As a whole, people with disabilities experience poorer health than their counterparts without disabilities (Campbell, Sheets, & Strong, 1999; Drum, Krahn, Culley, & Hammond, 2005; Turk, Scandale, Sambamoorthi and Mackleprang, & Weber, 2001). Persons with disabilities are more likely to experience difficulties or delays in accessing preventative health services (U.S. Department of Health and Human Services [DHHS], 1999). They are less likely to have had a Pap test or a mammogram within the recommended timeframe (Chevarley, Thierry, Gill, Ryerson, & Nosek, 2006; Wei, Findley, & Sambamoorthi, 2006). They have lower levels of physical activity, poorer nutrition, and higher levels of obesity (Draheim, Williams, & McCubbin, 2002), which are all factors highly related to chronic conditions such as diabetes, high blood pressure, and cardiovascular diseases.

HEALTHY PEOPLE 2020 OBJECTIVES

The significance of these problems have prompted the recognition and elimination of health disparities among people with disabilities as an important goal in both *Healthy People 2010* and *2020*, which provide a broad outline for public health activities. The "Disability and Health" chapter of *Healthy People 2020* emphasizes the following four areas for improvement and opportunities for persons with disabilities: (1) be included in public health activities, (2) receive well-timed interventions and services, (3) interact with their environment without barriers, and (4) participate in everyday life activities.

Healthy People 2020 provides an overview of 20 disability and health-related objectives. These objectives address critical public health areas, including systems and policies, barriers to health care, environment, and activities and participation. The first objective recommends the inclusion of a standardized set of questions that identify people with disabilities in population data systems (DHHS, 2010). This will enable the availability of baseline disability data to better determine the status and relationships of disability and health. The remaining systems and policies objectives call for an increase in public health surveillance and health-promotion programs for persons with disabilities and their caregivers, as well as an increase in graduate-level disability and health courses in our country's public health academic programs (DHHS, 2010).

Health care objectives identify barriers such as reducing the proportion of persons with disabilities who report delays in receiving primary and periodic preventive care, increasing the proportion of youth with special health care needs whose health care provider has discussed transition planning from pediatric to adult health care, increasing the proportion of people with epilepsy and uncontrolled seizures who receive appropriate medical care, and reducing the proportion of older adults with disabilities who use inappropriate medications (DHHS, 2010).

Objectives related to environment involve reducing the proportion of people with disabilities who report physical or program barriers to local health and wellness programs; encountering barriers to participating in home, school, work, or community activities; and reporting barriers to obtaining assistive devices, service animals, technology services, and accessible technologies that they need. Increasing the proportion of newly constructed and retrofitted U.S. homes and residential buildings that have visible features, as well as reducing the number of people with disabilities living in congregate care residences, are also identified (DHHS, 2010).

Finally, activities and participation-related objectives include the increase in the number of people who participate in social, spiritual, recreational, community, and civic activities to the degree that they wish as well as children and youth with disabilities who spend at least 80% of their time in regular education programs. Increasing employment among people with disabilities and people who report sufficient social and emotional support are listed. Another objective is to reduce the proportion of people with disabilities who experience nonfatal unintentional injuries that require medical care. Children with disabilities (birth through age 2 years) should receive increased early intervention services in home or community-based settings. An overview of the *Healthy People 2020* objectives related to disability is found in Appendix 9A.

EVOLVING FRAMEWORKS OF DISABILITY

There has been an evolution of thinking relative to how persons with disabilities are perceived in society over time, which is reflected in changing definitions and conceptual models. Initially, people with disabilities were perceived to be victims of "illness," as conceptualized by the medical model. This same approach also guided the development of several welfare schemes and long-term disability-type programs and policies. The expansion to incorporate the notion of rehabilitation and idea that people could consider alternatives to their lifestyles despite impairment or functional limitation originated post World War II, when returning servicemen expected that they could resume active lives in their communities, despite their disabling conditions.

Disability and the Environment

Saad Nagi's Disablement Model (1965) viewed disability as a limitation in performing socially defined tasks and roles expected of a person within his/her physical and sociocultural environment. This model includes the components of active pathology, impairment (loss or abnormality at organ and body system level), functional limitations (restrictions in basic performance of the person), and disability. Disability is demonstrated differently by people with similar diagnoses, impairments, and functional limitations by the reaction of others, self-perception, and the level of physical and sociocultural barriers (Nagi, 1991). The disability dimension, the final set of explanatory factors, includes physical barriers that may be considered the contextual location for conceptualizing environmental factors.

Extending this conceptual model, DeJong's independent living paradigm (1979) includes independent living and community-based options as the norm for persons living with impairments and disabilities. DeJong's contributions set the stage for inclusion, rather than exclusion, of people with impairments from society, and it was a response to civil rights activists who sought to ensure that the rights and lives of people with disabilities could be maintained within their communities (Wolfensburger, 1972).

Furthering the inclusion of the environment, "Enabling America," the landmark report published by the IOM in 1997, described disability as a dynamic process that is the outcome of the interactions of the individual and his/her environments (Pope & Brandt, 1997). This interactive model stated that enabling people with impairments could be accomplished by increasing the individual's functional capacity to perform an activity and/or improving access to his/her environment. The outcomes of the person and environment interactions form the basis for assessing the relative degree of disability. Environmental factors have the potential for expanding access to activities and enabling people with limitations to participate fully in their communities. However, no classification system or recommended measures of disability or environmental factors are described in the IOM model.

Strengths-Based Approach

Building upon these previously discussed models, there has been an important shift in public heath social work clinical practice approaches toward people with disabilities to a strengths-based and independence-oriented perspective. The European era of enlightenment from the mid-1970s conveyed the notion that people with disabilities could be perfected. Mackelprang and Salsgiver (1996) suggested that this era led to the development of a perspective that resulted in isolation rather than inclusion. This isolation was fueled by the "medicalization of disability," a model that works in direct contrast with a strengths perspective.

Components of the strengths-based approach include independence and least restrictive environment, two concepts extended from the civil rights and human rights movements of the 1960s (DeJong, 1979; Wolfensburger, 1972). Social workers generally view their clients or consumers from the vantage point of empowerment, with opportunities for self-determinism. Similarly, the independent-living perspective views the client-consumer from the vantage point of personal decision making rather than passivity, empowerment rather than powerlessness, and places a strong emphasis upon individual strength and control. It is this "strength and control" that has facilitated social and political change in society.

A strengths-based perspective to social work intervention recognizes that social workers and public health professionals focus on capabilities, capacities, and opportunities instead of impairments or disabilities (Cowger, 1994; Early & GlenMaye, 2000; Saleebey, 1992). Believing that people have the capacity for success despite their "impairment or disability," the strengths-based approach considers the strengths that individuals contribute to situations. Miley, O'Melia, and Dubois (1995) described the empowerment intervention mode to focus on three areas: (1) client strengths, (2) neighborhood/community resources that exist within one's own system, and (3) a vision that solutions are possible. The outcome of empowerment is to increase control over one's social and organizational environment, which should be a primary objective of effective interventions among public health social workers.

Disability Classifications: *ICF* and PIE Frameworks

In line with the strengths-based approach, two classification systems serve as essential frameworks and resources for understanding disability, identifying barriers and facilitators to persons with disabilities, and developing appropriate interventions. The first classification system is the *International Classification of Functioning, Disability, and Health* or *ICF* (World Health

Organization [WHO], 2001), and the second is the Person-in-Environment for Social Functioning Problems Model, or PIE (Karls & Wandrei, 1994).

The *ICF* was first published as the *International Classification of Impairments, Disabilities, and Handicaps*, or *ICIDH* (WHO, 1980). It retained this acronym despite changes in the name and the classification itself. The *ICIDH-2* attempts to provide a standard language and framework for describing the *functioning* (an umbrella term for body functions, activities, and participation) and *disability* (an umbrella term for impairments, activity limitations, and participation restrictions) associated with health conditions. It was designed for multiple uses across varying fields and disciplines, including education in designing curriculum, raising awareness, and undertaking social actions (WHO, 2001).

The PIE system was developed with the person-in-environment construct as its foundation. While many social work theorists advanced the concept of person-in-environment, Gordon (1981) believed that the social work profession should aim to produce person-in-environment transactions and improve environments for those who function within them. Integral to both the *ICF* and PIE classification systems is the environment, which plays a crucial role in understanding disability. The underlying concept involves viewing the person with a disability within his/her environmental context. The environment consists of attitudes, physical structures, and social contexts within a person's contextual setting.

Both classifications describe, classify, and code their respective areas of interest. Likewise, each system attempts to balance problems and strengths of the person as an interactive process. It is important to recognize this point since viewing the problems within the person only and not as the person–situation interaction has been a concern over the use of traditional classification systems (Northen, 1982). Moreover, the inclusion of environmental factors and strengths will enable the development and implementation of more effective and sustainable public health interventions.

CORE FUNCTIONS OF PUBLIC HEALTH AND DISABILITIES

As indicated by the Office on Disability and Health of the Centers for Disease Control and Prevention, which was created in 1988 in response to legislation by the National Council on Disability, the goal of the program is

> To promote the health and quality of life of people with disabilities and prevent the conditions that cause disabilities. Program objectives include increasing surveillance activities, developing effective preventative interventions, and building the capacity of the states to promote the health of people with disabilities. (Thierry, 1998, p. 505)

This goal links to the three core public health functions—assessment, policy development, and assurance—and their associated essential public health services that must include disability-related concerns that affect public health.

Regarding assessment, relevant services related to disability include monitoring and recognizing disability status as an important community health issue. Diagnosing and investigating issues related to disability and secondary conditions are crucial in public health as well as health-related problems experienced by persons with disabilities. A standardized set of operational definitions of disability and health are critical to meet this goal, as are surveillance systems, which include items that address disability. Finally, evaluating the effectiveness, accessibility, and quality of personal and population-based health services with regard to disability prevalence, epidemiology, and so forth may be considered an ongoing effort for public health social workers. These systems are not consistently addressed from state to state, or across countries.

In terms of policy development, key services involve the development of disability-friendly policies and plans that support both individuals with disabilities within their communities and overall community health efforts to support these population groups and their families. The enforcement of laws and regulations that protect health and ensure safety of persons with disabilities is needed regardless of the setting (home, work, or community). Additionally, research to discover new insights and innovations relevant to disability will continue to be important, especially in the expanding area of technology.

With regard to assurance, linking people with disabilities to needed health services and assuring the provision of the services are imperative in eliminating health disparities. Assuring a competent public health workforce to work with persons with disabilities is another necessary step. Raising awareness, educating, and empowering people with disabilities about their disabilities and secondary health conditions are critical. Facilitating community partnerships to help identify and address issues related to disability and problems faced by persons with disabilities are also extremely relevant.

PUBLIC HEALTH SOCIAL WORK STANDARDS AND COMPETENCIES

To enable the aforementioned core functions of public health social work, various key competencies and standards must be implemented and assessed with regard to disability. These core competencies address a theoretical base, methodological and analytical processes, leadership and communication, and policy and advocacy, as well as values and ethics. Some of the skills critical for public health social workers working with disability and secondary conditions will include principles of epidemiology, theories, and principles of community organization, planned changed and development, an understanding of health systems (including the dimensions of, use of, and access to health care), and macro-level public health social work practice methods. These skills will be useful in the detection and assessment of community and health care systems. In addition, public health social workers will need to utilize practice and epidemiologic theories to substantiate interventions and programming designed to promote health and behavioral change.

A number of methodological and analytical skills will also be essential for public health social workers, working to improve the status of people with disabilities and secondary conditions. These methodological skills include research design, sampling, measurement, and basic descriptive/inferential statistics to help with data interpretation. In addition, these skills will be useful in the design of public health social workers' practice trials to examine the impacts of interventions tailored to meet the needs of people with disabilities. Skills in the formulation of hypotheses or research questions in collaboration with internal or external resources for the development and implementation of an analytical strategy to influence health and social planned change are also useful competencies for public health social workers working in this arena.

Leadership and communication skills will also be key competencies for public health social workers taking the lead as community change agents. Some of these competencies will include skills in community organization and coalition building, especially directed toward addressing social and health disparities. Networking, multidisciplinary team building, and an understanding of group process will be critical when working with building a consensus for inclusion of people with disabilities and secondary conditions in community-based intervention efforts. Strategies for soliciting and maintaining consumer and other constituencies' input will strengthen the role that people with disabilities can play in community planning efforts, and help prevent this marginalized group from being considered "token" participants. Lastly, competencies in strategic planning, organizational development, performance outcome measures, and program evaluation activities will help facilitate long-term changes for people with disabilities and secondary conditions through assurance activities and policy development.

Public health social workers should be able to critically analyze health inequities based on disability and determine how disability contributes to health status, health behaviors, and program design. They should develop strategies to assure integrated service systems for disability populations to reduce risk for health and social issues. The use of public health laws and policies related to creating and promoting disability-based services and programs should be identified and implemented. Cultural competence within public health settings should include disability as a major comparison group along with gender, race, and ethnicity.

FUTURE ISSUES

The number of persons with disabilities, as well as the number of those with disabilities and secondary conditions, will continue to grow. As a result, the need to track and monitor disability at the national, state, and local levels will be heightened. In this regard, there must be consistent efforts in the tracking and monitoring systems. Hence, a standardized definition of disability must be established to enable effective tracking and monitoring of disability prevalence rates and other key disability-related indicators. At the current time not all states have a standardized set of questions in their surveillance strategy to identify people with disabilities. In addition, there is not a consistent set of operational definitions for identifying disability either. Public health social workers can be effective advocates in moving toward these *Healthy People 2020* goals.

In addition, *Healthy People 2020* objectives must be addressed by public health agencies at federal, state, and local levels. Otherwise, health disparities among persons with disabilities will most likely continue (DHHS, 2010). To accomplish these goals, funding from federal, state, private, and public entities must be increased to support public health research and program initiatives.

In order to effectively practice in public health and social work settings with people who have disabilities, public health social workers must be exposed to evidence-based practice, policy, and research regarding disability during their professional training and development (Chapin, 1995). Public health social workers can take the lead on defining, testing, and disseminating best practices.

Caregivers of people with disabilities tend to be a forgotten group, and they also comprise a group that needs to be addressed in efforts to meet the goals of *Healthy People 2020*. Health-promotion efforts also need to address the unique needs and accommodations that people with disabilities and their caregivers will present to public health agencies and to primary care providers.

Other future issues include the need for workforce development and preparation to work with people who have disabilities. Public health social workers and faculty teaching within this area will need to advocate for the inclusion of coursework and content within Master of Public Health and Master of Social Work programs in disability and public health. At a minimum, improved access and support for people with disabilities to receive accommodations and technology will be necessary. These accommodations will include assistive devices, service animals, technology services, and assistive technologies.

Last, public health social workers must adhere to the NASW standards for Social Work Practice in Health Care Settings (NASW, 2005). These standards include the need for cultural competence and the recognition of the unique issues that people with disabilities bring to the table.

SUMMARY AND FUTURE ISSUES

Although much progress has been made to recognize the importance of disabilities and secondary conditions, major gaps between people with and without disabilities are still evident within community and tribal settings. Although disabilities and secondary conditions have only recently been addressed within the *Healthy People* objectives (they were first introduced in 2010), much progress is still needed to bridge the gap between health disparities for people with and without disabilities and secondary conditions. There is much scope for the role of public health social workers in beginning to bridge this gap within policy, practice, and research arenas.

CLASSROOM EXERCISES

Discussion Questions

1. What are the similarities and differences between persons with disabilities and other marginalized groups (e.g., women, racial/ethnic minorities, immigrants) in terms of the health disparities experienced by these populations?
2. Discuss the role of the public health social worker in working with persons with disabilities. Is this expected to remain the same or change in the future? How so?
3. Identify current public health service systems at the federal, state, and local levels. Do they address the needs of persons with disabilities? What are the gaps?

Interactive Exercises

1. Famous People with Disabilities Exercise—Students should develop a list of famous people (celebrities, politicians, athletes, etc.) who have/had some type of disability and identify that specific disability. One by one, students can take turns announcing the name of the

person, and then the others must correctly identify the disability that affects the person. Students can brainstorm what kind of barriers need to be overcome in order to strengthen the public health arena for each of these individuals and list which are the common barriers and accommodations needed. Once listed, which of these are goals within the *Healthy People 2020* objectives?

INTERNET RESOURCES

Healthy People 2020—Disability and Health

(http://healthypeople.gov/2020/topicsobjectives2020/overview. aspx?topicId=9)

This chapter focuses on benchmarks associated with disability and health. Specific objectives related to disability and health are outlined and described.

Centers for Disease Control and Prevention (CDC)—Disability and Health

(www.cdc.gov/ncbddd/disabilityandhealth/index.html)

This section highlights the CDC's efforts in addressing disability and health. The CDC works to promote health and wellness among persons with disabilities as well as improve their quality of life. Information on types of disabilities, accessibility, disability data, and statistics are provided. Links to national disability organizations and funded programs are listed.

APPENDIX 9A

HEALTHY PEOPLE 2020 OBJECTIVES RELATED TO DISABILITIES AND SECONDARY CONDITIONS

- Include in the core of *Healthy People 2020* population data systems a standardized set of questions that identify "people with disabilities."
- Increase the number of tribes, states, and the District of Columbia that have public health surveillance and health promotion programs for people with disabilities and caregivers.
- Increase the number of State and the District of Columbia health departments that have at least one health promotion program aimed at improving the health and well-being of people with disabilities.
- Increase the number of State and the District of Columbia health departments that conduct health surveillance for caregivers of people with disabilities.
- Increase the number of State and the District of Columbia health departments that have at least one health promotion program aimed at improving the health and well-being of caregivers of people with disabilities.
- (Developmental) Increase the number of Tribes that conduct health surveillance for people with disabilities.
- (Developmental) Increase the number of Tribes that have at least one health promotion program aimed at improving the health and well-being of people with disabilities.
- (Developmental) Increase the number of Tribes that conduct health surveillance of caregivers of people with disabilities.
- (Developmental) Increase the number of Tribes that have at least one health promotion program aimed at improving the health and well-being of caregivers of people with disabilities.
- (Developmental) Increase the proportion of U.S. Master of Public Health programs that offer graduate-level courses in disability and health.
- (Developmental) Reduce the proportion of people with disabilities who report delays in receiving primary and periodic preventive care due to specific barriers.
- Increase the proportion of youth with special health care needs whose health care provider has discussed transition planning from pediatric to adult health care.
- (Developmental) Increase the proportion of people with epilepsy and uncontrolled seizures who receive appropriate medical care.
- (Developmental) Reduce the proportion of older adults with disabilities who use inappropriate medications.
- (Developmental) Reduce the proportion of people with disabilities who report physical or program barriers to local health and wellness programs.
- (Developmental) Reduce the proportion of people with disabilities who encounter barriers to participating in home, school, work, or community activities.
- (Developmental) Reduce the proportion of people with disabilities who report barriers to obtaining the assistive devices, service animals, technology services, and accessible technologies that they need.
- Increase the proportion of newly constructed and retrofitted U.S. homes and residential buildings that have visitable features.
- Reduce the number of people with disabilities living in congregate care residences.
- Reduce the number of adults with disabilities (aged 22 years and older) living in congregate care residences that serve 16 or more persons.

- Reduce the number of children and youth with disabilities (aged 21 years and under) living in congregate care residences.
- (Developmental) Increase the proportion of people with disabilities who participate in social, spiritual, recreational, community, and civic activities to the degree that they wish.
- Increase the proportion of children and youth with disabilities who spend at least 80% of their time in regular education programs.
- Reduce unemployment among people with disabilities.
- Increase employment among people with disabilities.
- Increase the proportion of adults with disabilities who report sufficient social and emotional support.
- (Developmental) Reduce the proportion of people with disabilities who report serious psychological distress.
- (Developmental) Reduce the proportion of people with disabilities who experience nonfatal unintentional injuries that require medical care.
- Increase the proportion of children with disabilities, birth through age 2 years, who receive early intervention services in home or community-based settings.

REFERENCES

Bradsher, J. E. (1995). Disability among racial and ethnic groups. *Disability Statistics Abstract, 10,* 1-4.

Campbell, M. L., Sheets, D., & Strong, P. S. (1999). Secondary health conditions among middle-aged individuals with chronic physical disabilities: Implications for unmet needs for services. *Assistive Technology, 11,* 105-122.

Centers for Disease Control and Prevention. (2010). DATA 2010 [Internet database]. Atlanta, GA: Author. Available from: http://wonder.cdc.gov/data2010/focus.htm.

Chapin, R. K. (1995). Social policy development: The strengths perspective. *Social Work, 40*(4), 506-514.

Chevarley, F. M., Thierry, J. M., Gill, C. J., Ryerson, A. B., & Nosek, M. A. (2006). Health, preventative health care, and health care access among women with disabilities in the 1994-1995 National Health Interview Survey, Supplement on Disability. *Women's Health Issues, 16,* 297-312.

Cowger, C. D. (1994). Assessing client strengths: Clinical assessment for client empowerment. *Social Work, 39*(3), 262-269.

DeJong, G. (1979). Independent living: From social movement to analytic paradigm. *Archives of Physical Medicine and Rehabilitation, 60,* 435-446.

Draheim, C., Williams, D., & McCubbin, J. A. (2002). Prevalence of physical inactivity and recommended physical activity in community-based adults with mental retardation. *Mental Retardation, 40,* 436-444.

Drum, C., Krahn, G., Culley, C., & Hammond, L. (2005). Recognizing and responding to the health disparities of people with disabilities. *California Journal of Health Promotion, 3*(3), 29-42.

Early, T. J., & GlenMaye, L. F. (2000). Valuing families: Social work practice with families from a strengths perspective. *Social Work, 45*(2), 118-130.

Fine, M., & Asch, A. (1988). Disability beyond stigma: Social interaction, discrimination, and activism. *Journal of Social Issues, 44*(1), 3-21.

Gordon, W. E. (1981). A natural classification system for social work literature and knowledge. *Social Work, 26,* 134–136.

Gray, D., & Hahn, H. (1997). Achieving occupational goals: The social effects of stigma. In C. Christiansen & C. Baum (Eds.), *Enabling function and well-being* (pp. 393–409). Thorofare, NJ: Slack.

Iezzoni, L. I., McCarthy, E. P., Davis, R. B., & Siebens, H. (2000). Mobility impairments and use of screening and preventative services. *American Journal of Public Health, 90,* 955–961.

Jurkowski, E., & Welch, P. (1999). *Status of disability content in social work curricula: A cross-national comparison.* International Federation of Social Workers and International Association of Social Work, Montreal, Canada. Retrieved from http://www. mun.ca/cassw-ar/papers2/Jurkowski.pdf

Jurkowski, E., & Welch, P. (2002). *Integrating curriculum content on disability within social work curricula: A model and tools for curriculum building.* International Association of Schools of Social Work, Montpellier, France. Retrieved from www. aforts.com/colloques_ouvrages/colloques/.../jurkowski_elaine.doc

Karls, J. M., & Wandrei, K. E. (1994). *Person-in-environment system: The PIE classification system for social functioning problems.* Washington, DC: National Association of Social Workers.

Kaye, S. (1997). *Disability watch. The status of people with disabilities in the United States.* Volcano, CA: Volcano Press.

Keefe, R. (2010). Health disparities: A primer for public health social workers. *Social Work and Public Health, 25,* 237–257.

Krahn, G., & Campbell, V. (2011). Evolving views of disability and public health: The roles of advocacy and public health. *Disability and Health Journal, 4*(1), 12–18.

Lollar, D. J. (2002). Public health and disability: Emerging opportunities. *Public Health Reports, 117,* 131–136.

Longmore, P. K. (1997). Conspicuous contribution and American cultural dilemmas: Telethon rituals of cleansing and renewal. In D. T. Mitchell & S. L. Snyder (Eds.), *The body and physical difference: Discourses of disability* (pp. 134–160). Ann Arbor, MI: University of Michigan Press.

Mackelprang, R., & Salsgiver, R. O. (1996). People with disabilities and social work: Historical and conceptual issues. *Social Work, 41*(1), 7–14.

Miley, K. K., O'Melia, M., & Dubois, B. L. (1995). *Generalist social work practice: An empowering approach.* Boston: Allyn & Bacon.

Nagi, S. Z. (1965). Some conceptual issues in disability and rehabilitation. In M. B. Sussman (Ed.), *Sociology and rehabilitation.* Washington, DC: American Sociological Association.

Nagi, S. Z. (1991). In A. M. Pope, & A. R. Tarlov (Eds.), *Disability in America: Toward a national agenda for prevention.* Washington, DC: National Academy of Sciences.

National Association for Social Workers. (2005). *Standards for social work practice in health care settings.* Washington, DC: Author.

Northen, H. (1982). *Clinical social work.* New York: Columbia University Press.

Parish, S. L., & Ellison-Martin, J. (2007). Health-care access of women Medicaid recipients. *Journal of Disability Policy Studies, 18*(2), 109–116.

Pope, A., & Brandt, E. (1997). *Enabling America: Assessing the role of rehabilitation science and engineering.* Washington, DC: National Academies Press.

Pope, A. M., & Tarlov, A. R. (1991). *Disability in America: Toward a national agenda for prevention.* Washington, DC: National Academies Press.

Rowland, K. (2011). *Defining secondary conditions*. Retrieved from http://www.ncpad. org/360/2050/Defining~Secondary~Conditions~for~People~with~Disabilities.

Saleebey, D. (Ed.). (1992). *The strengths perspective in social work practice*. New York: Longman.

Smart, J. F., & Smart, D. W. (1997). The racial/ethnic demography of disability. *Journal of Rehabilitation*, *63*(4), 9–15.

Tanenhaus, R. H., Meyers, A. R., & Harbison, L. A. (2000). Disability and the curriculum in U.S. graduate schools of public health. *American Journal of Public Health*, *90*(8), 1315–1316.

Thierry, J. (1998). Promoting the health and wellness of women with disabilities. *Journal of Women's Health*, *7*(5), 505–507.

Turk, M. A., Scabdale, J., Rosenbaum, P. F., & Weber, R. J. (2001). The health of women with cerebral palsy. *Physical Medicine and Rehabilitation Clinics of North America*, *12*, 153–168.

U.S. Bureau of the Census. (2000). *American community survey*. Washington, DC: U.S. Government Printing Office.

U.S. Department of Health and Human Services. (1999). *Healthy People 2000 review, 1998–1999*. Hyattsville, MD: National Center for Health Statistics.

U.S. Department of Health and Human Services (2000). *Healthy People 2010: Understanding and improving health* (2nd ed.). Washington, DC: U.S. Government Printing Office.

U.S. Department of Health and Human Services. (2010). *Healthy People 2020*. Retrieved from http://healthypeople.gov/2020/default.aspx

Waldrop, J., & Stern, S. M. (2003). *Disability status: 2000 [Census 2000 brief]*. Washington, DC: U.S. Department of Commerce, Census Bureau.

Wei, W., Findley, P., & Sambamoorthu, U. (2006). Disability and receipt of clinical preventative services among women. *Women's Health Issues*, *16*, 286–296.

Wolfensberger, W. (1972). *Citizen advocacy for the handicapped, impaired, and disadvantaged: An overview*. Washington, DC: President's Committee on Mental Retardation.

World Health Organization. (1980). *International classification of impairments, disability, and handicaps*. Geneva, Switzerland: Author.

World Health Organization. (2001). *International classification of functioning, disability, and health*. Geneva, Switzerland: Author.

CHAPTER 10

Chronic Health Conditions

Patricia Welch Saleeby and Elaine T. Jurkowski

INTRODUCTION

*R*ecent social, political, and demographic trends have resulted in increased opportunities for public health social workers to practice with people affected by chronic health conditions. Over 75% of our health care expenditures are designated for people affected by chronic conditions (Anderson, 2004). Common chronic diseases include asthma, cancer, diabetes, heart disease, HIV/AIDS, obesity, respiratory diseases, and stroke. Chronic conditions are considered the leading causes of death and disability in the United States. In fact, seven out of 10 deaths each year are attributed to chronic diseases (Kung, Hoyert, Xu, & Murphy, 2008).

Chronic conditions are those that are long lasting, generally exceeding 3 months. They differ from acute conditions, which are short course in nature, and from a recurrent course in which repeated relapses occur with remission periods in between. Acute diseases are usually isolated to one bodily area and respond to treatment. In contrast, long-term conditions frequently involve multiple systems and have an uncertain future (Murrow & Oglesby, 1996). Although acute injuries can lead to chronic conditions, such as pain, many never become chronic due to proper health care interventions. However, acute injuries do affect functioning in that one-fourth of people with chronic conditions have at least one daily activity limitation (Anderson, 2004).

Although many chronic diseases are costly, they are also preventable as compared to other health disorders and problems. According to the Centers for Disease Control and Prevention (CDC, 2011) there are four modifiable health risk behaviors: (1) poor nutrition, (2) lack of physical activity, (3) tobacco use, and (4) excessive alcohol consumption, that are responsible for much of the illness, suffering, and early death associated with chronic conditions. Consequently, it is essential that social workers not only understand the nature of chronic health conditions but also be competent in developing and implementing preventative public health strategies.

HEALTH DISPARITIES AND CHRONIC CONDITIONS

Certain population groups, including racial and ethnic minorities, persons with disabilities, women, immigrants, the elderly, and the poor, experience greater disparities with regard to chronic health conditions. Reasons for such health disparities reflect differences in health-related risk factors, socio-economic differences, and direct/indirect consequences of discrimination. Lack of insurance coverage, high prescription drug costs, and the absence of availability of usual sources of primary care all significantly affect access, especially among minority populations.

Health care access is one of the leading factors contributing to the existence of chronic conditions and health disparities. As defined by the Institute of Medicine (1998), *health care access* is considered the timely utilization of services to achieve the best possible health outcomes. Access to health care impacts the prevention of disease and disability, detection and treatment of health condition, life expectancy, preventable death, quality of life, and overall physical, social, and mental health status.

Individuals from racial and ethnic minority groups experience higher rates of chronic diseases compared to the general population (Mead et al., 2008). As reported by Keefe (2010), racial and ethnic minorities are less likely than Whites to have health insurance, have fewer choices of where to receive care, and are more likely to receive care in hospital emergency rooms. African Americans, Asian Americans, and Hispanic Americans face greater barriers to primary health care than Whites (Shi, 1999). African Americans experience higher rates of mortality from cancer compared to any other racial or ethnic group (American Cancer Society, 2009; DHHS, 2010). Asian Americans and Pacific Islanders have a greater risk for Type 2 diabetes (National Institute of Diabetes and Digestive and Kidney Diseases, 2000, 2002). Hispanic women face disproportionate rates of cervical cancer compared to White women (Mead et al., 2008). As stated by the Institute of Medicine (IOM, 2002), "evidence of racial and ethnic disparities in healthcare is, with few exceptions, remarkably consistent across a range of illnesses and health-care services" (p. 4).

Similarly, persons with disabilities report greater issues with accessing health care than persons without disabilities (Drainoni et al., 2006) and typically have elevated needs for health care services (Iezzoni, McCarthy, Davis, Harris-David, & O'Day, 2001). According to the National Organization on Disability (2002), "health care is less accessible to Americans with disabilities, who, ironically are often the citizens needing it the most." Generally, persons with disabilities experience poorer health and a higher prevalence of secondary conditions (Kinne, Patrick, & Doyle, 2004). People with disabilities frequently underutilize basic preventative services (Schopp, Sanford, Hagglund, Gay, & Coatney, 2001). For example, women with disabilities are less likely to receive routine breast and cervical cancer screenings than women without disabilities (Chevarley, Thierry, Gill, Ryerson, & Nosek, 2006; Havercamp, Scandlin, & Roth, 2004). Moreover, other personal characteristics, including age, gender, socioeconomic status, ethnicity, and sexual orientation, may further contribute to increased health disparities among persons with disabilities (Johnson & Woll, 2003).

While individual risk factors play a role in health disparities across chronic conditions, socioeconomic factors are positively associated with health status; specifically, individuals with higher incomes have better outcomes, whereas individuals with lower incomes have worse outcomes. Minorities represent a disproportionate number of individuals of lower socioeconomic status (IOM, 2002; Kaplan, Everson, & Lynch, 2000), and suffer more from hunger and malnutrition and in turn have worse health status and health outcomes (Kaiser Family Foundation, 2004). According to the IOM (2002), lower socioeconomic status is more important than race in determining medical care for women with breast cancer.

HEALTHY PEOPLE 2020

Specific chronic conditions, including arthritis, cancer, chronic back conditions, diabetes, heart disease, HIV, kidney disease, obesity, oral health, osteoporosis, respiratory diseases, and stroke, are addressed in *Healthy People 2020*. For each condition, an overview is provided along with emerging issues. Information related to disparities and barriers to care is also highlighted for certain chronic diseases across relevant demographic variables.

Goals and objectives are outlined for each chronic condition. A sample of these objectives include the improvement of cardiovascular health and quality of life through prevention, detection, and treatment of risk factors for heart attack and stroke; early identification and treatment of heart attacks and strokes; the prevention of repeat cardiovascular events; the reduction of the number of new cancer cases, as well as the illness, disability, and death caused by cancer; the reduction of the disease and economic burden of diabetes mellitus (DM) and improvement of the quality of life for all persons who have, or are at risk for DM; and the promotion of respiratory health through better prevention, detection, treatment, and education efforts.

Highly related to the prevalence of chronic health conditions is access to health services. *HP2020* includes, as one of its goals, to improve access to comprehensive, quality health care services and focuses on four components of access to care: (1) coverage, (2) services, (3) timeliness, and (4) workforce. Although space does not allow all benchmarks to be documented in detail here, it does allow for some brief descriptions. Appendix A outlines specific *Healthy People 2020* objectives and their associated benchmarks. Some of these benchmarks to be met by *Healthy People 2020* include benchmarks for diabetes, heart and stroke, and respiratory health conditions.

In 2008, The National Health Interview Survey (2008) reported that eight of every 1,000 people in the population were identified as new cases with diabetes. In a population of 100,000 people, 73.1 died due to diabetes (CDC, 2008). *HP2020* strives to reduce these numbers by 10%. Other goals include the increase in dilated eye, oral health and foot examinations for people living with diabetes, and a decrease in the number of people who require amputations due to complications associated with their diabetes. From a prevention point of view, *HP2020* strives to increase the amount of preventative health education that is provided to people in an effort to help them address the potential to acquire diabetes. Benchmarks also target preventative health education for people who are prediabetic, in efforts to control the onset of the disease (CDC, 2010).

Stroke and heart disease are other leading chronic health conditions. In 2008, the CDC's Center for Vital Statistics reported that there were 126 per 100,000 deaths due to heart disease, and 42.2 deaths per 100,000 due to stroke (CDC, 2010). *HP2020* strives to reduce these numbers by 10%, by the year 2020. In efforts to meet these targets, *HP2020* has established benchmarks to reduce the proportion of hypertension in youths, adolescents, and adults. It also calls for an increase in the proportion of adults who have their blood pressure under control through a range of prevention strategies, to include a cholesterol reduction diet, reduced sodium intake, moderate alcohol consumption, blood glucose monitoring, and a low-cholesterol diet. From a prevention perspective, some *HP2020* goals include making the general population aware of the signs of stroke and heart attacks, and how to access emergency services through by calling 9-1-1. In terms of care and treatment, *HP2020* goals also strive to increase the number of people who are referred to rehabilitation centers following the diagnosis of a heart attack or stroke.

Health insurance coverage is crucial since the uninsured are less likely to obtain necessary medical care, more likely to have poor health status, and more likely to die early (Hadley, 2007). Increasing access to and use of both a primary care provider as a usual source of care as well as evidence-based preventive services are important (National Commission on Prevention Priorities, 2007; U.S. Department of Health and Human Services, 2000).

CORE FUNCTIONS OF PUBLIC HEALTH

It is imperative that the core functions of public health—assessment, policy development, and assurance—continue to address chronic conditions since they affect a significant percentage of the U.S. population. Essential public health services must increase services related to chronic diseases at the national, state, and local levels.

In terms of monitoring health status to identify and solve community health problems, screening for chronic diseases like diabetes and testing for HIV should be made available to people who need them, most especially the uninsured. The focus of data collection efforts on the multitude of chronic conditions should be increased and coordinated to facilitate a better understanding of these diseases as well as the development of effective public health interventions. Personal and population-based health services should be evaluated across key indicators such as their accessibility, effectiveness, and quality.

Some specific examples of how assessment activities that address chronic health conditions are carried out in the community include the process of monitoring health status through the use of vital statistics to identify community health problems and local health planning that assess community health needs. An understanding of the rates, risk factors, and epidemiology of chronic health conditions can also help public health social workers diagnose specific community health problems. Hand in hand with the detection of health care resources and issues is the importance of evaluating existing resources to address chronic health issues including the availability, accessibility, and quality of publicly available health care.

Monitoring of the health status of individuals also includes immunizations (e.g., polio), sexually transmitted disease/HIV counseling, and screening activities for conditions such as diabetes and hypertension. Public health departments often prioritize which of these areas will take precedence through Local Area Plan for Assessment strategies. Public health social workers are often at the helm of these activities.

Regarding policy development, policies and plans should support individual and community health efforts addressing chronic health conditions. Activities by state and local public health agencies should involve tobacco-free coalitions, referrals to health care providers, and collaboration with special population advocates. Research into new insights on chronic diseases and innovative solutions to chronic health conditions is necessary, including the implementation of ongoing health needs assessment. Public health social workers also take a lead role in enforcing laws and regulations designed to protect the health and ensure the safety of people living in communities, particularly when health hazards are involved. Customer service evaluations with chronic-condition indicators and the study of successful public health programs addressing chronic diseases are also activities which are carried out through this core function.

Assurance activities link people to needed personal health services and promise the provision of health care when otherwise unavailable. Assurance functions also include the development and regulation of a competent public health social worker workforce. The importance of informing, educating, and empowering people about chronic health care issues and working toward moving the community and community partnerships to identify and solve health problems are also functions that public health social workers will be confronted with when working to impact chronic health conditions.

A number of community-based coalitions have emerged to address chronic health conditions in local communities. Public health social workers can have an impact on addressing and building effective community interventions through their assurance function. In addition, they can inform and educate through community-health education strategies that include health fairs and community-education events and through the use of print media, social networking, public presentations, and the radio and television. Chronic health conditions such as diabetes, hypertension, and HIV/AIDS can also be addressed by public education and risk reduction curricula delivered by public health social workers.

Public health social workers often spearhead community partnerships and coalitions, such as Healthy Communities Coalitions and Tobacco-Free Coalitions that address the chronic health care needs of people in communities. Likewise, public health social workers address chronic health care needs of various groups by advocating for the groups' needs. Other examples of strategies used to promote community interventions include arthritis support groups, community-wide walking programs, and physical fitness programs for people with disabilities.

Although there are myriad activities that public health social workers can participate in to impact the chronic health conditions of people living in communities, this section addresses a number that fall within the three core functions of assessment, policy development, and assurance. Hand in hand with the core functions are a series of public health social work competencies that are necessary to effectively carry out these core functions.

PUBLIC HEALTH SOCIAL WORK STANDARDS AND COMPETENCIES

Effective assessment, policy development, and assurance of services to meet the chronic health care needs in communities cannot happen without the mastery of several core competencies germane to public health social workers. These competencies can be found within the realm of theory, methodology, leadership/communication, policy/advocacy, and values and ethics.

Theoretical skills necessary for public health social workers include an understanding of epidemiologic principles to help identify patterns of disease and rates and ratios across various population and ethnic groups. The application of macro-level public health social work methods (e.g., social planning, community organization and development, and social marketing) will be effective tools to address the chronic health care needs of communities. The ability to conduct, interpret, address, and analyze inequities in health status based on race/ethnicity, socioeconomic position, and gender are skills that will also require a theoretical foundation.

In concert with these skills is the ability to recognize various strengths, needs, values, and practices of diverse cultural, racial, ethnic, and socioeconomic groups to determine how these factors affect health status, health behaviors, and program design. Lastly, the ability to apply primary, secondary, and tertiary strategies to address the heath, social, and economic issues of individuals, families, and communities will help equip public health social workers with the skills necessary to build effective interventions that address chronic health conditions.

A series of methodological and analytical skills can also be an asset for public health social workers combating chronic health conditions. Some of these skills should include the collection and interpretation of data from vital statistics, censuses, surveys, service utilization, and other relevant reports on social and health status for all, especially vulnerable and underserved populations. In addition, the detection of meaningful inferences from data and the translation of data into information for community assessment (gaps, barriers, and strengths analysis), program planning, implementation, and evaluation would also be an asset in the process of understanding and responding to chronic diseases. The ability to formulate research questions for the development and implementation of strategies to influence health and social planned change will also prove to be of vital importance.

Public health social workers working in the area of chronic conditions will also need competencies and skills in leadership and communication. Some specific competencies include the need to understand organizational culture and change and the ability to provide leadership and communicate across diverse groups. Some specific skills will include the ability to develop, implement, monitor, and evaluate grant-funded programs.

Hand in hand with these skills is the application of management and organizational theories and practices to the development, planning, budgeting, staffing, administration, and evaluation of public health programs, including the implementation of strategies promoting integrated service systems, especially for vulnerable populations. Given that health promotion projects often include a variety of community partners, it will also be important for public health social workers to have skills to communicate effectively with diverse and multicultural organizations and community and consumer boards and coalitions.

Competencies and skills in policy and advocacy will also be essential if the vision for effective interventions will include the institutionalization of new programs and services. Competencies critical to meeting this goal will include an understanding of federal and state mandates that guide the funding and implementation of health and social service programs and an understanding of legislative, administrative, and judicial processes at the national, state, and local levels. Skills essential to meet the needs of policy development and advocacy will include the application of critical thinking to every stage of policy development and practice and the identification of public health laws, regulations, and policies related to specific programs. In addition, skills in collecting and summarizing data relevant to a particular policy and problem will also bolster the success of public health social workers in the area of policy and advocacy.

Lastly, as public health social workers, we have a responsibility to ethical social work practice. Ethics as prescribed by the National Association of Social Workers code of ethics and the American Public Health Association guide our practice across all fields of public health social work, particularly when working with micro-, mezzo- and macro-level interventions to alleviate the negative effects of chronic conditions.

FUTURE ISSUES AND IMPLICATIONS FOR PUBLIC HEALTH SOCIAL WORK PRACTICE

Chronic diseases and disease prevention will likely be on the rise in the future due to the increased levels of stress and contaminants in our communities. Nearly two-thirds of adults believe that the U.S. health care system should emphasize more prevention of chronic conditions than is currently provided (National Association of Chronic Disease Directors, 2008). Public health social workers should promote regular preventive care, especially for those minority groups experiencing health disparities.

Innovative and preventive health-promotion strategies aimed at reducing the incidence of chronic diseases will also be essential. Children, teens, and young adults are groups that will be targeted. Social networking sites, e-health literacy, and intergenerational health promotion strategies, will be useful in an effort to help reduce the incidence and prevalence of chronic health care conditions. School health programs will look toward partnering students, their parents and grandparents, and e-health literacy strategies in efforts to educate each generation about the causes and health promotion strategies to curtail and combat chronic health conditions. Health promotion efforts will also make use of innovative ways to reach people across the life span.

SUMMARY

Recent social, political, and demographic trends have resulted in increased opportunities for public health professionals to work with people affected by chronic health conditions. As a result, the need for trained public health professionals familiar with issues related to chronic health conditions has heightened. This chapter explored the core public health functions relevant to practicing with chronically ill individuals. Public health social work standards and competencies were discussed. Recommendations for future practice were provided to improve public health social work practice with people with chronic health conditions.

CLASSROOM EXERCISES

Discussion Questions

1. What are the short-term and long-term consequences of chronic health conditions for individuals, families, and communities?
2. How do chronic diseases differently affect individuals by age, gender, race, ethnicity, disability, and socioeconomic status?
3. In what clinical and community-based settings would you expect public health social workers to be practicing? Describe their roles, tasks, and activities.
4. You have been deployed to work with your local health department to develop a community-based intervention for chronic diseases.
   - Where would you begin?
   - Which stakeholders would be included?
   - What would you include in your plan of action?

INTERNET RESOURCES

Healthy People 2020

(http://healthypeople.gov/2020/default.aspx)

Healthy People outlines science-based, 10-year national objectives for improving the health of all Americans. For 3 decades, Healthy People has established benchmarks and monitored progress over time in order to (1) encourage collaborations across sectors, (2) guide individuals toward making informed health decisions, and (3) measure the impact of prevention activities. *HP2020* provides an overview, objectives, and interventions for specific chronic conditions, including arthritis, cancer, diabetes, heart disease, respiratory diseases, and stroke. Information regarding access to health services is provided as well.

Centers for Disease Control and Prevention (CDC)

(www.cdc.gov/chronicdisease/resources/publications/index.htm)

This main section highlights the CDC's efforts in addressing chronic diseases through its National Center for Chronic Disease Prevention and Health Promotion (NCCDPHP). Its mission focuses on efforts that promote health and well-being through prevention and control of chronic diseases. Information on specific chronic conditions is provided.

CDC Racial and Ethnic Approaches to Community Health

(www.cdc.gov/reach/)

Racial and Ethnic Approaches to Community Health is a national program that serves as the cornerstone of the CDC's efforts to eliminate racial and ethnic disparities in health. The CDC supports grantee partners that establish community-based programs and culturally appropriate interventions to eliminate health disparities among African Americans, American Indians, Hispanics/Latinos, Asian Americans, Alaska Natives, and Pacific Islanders.

REFERENCES

American Cancer Society. (2009). *Cancer facts & figures for African Americans 2009-2010.* Atlanta, GA: American Cancer Society.

Anderson, G. (2004). *Chronic conditions: Making the case for ongoing care.* Baltimore, MD: John Hopkins University.

Centers for Disease Control and Prevention. (2011). *Chronic diseases and health promotion.* Atlanta, GA: U.S. Department of Health and Human Services. Available from http://www.cdc.gov/chronicdisease/overview/index.htm

Chevarley, F. M., Thierry, J. M., Gill, C. J., Ryerson, A. B., & Nosek, M. A. (2006). Health, preventive health care, and health care access among women with disabilities in the 1994-1995 National Health Interview Survey, Supplement on Disability. *Women's Health Issues, 16,* 297-312.

Drainoni, M. L., Lee-Hood, E., Tobias, C., Bachman, S., Andrew, J., & Maisels, L. (2006). Cross-disability experiences of barriers to health-care access. *Journal of Disability Policy Studies, 17*(2), 101-115.

Hadley, J. (2007). Insurance coverage, medical care use, and short-term health changes following an unintentional injury or the onset of a chronic condition. *Journal of the American Medical Association, 297*(10), 1073–1084.

Havercamp, S. M., Scandlin, D., & Roth, M. (2004). Health disparities among adults with developmental disabilities, adults with other disabilities, and adults not reporting disability in North Carolina. *Public Health Reports, 100*, 418–427.

Iezzoni, L. I., McCarthy, E. P., Davis, R. B., Harris-David, L. H., & O'Day, B. (2001). Use of screening and preventative services among women with disabilities. *American Journal of Medical Quality, 16*, 135–144.

Institute of Medicine. (1998). *Medicare: A strategy for quality assurance* (Vol. 1). Washington, DC: National Academies Press.

Institute of Medicine. (2002). *Unequal treatment: Confronting racial and ethnic disparities in health care*. Washington, DC: National Academies Press.

Johnson, J., & Woll, J. (2003). A national disgrace: Health disparities encountered by persons with disabilities. *Disability Studies Quarterly, 23*(1), 61–74.

Kaiser Family Foundation. (2004). Health care priorities. In *Kaiser Health Poll Report*. Available from http:www.kff.org/healthpollreport/CurrentEdition/about.cfm

Kaplan, G., Everson, S., & Lynch, J. (2000). The contribution of social and behavioral research to an understanding of the distribution of disease: A multilevel approach. In B. Smedley & S. Syme (Eds.), *Promoting health: Intervention strategies from social and behavioral research*. Washington, DC: National Academies Press.

Keefe, R. H. (2010). Health disparities: A primer for public health social workers. *Social Work in Public Health, 25*, 237–257.

Kinne, S., Patrick, D. L., & Doyle, D. L. (2004). Prevalence of secondary conditions among people with disabilities. *American Journal of Public Health, 94*(3), 443–445.

Kung, H. C., Hoyert, D. L., Xu, J. Q., & Murphy, S. L. (2008). Deaths: Final data for 2005. *National Vital Statistics Reports, 56*(10). Hyattsville, MD: National Center for Health Statistics.

Mead, H., Cartwright-Smith, L., Jones, K., Ramos, C., Siegel, B., & Woods, K. (2008). *Racial and ethnic disparities in U.S. healthcare: A chartbook*. New York: The Commonwealth Fund.

Murrow, E. J., & Oglesby, F. M. (1996). Acute and chronic illness: Similarities, differences and challenges. *Orthopaedic Nursing, 15*(5), 47–51.

National Association of Chronic Disease Directors. (2008). *Two-thirds of adult Americans believe more money needs to be spent on chronic disease prevention programs, and they're willing to pay higher taxes to fund them, survey finds* [Press release]. Available from http:www.chronicdisease.orgfilespublicPressRelease_ NACDD_Publi cHealthSurvey_August2008.pdf

National Commission on Prevention Priorities. (2007). *Preventive care: A national profile on use, disparities, and health benefits*. Washington, DC: Partnership for Prevention.

National Institute of Diabetes and Digestive and Kidney Diseases. (2000). *National diabetes statistics fact sheet: General information and national estimates on diabetes in the United States*. Available from www.niddk.nih.gov/health/diabetes/pubs/dmstats/dmstats.htm

National Institute of Diabetes and Digestive and Kidney Diseases. (2002). *Diabetes in Asian and Pacific Islander Americans*. Bethesda, MD: Author. Avaiable from: http://diabetes.niddk.nih.gov/index.htm

Schopp, L. H., Sanford, T. C., Hagglund, K. J., Gay, J. W., & Coatney, M. A. (2001). Removing service barriers for women with physical disabilities: Promoting accessibility in the gynecologic care setting. *Journal of Midwifery & Women's Health*, 47(2), 74-79.

Shi, L. (1999). Experience of primary care by racial and ethnic groups in the United States. *Medical Care, 37*, 1068-1077.

U.S. Department of Health and Human Services. (2000). *Healthy People 2010* (2nd ed.). Washington, DC: U.S. Government Printing Office. Available from: http://www.healthypeople.gov

U.S. Department of Health and Human Services. (2010). *Healthy People 2020*. Washington, DC: U.S. Government Printing Office. Available from http://healthypeople.gov/2020/default.aspx

CHAPTER 11

Substance Abuse

*Patricia A. Ely, Tammie L. Scamell, and
Elaine T. Jurkowski*

INTRODUCTION

S ubstance abuse affects every segment of our society. According to the National Institute on Drugs and Alcohol, the annual estimated cost of the treatment of substance abuse disorders to the health care system exceeded $600 billion. It has been estimated that $181 billion is spent on illicit drugs, while $193 billion is spent on tobacco (Centers for Disease Control and Prevention, 2007; Office of National Drug Control Policy, 2004; National Center for Chronic Disease Prevention and Health Promotion, 2007). In addition, $235 billion is spent on alcohol (Centers for Disease Control and Prevention, 2007; National Center for Chronic Disease Prevention and Health Promotion, 2007). The Substance Abuse and Mental Health Services Administration (SAMHSA, 2009) estimates that over half of all incarcerations in the United States are related to substance abuse.

As significant as these numbers appear to be, they do not address the integral place alcohol and drugs have in the entire economy and on public health. These public health impacts affect numerous target population groups and health issues, such as domestic violence/sexual assault, mental illness, gay and lesbian sexual assault, physical diseases caused by substance abuse and alcohol, family dysfunction, child abuse, loss of employment, and failure in school. As the U.S. population ages, people born from 1946 to 1964, the "boomers," are the most recent group being added to the population affected by substance abuse.

193

SUBSTANCE ABUSE AND SEXUAL ASSAULT

Increasingly, we are seeing a connection between substance use/abuse and sexual assault. This connection is prevalent in male, female, heterosexual, homosexual, and transsexual groups. Substance abuse/use is also directly correlated with domestic violence. McCarroll, ZiZhong, and Bell (2009) conducted a longitudinal study using a sample from the U.S. Army over a 6-year period from 1998 to 2004, and found a direct correlation between increased domestic violence when alcohol was involved. Alcohol use during incidents of sexual assault has a direct correlation on the victim's recovery and future alcohol abuse (Bedard-Gilligan, Kaysen, Desai, & Lee, 2011). The authors found that the impact was more severe with prolonged use, and the recovery time longer. Karila et al. (2009) found that sexual assault among gays and lesbians is also correlated with substance abuse.

Sexual assault perpetrators' alcohol or substance abuse during the assault resulted in a greater incidence of gamma-hydroxybutyric acid battery during the incident. "The reported prevalence of men's sexual aggression varied widely depending on the methods used and the population studied: Some populations (e.g., veterans, prison inmates, and gay and bisexual men) reported higher rates of adult sexual assault than men in the general population" (Peterson, Voller, Polusny, & Murdoch, 2011). Although use of this drug is illegal in many countries, its legal status has not impacted its usage. Using the drug has resulted in assault victims experiencing more time off of work, school, and attending to home duties and recreation. Both the assault and the concurrent battery happened when alcohol of other substances were involved no matter what relationship the perpetrator had with the victim. Neither the location of the sexual assault, nor the victim's ethnic background, influenced the correlation between alcohol consumption (and other substances) and assault and battery (Busch-Armendariz, DiNitto, Bell, & Bohman, 2010). Perpetrators consistently use alcohol while involved in sexual assault (Berensen, Wiemann, & McCombs, 2011).

INTEGRATED CARE

Older models of substance abuse, and current public sentiment, have addressed substance abuse as a personal decision and therefore not deserving of the same attention the medical profession gives major diseases such as cancer and heart disease. Consequently, there are antiquated modalities of substance abuse treatment and prevention that have isolated substance dependence and abuse from other physical and mental health problems. Today, medical, mental, and substance abuse treatment is integrally interwoven in individuals with comorbid conditions. In fact, individuals with medical and mental health diagnoses have related substance abuse or dependence issues affecting their mental and physical health; thus, we question the effectiveness of modalities that isolate substance abuse treatment from medical and mental health care.

ALCOHOL CONSUMPTION IN COLLEGE STUDENTS

According to SAMHSA (2010), substance abuse treatment admissions for 18- to 24-year-olds, both college students and nonstudents, primarily select alcohol as their main substance of choice. Over 45.5% of college students admitted for substance abuse stated that alcohol was their main substance of abuse compared to 30% of non-students who chose alcohol as their substance of choice. Alcohol abuse appears to be more accepted among college students, and a part of the college culture. Both college students' and nonstudents' second choice for substance of abuse was marijuana. The third main substance of abuse for both groups was heroin; however, for college students, the cases of heroin abuse were less than the cases for noncollege students (6% and 16%, respectively). The high levels of heroin abuse among nonstudents and alcohol abuse among college students is probably a result of economic and financial means. Other opiates, cocaine, and methamphetamine use, ranked 4th, 5th, and 6th, respectively, for the main abused substance identified among 18- to 22-year-olds in 2010 (SAMHSA, 2010).

Co-occurring disorders reported in 2010 revealed that there were 9.2 million Americans reporting both a substance abuse disorder and a mental illness (SAMHSA, 2010). Among the 20.3 million people who reported a substance abuse disorder in 2010, 45.3% had a mental health disorder as well, further indicating that co-occurring disorders are rampant among those with substance abuse disorders (SAMHSA, 2010; see Figures 11.1 and 11.2).

One of the main shortcomings in these prevalence data is that data collected by SAMHSA do not contain the new wave of designer drugs, such as bath salts and synthetic marijuana. The Department of Justice, which labels and categorizes illegal drugs, requires time to analyze and process the chemical in question, collect data, and officially label the substance as a "drug of interest." Designer drugs are much more economical options available to people in communities that lack financial means to purchase other drugs, and given that designer drug use data remain unreported, the actual perception of drug use may be negatively skewed.

Figure 11.3 provides a comparison of age groups and illicit drug use among persons 12 and older during 2009 and 2010. Clearly, the highest illicit drug use among groups occurs in those 18 to 20 years old.

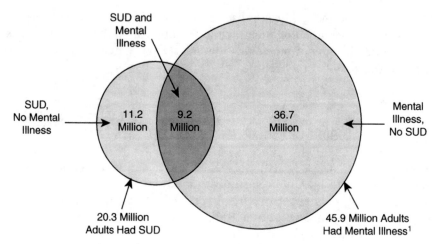

FIGURE 11.1   Past year substance use dependence (SUD) or abuse and mental illness among adults aged 18 or older: 2010. From SAMHSA (2010).

SAMHSA data from 2009 to 2010 reveal, in most areas, that substance abuse is on the rise. Availability of services for screening, assessment, and treatment is shrinking due to fiscal and economic crises within the human services sector, while the need for these services is growing.

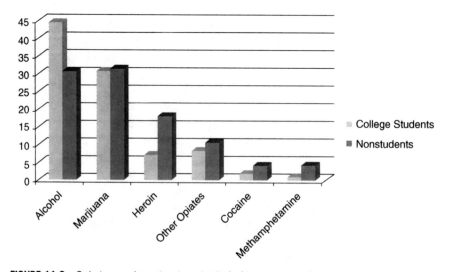

FIGURE 11.2   Substance abuse treatment admissions among college students and nonstudents aged 18 to 24, by primary substance of abuse, 2009. From SAMHSA (2010).

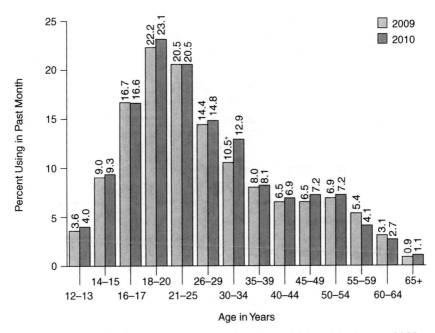

FIGURE 11.3 Past month illicit drug use among persons aged 12 or older, by age: 2009 and 2010. From SAMHSA (2010).

SUBSTANCE ABUSE ISSUES AND WOMEN

In previous years, clinicians believed that substance abuse and post-traumatic stress disorder (PTSD) were problems independent of one another and believed that these diagnoses should be dealt with separately (Henslee & Coffey, 2010; Killeen et al., 2008; McGovern et al., 2009). Research now indicates that women in substance abuse treatment have a high prevalence of trauma in their history and that these issues are found to be interrelated and co-occurring (Brown et al., 2007; Henslee & Coffey, 2010; Hien et al., 2010; Killeen et al., 2008; McGovern et al., 2009; Norman, Tate, Wilkins, Cummins, & Brown, 2010; Staiger, Melville, Hides, Kambouropoulos, & Lubman, 2009). Studies indicate a need for trauma-related treatment in substance abuse facilities to enhance the likelihood for long-term sobriety and recovery from previous trauma (Henslee & Coffey, 2010; Hien et al., 2010; Killeen et al., 2008; McGovern et al., 2009).

Over the years, several methods for addressing PTSD and substance abuse have been researched and developed (Brown et al., 2007; Ford & Russo, 2006; Henslee & Coffey, 2010; Hien et al., 2009, 2010; Killeen et al., 2008; McGovern et al., 2009; Norman et al., 2010; Staiger et al., 2009). Despite the completed research, there still appears to be a need for further studies regarding trauma-based treatment programs during substance abuse interventions to prove overall efficacy (Brown et al., 2007; Hien et al., 2009, 2010; Killeen et al., 2008; McGovern et al., 2009; Norman et al., 2010; Staiger et al., 2009). Methods focusing on substance abuse and PTSD, such as the "Seeking Safety" program, have yet to show a significant difference in outcomes when compared with education-based interventions; however, qualitative data indicate that both clinicians and clients approve this approach (Brown et al., 2007; Hien et al., 2009, 2010; Killeen et al., 2008).

According to Brady and Ashley (2005), female individuals are more likely to suffer greater social stigmatization due to substance abuse than male individuals. Fear of this stigma, along with other factors, such as economic hardship, a lack of child care, and social support, deter women from seeking treatment for their addictions (Brady & Ashley, 2005; Finkelstein, 1994; Taylor, 2010). Along with social effects, physiological and psychological effects for women are also more severe than those for men (Piazza, Vebeka, & Yaeger, 1989). Physiologically, women become addicted to drugs and alcohol faster than men, suffer harsher side effects, and develop more chronic medical conditions due to substance use as well (Back, Sonne, Killeen, Dansky, & Brady, 2003; Brady & Ashley, 2005; Piazza et al., 1989).

The Transtheoretical Model of Change seems to be popular when taking an in-depth look at the client. It appears that clients' readiness to change plays a significant role in recovery from addictions (DiClemente, Schumann, Greene, & Earley, 2011). Therefore, using this framework seems to be imperative to understanding policy within substance abuse treatment.

According to Kennedy and Gregoire (2009), persons entering treatment with higher levels of internal motivation (in the Action stage) have a higher likelihood for a longer length of sobriety following discharge than a person entering treatment with a lower level of internal motivation (e.g., in the Pre-contemplation). Other research has suggested that a client's readiness to change is crucial to the recovery and treatment process and, if they fail to address clients' readiness, clinicians may be neglecting a vital piece of information necessary to assist in the process. Little is known, however, and more research is needed, to uncover how social workers should help the client move from one stage to the next in such a limited time frame (DiClemente, Nidecker, & Bellack, 2008). As mentioned in Velasquez, Von Sternberg, Dodrill, Kan, and Parsons (2005), self-efficacy is also an important construct to consider in substance abuse treatment. Finding a method to intertwine counseling or education that would promote self-efficacy, especially when treating women with substance addictions, is a key for long-term sobriety (Davis & Jason, 2005).

SUBSTANCE ABUSE ISSUES AND OLDER ADULTS

Demographically, in North America and most industrialized countries, the population is shifting toward a graying/aging society. Although the general population may carry a stereotype of an older adult as being white or gray-haired, jovial, meek, or frail, we seldom think of older adults as "substance abusers" or "out of control" drinkers, or at-risk for these conditions. Recent analyses of data examining alcohol consumption practices in older men and women drawn from sources such as the National Health Interview Survey (NHIS, 2010), the Behavioral Risk Factor Surveillance System (CDC, 2008; BRFSS, 2010), and the National Household Survey on Drug Abuse (SAMHSA, 2010) have shed light on the prevalence of alcohol consumption among older adults. In fact, these data suggest that older adults in the 65+ age category found 56.8% of the population to be at risk for drinking in the past 30 days when surveyed. On the days these same older adults reported that they drink, 32.1% said they have two or more drinks (NHIS, 2010). Brelow, Faden, and Smothers (2003) found in their secondary analyses of these data that about one-third of the U.S. elderly population consumes alcohol, regardless of risk to themselves. These authors concluded that, as we see our population "graying" over the upcoming decades, practitioners and public health officials will need to be more aware of dealing with this segment of the population.

Mental health issues and substance abuse disorders often co-occur for both adults and children (Regier et al., 1990; Wallace, 2010; Wu & Blazer, 2010). Despite this awareness, and evidence-based practices that have been established for treating these co-occurring disorders (Drake et al., 2001; Vannoy, Arean, & Unutzer, 2010), a limited amount of work and research has examined both the etiology and treatment of these disorders, either individually or as co-occurring within rural areas. The field appears to lack an understanding of both the need for and how to tailor evidence-based approaches to treat people with co-occurring disorders in rural areas (U.S. Department of Health and Human Services [DHHS], 2005; Kalapatapu & Sullivan, 2010).

Although older adults may be at increased risk of or vulnerability to experiencing mental health-related problems, they often do not seek, or are not successful at linking with the necessary mental health services (DHHS, 1999). A variety of factors can account for this outcome, including the stigma of mental illness; ageism; complexity and fragmentation of services; lack of coordination among medical, mental health, and aging systems of care; lack of professional staff trained in geriatric mental health; and inadequacy of health insurance coverage (DHHS, 1999; Han, Gfroerer, Colpe, Barker, & Colliver, 2011; Kaskie & Buckwalter, 2010; Rothrauff, Abraham, & Roman, 2011). Symptoms of depression, existing and

undetected, within the older adult population have been noted in the literature (Bland, Newman, & Orn, 1988, Blazer, 1999; Dorfman et al., 1995;
Proctor, Morrow-Howell, Rubin, & Ringenberg, 1999; Rogers & Barusch,
2000; Vannoy, Arean, & Unitzer, 2010). Consequently, a poorly coordinated
system of care and lack of integration between systems (especially aging,
mental health, and primary care) contributes to this problem (DHHS,
1999). This problem becomes magnified when layered with the issues of substance use and abuse for older adults, whether the use and abuse are via prescription or over-the-counter medication.

Schonfield et al. (1993) examined prevalence estimates of alcohol use
and misuse among older adults through surveying staff providing services
to older adults. They found that few staff had received in-service training
on substance abuse issues, but conversely saw substance abuse issues as
being of high priority in their day-to-day work. This study is dated; little
recent research has been conducted in this area.

This issue is further illustrated by the work of Hanson and Guthiel
(2004), who prepared the case for brief motivational interviewing as a successful intervention when working with older adults. They argued that
social workers and other health professionals do not adequately address
problem-related drinking with older adults. These authors suggested that
issues such as inadequate knowledge about addictive behaviors, limited
development in assessment tools, and limited evidence-based treatment
options account for social work practitioners' limitations when dealing
with these issues. The findings build on the work of Klein and Jess (2002),
who found that staff training and education issues were identified as
limited, despite a clear awareness that alcohol posed a problem for people
who were residing in intermediate care facilities. Klein and Jess interviewed
directors of intermediate care facilities ($n = 111$) in the United States to learn
that, although alcohol use was common in such facilities, comfort level on
the part of the staff related to alcohol use among older adults was limited.

Emlet, Hawks, and Callahan (2001), in their retrospective chart study of
community dwelling older adults ($n = 148$), found that functional status was
not a predictor of alcohol use and abuse among older persons; however,
gender played a specific role in that men were 3 times more likely to drink
than women (Emlet et al., 2001). Moreover, the authors illuminated the
growing problem of substance abuse/use among older adults and articulated
the need for intervention with this population.

Wu and Blazer (2010), along with Memmet (2003), argued that older
adults in general are at risk for the development of poly drug problems
due to the interactive effects of alcohol and prescription or over-the-counter
medications. The importance of screening elderly clients for substance abuse
is a critical factor in the detection and treatment of substance use issues
among this population. Kalapatapu and Sullivan (2010) also estimated that

the number of older adults needing substance abuse treatment will increase over the next several decades. This epidemic will include the use of opioids, stimulants, and benzodiazepines.

Although minimal research has been conducted in rural areas, Musnick, Blazer, and Hays (2000) examined a sample of elderly people affiliated with the Baptist church and who live in the rural area of central North Carolina. They found a strong relationship between religiosity (being Baptist) and the nonuse of alcohol. They also found a relationship between symptoms of depression and alcohol use among Baptists who did not attend church services regularly.

Frissel (1992) found that older adults are at risk of alcohol abuse and argued for treatment for older adults. However, LaGreca, Akers, and Dwyer (1988) found in the sample of older adults (more than 60 years) living in retirement communities ($n = 1,410$) that problem drinking was not linked to members of the communities or to life transitions. Conversely, social support networks did not serve as mediators for the impact of life events on alcohol use. LaGreca et al.'s work extends the work of Alexander and Duff (1988), who discovered, after surveying three retirement communities, that drinking was an integral part of the leisure subculture.

Although Brody (1982) suggested that developing an understanding of alcohol-related issues with older adults is critical, especially in the areas related to detection and treatment, little progress appears to have been made in the last 20 years in this area. This seems to also have been argued in several of the preceding studies. Moreover, there is a dearth of studies that have examined the prevalence of alcohol use among older adults in rural communities, issues that providers face, and barriers to solutions/interventions within a rural context. This problem will increase as more older adults migrate to rural areas to escape the expense and challenges of urban lifestyles. Consequently, answers to these questions will become more critical.

POLICY DEVELOPMENT

On January 1, 2012, the Department of Labor's "Report to Congress on Compliance with the Mental Health Parity and Addiction Equity Act of 2008" (MHPAEA) set September 23, 2012, as a deadline for insurance companies to comply nationwide. This piece of legislation requires all insurers to provide substance abuse treatment in the same manner that they provide other medical treatments.

Nationally implementing this policy in the current economic crisis is now mandated. This requires restructuring and educating medical health, mental health, and substance abuse providers to integrate diagnosis and treatment of medical, mental health, and substance abuse disorders. Equal funding distribution has been allotted for other medical diagnoses and surgical procedures as is allotted for mental health and substance abuse disorders. Practically, this means restructuring primary care, mental health care, and substance abuse care into an integrated format for best patient care. Integrated multidisciplinary teams of medical, mental health, and substance abuse providers will become essential for compliance as identified in the legislation.

ESSENTIAL SERVICES FOR PUBLIC HEALTH AND SUBSTANCE ABUSE

SAMHSA (2010) outlined the following eight strategic initiatives to address the MHPAEA implementation in the following years: The strategic initiatives include:

1. *Prevention of Substance Abuse and Mental Illness*: Creating communities where individuals, families, schools, faith-based organizations, and workplaces take action to promote emotional health and reduce the likelihood of mental illness and substance abuse, including tobacco, as well as suicide. This initiative will include a focus on the nation's high-risk youth, youth in tribal communities, and military families.
2. *Trauma and Justice*: Reducing the pervasive, harmful, and costly health impacts of violence and trauma by integrating trauma-informed approaches throughout health, behavioral health, and related systems and addressing the behavioral health needs of people involved in or at risk of involvement in the criminal and juvenile justice systems.
3. *Military Families*: Supporting America's servicemen and women—active duty, National Guard, reserve, and veteran—together with their families and communities by leading efforts to ensure that needed behavioral health services are accessible and that outcomes are positive.
4. *Recovery Support*: Partnering with people in recovery from mental health and substance use disorders and family members to guide the behavioral health system and promote individual-, program-, and system-level approaches that foster health and resilience; increase permanent housing, employment, education, and other necessary supports; and reduce discriminatory barriers.
5. *Health Reform*: Increasing access to appropriate high-quality prevention, treatment, and recovery services; reducing disparities that currently exist between the availability of services for mental health and substance use disorders compared with the availability of services for other medical conditions; and supporting integrated, coordinated

care, especially for people with behavioral health and other co-occurring health conditions, such as HIV/AIDS.

6. *Health Information Technology*: Ensuring that the behavioral health system, including states, community providers, and peer and prevention specialists fully participates with the general health care delivery system in the adoption of health information technology and interoperable electronic health records.

7. *Data, Outcomes, and Quality*: Realizing an integrated data strategy and a national framework for quality improvement in behavioral health care that will inform policy; measure program impact; and lead to improved quality of services and outcomes for individuals, families, and communities.

8. *Public Awareness and Support*: Increasing the understanding of mental and substance use disorders and the many pathways to recovery to achieve the full potential of prevention, help people recognize mental and substance use disorders and seek assistance with the same urgency as any other health condition, and make recovery the expectation.

According to SAMHSA's chief administrator, Pamela S. Hyde, JD, "the strategic initiatives paper provides a clear roadmap for SAMHSA's immediate and longer term priorities for reaching our essential public health mission." Hyde continued, "these initiatives are data driven, overarching in purpose and will help SAMHSA work in an unprecedented way across health, justice, social service, education and other systems to improve health care services to all Americans" (SAMHSA, 2010).

HEALTHY PEOPLE 2020 OBJECTIVES

The area of substance abuse has been the most perplexing for intervention due to its low success rate in prior years and high recidivism rate. Within the *Healthy People 2020* goals outlined, this segment probably has the most objectives identified. Appendix A details the specific goals identified within this topical area.

EMERGING ISSUES

Brain Imaging and Addiction and Medication-Assisted Treatment, MHPAEA

We now understand how drugs affect the brain. We also know, based on brain imaging, which individuals are more vulnerable to addiction. This technology allows us to determine and develop more effective prevention and treatment strategies in the future (Amen, 2010). Evolving technology in brain imaging has also allowed us to develop a new generation of medications for specific addictions. Medication-assisted treatment for severe, chronic addictions is facilitating the recovery of substance abusers who were unable in the past to sustain recovery (Rieckmann, Kovas, & Rutkowski, 2010). With the implementation of MHPAEA in 2012, general practitioners and social workers can develop new strategies to effectively treat more substance abuse cases. Substance abuse treatment and recovery programs can be offered by family doctors and social workers in neighborhood medical practices, thus eliminating the barriers to care (Rieckmann, Kovas, & Rutkowski, 2010).

Designer Drugs

Designer drugs are the most current rage in substance use/abuse. The Centers for Disease Control and Prevention reported in 2010 that they received 304 calls to poison control centers about bath salts. In the first 3 months of 2010 alone, they averaged 25.3 calls per month. The U.S. Center for Poison Control received 1,511 calls during the first 3 months of 2011, averaging 503.6 calls per month (Wehrman, 2010), which represented a 1,991% increase from 2010 to 2011. The American Association of Poison Control Centers (AAPCC) monitor emergency calls to all poison control centers nationally. According to Canton (2010), the AAPCC first documented bath salts in July, 2010, and documented an average of 60.8 calls per month in the following 5-month period. In 2011, the AAPCC documented 6,138 calls related to bath salt poisoning, averaging 511.5 calls per month. This illustrates a greater than 800% increase from 2010 to 2011 in calls made that were specifically related to bath salt consumption. The increase in use could be due to heightened awareness of public health personnel contributing to an increase in reporting from 2010 to 2011, or it could be directly correlated to a new emerging public health issue (Ely, 2012).

Bath salts mimic some of the effects of methamphetamines and do not always show up in drug tests (U.S. Department of Justice Drug Enforcement Administration, 2011). Consequently, users may be able to "get high" without testing positive for drugs in their blood stream. Individuals who are in drug rehabilitation treatment, on parole or probation and required to take a drug test at regular intervals will be attracted to the use of bath salts as a drug option. Professionals with no drug record but required to comply with drug testing for employment purposes can use a designer drug such as bath salts to get high and still test clean. The AACPC received 2,906 calls on synthetic marijuana in 2010 and 6,959 calls in 2011—a 400% increase (AAPCC, 2012). Once a drug is recognized as a Schedule 1 drug and, consequently, carries penalties for use, chemists are able to slightly reconfigure the molecular structure of the drug, creating a designer drug that is "legal." Then the process of distribution starts over with the slightly altered substance. Each time a drug is altered, the lengthy process of chemically labeling it, evaluating its use and chemical effects, and eventually making it illegal starts over again.

Once the MHPAEA is effectively integrated into health care nationally, medical professionals can provide care immediately for clients without being required to wait for the drug to appear in a urine test, or for the drug to be classified legally as a drug. Currently, many individuals using these substances are unable to receive services because services are restricted to drugs that have been authorized to receive funding for drug treatment. SAMHSA's initiatives allow the maintenance of the separated approach to mental health substance abuse and medical health care.

Segregated Treatment Options for Women, People With Disabilities, and Older Adults

Increasingly, there is a trend toward differences in screening, assessment, and treatment needs for different population groups. No longer is a cookie-cutter or one-size-fits all approach to substance abuse treatment the norm. As these differences emerge, there will be an increasing growth in specialized services developed and necessary to impact the specific and unique needs that specialized groups bring to treatment.

Harm Reduction Approaches to Treatment

Traditional treatment approaches have focused upon "abstinence only" directives, and have made total abstinence the treatment goal for people seeking treatment for substance use issues. Increasingly, goals for treatment will focus on the reduction of harm to the individual as opposed to direct abstinence as a treatment option. Intervention will also focus on moving people from one stage of treatment to another through the "Stages of Change" continuum (Prochaska & DiClemente, 1988).

Recommendations for Essential Services Addressing Public Health and Substance Abuse

This chapter has addressed a number of issues impacting substance abuse within the field of public health. In an effort to meet the HP2020 goals, the following recommendations should be considered (SAMHSA, 2010):

- Identify providers who integrate medical, mental, and substance abuse services
- Determine which providers will need to integrate care

- Monitor care of patients needing medical, mental health, and substance abuse treatment
- Identify providers not addressing integrated care
- Develop public health education forums to assist in the MHPAEA transition required in 2012
- Identify insurance providers not complying with the MHPAEA after the September 2012 deadline
- Form integrated-care coalitions
- Develop collaborative efforts between private industry and public health services
- Formulate systems to integrate treatment through referrals, and collaboration of health care providers
- Develop programming to educate the public about the connection between physical and mental health and substance abuse
- Promote access to mental health substance abuse and medical health care under one roof whenever possible to facilitate integrated care
- Develop policies and plans that support individual and community health care efforts integrating medical, mental, and substance abuse care.

SUMMARY

This chapter has addressed a number of issues related to substance use and abuse that are essential for public health social workers to be aware of when working with people, families, and communities in efforts to address substance use and abuse. Women, people with disabilities, and older adults are all groups with needs whose incidence and prevalence of substance use/abuse problems are on the rise. Each of these groups will need specialized options in assessment and treatment of their issues. Community-based treatment will continue to be an issue in the future due to economic and fiscal restraints.

CLASSROOM ACTIVITIES

1. Discuss the similarities and differences in screening, intervention, and treatment needs between different cohorts of people, such as teenagers, college-aged students, young adults, middle-aged adults, older adults, and women. How can we tailor substance use programs to meet the needs of each specific group?
2. You are responsible for developing a community education strategy that will target community awareness about specific drug and

substance use/abuse issues. The strategy includes building awareness at various stages of change (see Prochaska and Diclemente's [1988] Stages of Change Theory). What will you do in this effort and identify the stage you are addressing.

3. You and a team of colleagues are asked to sit on a task force to build an intervention project to target the increasing use of synthetic drugs in your community. What will you do to intervene? How will you address this issue from the perspectives of the three core functions, assessment, policy development, and assurance?

4. You and a team of colleagues are asked to work with the local Area Agencies on Aging to build an educational and treatment-oriented program to help meet the needs of older adults. How will you go about identifying and addressing the needs of the community, especially in the areas of alcohol consumption, drug use, and prescription drug use/overuse? How will you address the core functions of assessment, policy development, and assurance?

5. Identify the skills and competencies you would need to work in the area of substance use/abuse as a public health social worker.

INTERNET RESOURCES

Substance Abuse and Mental Health Services Administration

(www.SAMHSA.gov)

This website is maintained by the federal government and serves as a repository for publications, grant funding opportunities, data about substance use-related topics, evidence-based interventions, and topical discussions.

Substance Abuse Treatment Locator

(http://findtreatment.samhsa.gov/TreatmentLocator/faces/quickSearch. jspx)

This site provides consumers and professionals the opportunity to locate treatment facilities for substance abuse in all 50 states.

National Institute on Alcohol and Alcohol Abuse and Alcoholism

(www.niaaa.nih.gov/Pages/default.aspx)

This site, funded by the National Institutes of Health, provides information about current trends in alcohol and alcohol abuse-related topics. It provides links to publications, funding information, clinical trial studies, resources, and data. The site also provides the reader a host of additional useful links.

Office of National Drug Control Policy

(www.whitehouse.gov/ondcp)

This site provides information on drug control policies, which have been enacted in the United States. It covers policies related to drug abuse, prescription drug misuse and abuse, and alcohol-related issues (driving under the influence, etc.). The site also has links to treatment modalities, international partnerships, and resources.

REFERENCES

Alexander, F., & Duff, R. W. (1988). Social interaction and alcohol use in retirement communities. *The Gerontologist, 28*(5), 632–636.

Amen, D. (2010). High resolution brain SPECT imaging in a clinical substance abuse practice. *Journal of Psychoactive Drugs, 42*(2), 153–160.

American Association of Poison Control Centers. (2012, February 8). Synthetic marijuana (Data file). Retrieved from http://www.aapcc.org/dnn/Portals/0/Synthetic%20Mari juana%20Data%20for%20 ebsite%202.8.2012.pdf

Back, S., Sonne, S., Killeen, T., Dansky, B., & Brady, K. (2003). Comparative profiles of women with PTSD and comorbid cocaine or alcohol dependence. *American Journal of Drug & Alcohol Abuse, 29*(1), 169.

Bedard-Gilligan, M., Kaysen, D., Desai, S., & Lee, C. (2011). Alcohol-involved assault: Associations with post trauma alcohol use, consequences, and expectancies. *Addictive Behaviors, 36*(11), 1076–1082.

Behavioral Risk Factor Surveillance System (2010). Retrieved August 25, 2011, from http://www.cdc.gov/brfss/index.htm

Berensen, A., Wiemann, C. M., & McCombs, S. (2011). Exposure to violence and associated health risk behaviors among adolescent girls. *Archives of Pediatric Adolescent Medicine, 155*(11), 1238–1242.

Bland, R. C., Newman, S. C., & Orn, H. (1988). Prevalence of psychiatric disorders in the elderly in Edmonton. *Acta Psychiatrica Scandinavica Supplement, 338*, 57–63.

Blazer, D. (1999). Depression in the elderly. *New England Journal of Medicine, 320*, 164–166.

Brady, T. M., & Ashley, O. S. (Eds.). (2005). *Women in substance abuse treatment: Results from the Alcohol and Drug Services Study* (DHHS Publication No. SMA 04-3968, Analytic Series A-26). Rockville, MD: Substance Abuse and Mental Health Services Administration, Office of Applied Studies.

Brelow, R. A., Faden, V. B., & Smothers, B. (2003). Alcohol consumption by elderly Americans. *Journal of Studies on Alcohol, 64*(6), 884–892.

Brody, J. A. (1982). Aging and alcohol use. *Journal of the American Geriatrics Society, 30*(2), 123–126.

Brown, V., Najavits, L., Cadiz, S., Finkeistein, N., Heckman, J., & Rechberger, E. (2007). Implementing an evidence-based practice: Seeking safety group. *Journal of Psychoactive Drugs, 39*(3), 231–240.

Busch-Armendariz, N., DiNitto, D. M., Bell, H., & Bohman, T. (2010). Sexual assault perpetrators' alcohol and drug use: The likelihood of concurrent violence and post sexual assault outcomes for women victims. *Journal of Psychoactive Drugs, 42*(3), 393–399.

Centers for Disease Control and Prevention (2007). *Best practices for comprehensive tobacco control programs—2007*. Available at: http://www.cdc.gov/tobacco/sta teandcommunity/best_practices/pdfs/2007/bestpractices_complete.pdf

Centers for Disease Control and Prevention (CDC). (2008). *Behavioral risk factor surveillance system (BRFSS) survey data*. Atlanta, GA: U.S. Department of Health & Human Services, Centers for Disease Control and Prevention.

Davis, M., & Jason, L. (2005). Sex differences in social support and self-efficacy within a recovery community. *American Journal of Community Psychology, 36*(3/4), 259–274.

DiClemente, C., Nidecker, M., & Bellack, A. (2008). Motivation and the stages of change among individuals with severe mental illness and substance abuse disorders. *Journal of Substance Abuse Treatment, 34*(1), 25–35.

DiClemente, D. C., Schumann, K., Greene, P. A., & Earley, M. D. (2011). A transtheoretical model perspective on change: Process-focuses intervention in mental health-substance use. In D. Cooper (Ed.), *Intervention in mental health-substance use* (pp. 69–87). Milton Keynes, UK: Radcliffe Publishing.

Dorfman, R. A., Lubben, J. E., Mayer-Oakes, A., Atchison, K., Schweitzer, S. O., DeJong, F. J., et al. (1995). Screening for depression among a well elderly population. *Social Work, 40*(3), 295–304.

Drake, R. E., Essock, S. M., Shaner, A., Carey, K., Minkoff, K., Kola, L., et al. (2001). Implementing dual diagnosis services for clients with severe mental illness. *Psychiatric Services, 52*(4), 469–476.

Ely, P. (2012, February 14). Personal interview Loreeta Canton from American Association of Poison Control Centers. http://www.aapcc.org/dnn/Portals/0/Bath%20Salts%20 Data%20for%20Website%202.8.2012.pdf

Emlet, C., Hawks, H., & Callahan, J. (2001). Alcohol use and abuse in a population of community dwelling, frail older adults. *Journal of Gerontological Social Work, 35*(4), 21–33.

Finkelstein, N. (1994). Treatment issues for alcohol- and drug-dependent pregnant and parenting women. *Health and Social Work, 19*. Retrieved from http://www. questia.com/googleScholar.qst?docId=5001659216

Ford, J., & Russo, E. (2006). Trauma-focused, present-centered, emotional self-regulation approach to integrated treatment for posttraumatic stress and addiction: Trauma Adaptive Recovery Group Education and Therapy (TARGET). *American Journal of Psychotherapy, 60*(4), 335–355.

Han, B., Gfroerer, J. C., Colpe, L. J., Bakker, P. R., & Collier, J. D. (2011). Serious psychological distress and mental health service use among community dwelling older adults. *Psychiatric Services, 62*(3), 291–298.

Hanson, M., & Guthiel, L. A. (2004). Motivational strategies with alcohol involved older adults: Implications for social work practice. *Social Work, 49*(3), 364–372.

Henslee, A., & Coffey, S. (2010). Exposure therapy for posttraumatic stress disorder in a residential substance use treatment facility. *Professional Psychology: Research & Practice, 41*(1), 34–40.

Hien, D., Jiang, H., Campbell, A., Hu, M., Miele, G., Cohen, L. et al. (2010). Do treatment improvements in PTSD severity affect substance use outcomes? A secondary analysis from a randomized clinical trial in NIDA's clinical trials network. *American Journal of Psychiatry, 167*(1), 95–101.

Hien, D., Wells, E., Jiang, H., Suarez-Morales, L., Aimee, N. C., Cohen, L., et al. (2009). Multisite randomized trial of behavioral interventions for women with co-occurring PTSD and substance use disorders. *Journal of Consulting and Clinical Psychology*, 77(4), 607–619.

Kalapatapu, R. K., & Sullivan, M. A. (2010). Prescription use in older adults. *The American Journal on Addictions*, 19(6), 515–522.

Karila, L., Novarin, J., Megarbane, B., Cottencin, O., Dally, S., Lowenstein, W., & Reynaud, M. (2009). Gamma-hydroxybutyric acid (GHB): More than a date rape drug, a potentially addictive drug. *PresseMédicale (Paris, France: 1983)*, 38(10), 1526–1538.

Kaskie, B. P., & Buckwalter, K. C. (2010). The collaborative model of mental health care for older Iowans. *Research in Gerontological Nursing*, 3(3), 20–208.

Kennedy, K., & Gregoire, T. K. (2009). Theories of motivation in addiction treatment: Testing the relationship of the transtheoretical model of change and self-determination theory. *Journal of Social Work Practice in Addiction*, 9(2), 163–183.

Killeen, T., Hien, D., Campbell, A., Brown, C., Hansen, C., Jiang, H., et al. (2008). Adverse events in an integrated trauma-focused intervention for women in community substance abuse treatment. *Journal of Substance Abuse Treatment*, 35(3), 304–311.

Klein, W. C., & Jess, C. (2002). One last pleasure? Alcohol use among elderly people in nursing homes. *Health and Social Work*, 27(3), 193–203.

LaGreca, A. J., Akers, R. L., & Dwyer, J. W. (1988). Life events and alcohol behavior among older adults. *The Gerontologist*, 28(4), 552–558.

Library of Congress. (2009). *Family-based meth treatment access act of 2009 (introduced in house)* (H.R.439). 111th Congress, 1st Session: Retrieved from http://thomas.gov/cgi-bin/query/z?c111:H.R.439

Library of Congress. (2010). *Methamphetamine education, treatment, and hope act of 2010 (engrossed in house, passed house)* (H.R.2818). 111th Congress, 2nd Session: Retrieved from http://thomas.loc.gov/cgi-bin/query/z?c111:H.R.2818.EH

McCarroll, J. E., ZiZhong, F., & Bell, N. S. (2009). Alcohol use in non mutual and mutual domestic violence in the U.S. Army: 1998–2004. *Violence & Victims*, 24(3), 364–379.

McGovern, M., Lambert-Harris, C., Acquilano, S., Xie, H., Alterman, A., & Weiss, R. (2009). A cognitive behavioral therapy for co-occurring substance use and posttraumatic stress disorders. *Addictive Behaviors*, 34(10), 892–897.

Memmet, J. L. (2003). Alcohol consumption by elderly Americans. *Journal of Studies on Alcohol*, 64(6), 884–892.

Musnick, M. A., Blazer, D. G., & Hays, J. C. (2000). Religious activity, alcohol use, and depression in a sample of elderly Baptists. *Research on Aging*, 22(2), 91–116.

National Health Interview Survey. (2010). Retrieved from http://www.cdc.gov/nchs/about/major/nhis/quest_data_related_1997_forward.htm

National Institute on Drug Abuse. (2011, April). *Info facts understanding drugs and addiction*.

National Institute on Drug Abuse. (2010). *March drug facts. Understanding drug fats*. Retrieved from http://www.drugabuse.gov/publications/drugfacts/understanding-drugabuse-addiction

Norman, S., Tate, S., Wilkins, K., Cummins, K., & Brown, S. (2010). Posttraumatic stress disorder's role in integrated substance dependence and depression treatment outcomes. *Journal of Substance Abuse Treatment*, 38(4), 346–355.

Office of National Drug Control Policy. (2004). *The economic costs of drug abuse in the United States, 1992–2002*. (Publication No. 207303). Available at www.ncjrs.gov/ondcppubs/publications/pdf/economic_costs.pdf

Peterson, Z., Voller, E., Polusny, M., & Murdoch, M. (2011). Prevalence and consequences of adult sexual assault of men: Review of empirical findings and state of the literature. *Clinical Psychology Review, 31*(1), 1-24.

Piazza, N. J., Vrbka, J. L., & Yeager, R. D. (1989). Telescoping of alcoholism in women alcoholics. *The International Journal of the Addictions, 24*, 19-28.

Prochaska, J. O., & DiClemente, C. C. (1988). Stages and processes of self-change of smoking: Toward an integrative model of change. *Journal of Consulting and Child Psychology, 51*, 390-395.

Proctor, E. K., Morrow-Howell, N., Rubin, E., & Ringenberg, M. (1999). Service use by elderly patients after psychiatric hospitalization. *Psychiatric Services, 50*(4), 553-555.

Regier, D. A., Farmer, M. E., Rae, D. S., Locke, B.Z., Keith, S. J., Judd, L., et al. (1990). Co-morbidity of mental disorders with alcohol and other drug abuse. Results from the Epidemiologic Catchment Area (ECA) Study. *Journal of the American Medical Association, 264*(19), 2511-2518.

Rieckmann, T., Kovas, A., & Rutkowski, B. (2010). Adoption of medications in substance abuse treatment: Priorities and strategies of single state authorities. *Journal of Psychoactive Drugs, Suppl. 6*, 227-238.

Rogers, A., & Barusch, A. (2000). Mental health service utilization among frail, low income elders: Perceptions of home service providers and elders in the community. *Gerontological Social Work, 34*(2), 23-38.

Rothrauff, T. C., Abraham, A. J., Bride, B. E., & Roman, P. M. (2011). Substance abuse treatment for older adults in private centers. *Substance Abuse, 32*(1), 7-15.

Schonfeld, L., Rohrer, G. E., Zima, M., & Spiegel, T. (1993). Alcohol abuse and medication misuse in older adults as estimated by service providers. *Journal of Gerontological Social Work, 21*, 113-125.

Shetty, P. (2011). Nora Volkow—Challenging the myths about drug addiction. *Lancet, 378*(9790), 477.

Staiger, P., Melville, F., Hides, L., Kambouropoulos, N., & Lubman, D. (2009). Can emotion-focused coping help explain the link between posttraumatic stress disorder severity and triggers for substance use in young adults? *Journal of Substance Abuse Treatment, 36*(2), 220-226.

Substance Abuse and Mental Health Services Administration. (2009). *Results from the 2008 National Survey on Drug Use and Health: National findings* (HHS Publication No. SMA 09-4434). Rockville, MD: Author.

Substance Abuse and Mental Health Services Administration (2010). *Results from the 2009 National Survey on Drug Use and Health: Volume 1: Summary of national findings.* Office of Applied Studies, NSDUH Series H-38A, HHS Publication No. SMA 104586 Findings. Rockville, MD: Author.

Substance Abuse and Mental Health Services Administration (2011). *Results from the 2010 National Survey on Drug Use and Health: Summary of national findings.* Retrieved February 7, 2012, from http://www.samhsa.gov/data/NSDUH/2k10NSDUH/2k10Results.htm#Ch7

Taylor, O. D. (2010). Barriers to treatment for women with substance use disorders. *Journal of Human Behavior in the Social Environment, 20*(3), 393-409.

U.S. Department of Health and Human Services. (1999). Mental health and older adults. *In Report of the Surgeon General on Mental Health Needs.* Washington, DC: U.S. Government Printing Office.

U.S. Department of Health and Human Services. (2001). *Mental health: Culture, race and ethnicity, a supplement to mental health: A report of the Surgeon General.* Washington, DC: U.S. Government Printing Office.

U.S. Department of Health and Human Services. (2005). *Mental health and rural America: 1994–2005. An overview and annotated bibliography.* Rockville, MD: DHHS, HRSA, Office of Rural Health Policy.

U.S. Department of Justice, Drug Enforcement Administration. (2011, August). *Background, data and analysis of synthetic cathinones.* Retrieved from http://www.deodi version.usdoj.gov/fed_regs_/rules12011/HHS PDF/background

Vannoy, S. D., Arean, P., & Unutzer, J. (2010). Advantages of using estimated depression free days for evaluating treatment efficacy. *Psychiatric Services, 61*(2), 160–163.

Velasquez, M., von Sternberg, K., Dodrill, C., Kan, L., & Parsons, J. (2005). The transtheoretical model as a framework for developing substance abuse interventions. *Journal of Addictions Nursing, 16*(1–2), 31–40.

Wallace, C. (2010). Integrated assessment of older adults who misuse alcohol. *Nursing Standard, 24*(33), 51–57.

Wehrman, J. (2010, April 6). *U.S. poison centers raise alarm about toxic substances marketed as bath salts.* Retrieved from http:// www.aapcc.org/dnn/portals/o/prrea/bath salts-final.pdf

Wu, L. T., & Blazer, D. G. (2011). Illicit and nonmedical drug use among older adults: A review. *Journal of Aging and Health, 23*(3), 481–504.

CHAPTER 12

Global Health

Karun Karki, Mizanur Miah, and Elaine T. Jurkowski

INTRODUCTION

*I*ncreasingly, social work, as a profession, recognizes that it meets no borders in its interventions and the needs to which it responds. This is also true for public health social work practice. As a profession, social workers are regularly called to mediate in crises abroad or intervene in situations that may surface domestically, but originated in some other global location. This chapter will focus on public health social work within the global arena, discuss some of the challenges for public health social work, and provide an overview of some of the current practices and opportunities. These themes will be explored through the lens of the core functions of public health, *Healthy People 2020* objectives, and public health social work standards and competencies.

WHAT IS GLOBAL HEALTH?

The term *global health* has been used broadly, but it is important to understand when the term is used and what it is referring to. *International health* had previously been used to describe issues within the global context (Brown, Cueto, & Fee, 2006). It is essential to have a common understanding of what global health is in order to assure that there are consistent perceptions of global health issues and ways to address these (Koplan et al., 2009). Koplan and his colleagues (2009) also argued that the definition of global health should be broad, with a focus on health improvement and health equity. Other authors define global health as "those issues that transcend national boundaries and governments and call for actions on global forces that determine the health of people" (Kickbush, 2006). This definition is broad and lacks a clear goal, passion for research, and action. Macfarlane, Jacobs, and Kaaya (2008) provided a definition of global health which includes the "worldwide improvement of health, reduction of disparities, and protection against global threats that disregard national borders" (p. 5142). Beaglehole and Bonita (2010) synthesized these definitions and provided a crisper description, which suggests that "global health builds on national public health efforts and institutions. In many countries, public health is equated primarily with population-wide interventions; global health is concerned with all strategies for health improvement" (p. 5142).

If social workers consider that global health is not just a function of health, well-being, and health status, but broaden the definition to examine how other factors within the ecosystem contribute to health, it becomes easier to understand why health disparities exist. Factors such as literacy rate; per capita spending on health; overall gross domestic product (GDP); overall gross national product (GNP); and access to primary, secondary, and tertiary health care all play roles in the health status of specific nations. These factors need to be considered when examining a country's public health status.

The concept of global or international health also appears to be of more interest to high-income nations. Beaglehole and Bonita (2010) provided an explanation for these differences; they suggested that low-income countries may not be as concerned about the issues of global health as they are about their own health care systems because they have more pressing issues. Second, these issues are often taken up not by governments in low-income countries but by nongovernmental organizations, which advocate for specific health issues. An example is the National Lung Foundation, which advocates for treatments for tuberculosis in low-income countries. Finally, low-income countries collaborate with public health authorities to assist with the development of resources to meet the health care needs of their countries, whereas higher income countries consider global health to be an interest of strong national health systems. These networks of health care systems may not exist in low-income countries (Beaglehole & Bonita, 2010).

GLOBAL HEALTH STATUS AND HEALTH DISPARITIES

It is often difficult to conceptualize what contributes to the differences or disparities in health from country to country and between industrialized versus agrarian or nonindustrialized countries. People who travel often from country to country can probably contrast the standard of living, as well as GDP/GNP differences across high-income versus low-income countries. Visually, one may be able to see aesthetic differences, which may lead to clues on differences in the standards of living; however, other indicators can help identify some specific differences. Indicators such as incidence and prevalence of tuberculosis, average life span, maternal mortality rate, and infant mortality rate are most helpful. Other indicators which provide understanding of the health status of different countries include private health plans as a percentage of private expenditures on health and per capita expenditures on health in U.S. dollars.

As illustrated in Table 12.1, one can see that industrialized countries such as the United States, Canada, the United Kingdom, and Finland have higher expenditures on health care as opposed to countries which are economically less well off, such as Niger, Nepal, and Kenya. These differences in health expenditures also are directly correlated with rates of tuberculosis, HIV, and life expectancy.

Investment in health also promotes a longer life span, and impacts infant and child mortality. Table 12.2 provides a comparison of these areas, among high-income countries, middle-income countries, and lower-income countries, with data reported from the year 2010.

Social determinants of health also play a critical role in understanding and building a health and public health infrastructure. Originally conceptualized by Lalonde (1974) as a strategy to promote the capacity and health for Canadians, the model has been adopted by the World Health Organization (WHO), and includes human biology, environment, lifestyle, social support, and health care delivery systems as social determinants of health. All of these factors need to be taken into consideration when contemplating the public health status of countries within the global context.

TABLE 12.1 A Comparison Among Health Expenditures, Tuberculosis Rates, HIV prevalence, and Life Expectancy

COUNTRY	HEALTH EXPENDITURES (US$ 2009)	INCIDENCE OF TUBERCULOSIS (PER 100,000)	PREVALENCE OF TUBERCULOSIS (PER 100,000)	NUMBER OF PEOPLE LIVING WITH HIV	LIFE EXPECTANCY AT BIRTH (M/F)
United States	3,602	4.10	4.50	1,200,000	76/81
Canada	3,009	4.80	5.80	68,000	79/83
United Kingdom	2,747	12	15	85,000	78/82
Finland	3,105	8.8	12	2,600	77/83
Niger	12	181	328	61,000	57/58
Nepal	9	163	240	64,000	65/69
Kenya	11	305	282	1,500,000	58/62
China	85	96	138	740,000	72/76
Argentina	485	28.0	40.0	2,900	72/79

Source: World Health Organization. (2011).

TABLE 12.2 Comparison Among Select Countries' Infant Mortality, Child Mortality, and Life Expectancy Rates With Health Expenditures

INDICATORS	TP	GROSS NATIONAL INCOME PER CAPITA (PPP INTERNATIONAL $)	LIFE EXPECTANCY AT BIRTH M/F (YEARS)	PROBABILITY OF DYING UNDER FIVE (PER 1000 LIVE BIRTHS)	PROBABILITY OF DYING BETWEEN 15 AND 60 YEARS M/F (PER 1000 POPULATION)	TOTAL EXPENDITURE ON HEALTH PER CAPITA (INTL $, 2009)	TOTAL EXPENDITURE ON HEALTH AS % OF GDP (2009)
China	1,353,311,000	6,010	72/76	19	142/87	309	4.6
India	1,198,003,000	2,930	63/66	66	250/169	132	4.2
Nepal	29,331,000	1,120	65/69	48	234/159	69	5.8
Finland	5,326,000	35,940	77/83	3	124/56	3,357	9.7
Turkey	74,816,000	13,420	72/77	20	134/73	965	6.7
United Kingdom	61,565,000	36,240	78/82	5	95/58	3,399	9.3
Kenya	39,802,000	1,560	58/62	84	358/282	68	4.3
Niger	15,290,000	680	57/58	160	229/224	40	6.1
S. Africa	50,110,000	9,790	54/55	62	521/479	862	8.5
Canada	33,573,000	38,710	79/83	6	87/53	4,196	10.9
Haiti	10,033,000	not available	60/63	87	278/227	71	6.1
USA	314,659,000	46,790	76/81	8	134/78	7,410	16.2
Argentina	40,276,000	14,000	72/79	15	160/88	1,387	9.5
Brazil	193,734,000	10,080	70/77	21	205/102	943	9
Chile	16,970,000	13,250	76/82	9	116/59	1,172	8.2
Australia	21,293,000	37,250	80/84	5	79/45	3,382	8.5
New Zealand	4,266,000	25,200	79/83	6	86/57	2,667	9.7

Source: Retrieved from: http://www.who.int/countries/en/ on January, 18, 2012.

Healthy People 2020 Objectives Related to Global Health

Healthy People 2020 (U.S. Department of Health and Human Services (DHHS), 2010) is the first edition in which global health objectives have been incorporated, as previous editions of Healthy People objectives for the nation have not included objectives for global health. Some of the areas addressed include reducing the incidence rates of malaria and tuberculosis (within the United States), and the development of additional resources for global disease detection as specific benchmarks/goals to be reached by the year 2020. Although the benchmarks for malaria and tuberculosis are identified for the United States, it becomes clear that global disease detection centers are important because people from the United States travel to countries worldwide, and people from foreign countries will migrate to the United States.

Currently, the benchmark is reducing the number of cases of malaria reported in the United States by 10%, and this will be monitored by the National Malaria Surveillance Project, Centers for Disease Control and Prevention. The *Healthy People 2020* goal for tuberculosis calls to decrease the tuberculosis case rate for foreign-born persons living in the United States also by 10%. The actual numbers of cases are still reported as an estimate, developed through probability modeling on cases and provided by the National Tuberculosis Indicators Project, Centers for Disease Control and Prevention.

The third goal within the global health scheme of *Healthy People 2020* is related to Global Disease Detection Regional Centers (GDDs). Three specific objectives related to GDDs are as follows:

- Increase the number of GDDs worldwide to detect and contain emerging health threats from 7 to 13 by the year 2020.
- Increase the number of public health professionals trained by GDD programs worldwide from 37,132 to 144,132 by the year 2020.
- Increase diagnostic testing capacity in host countries and regionally through the GDDs from 154 tests to 264 tests.

These goals and figures related to the GDDs were developed and supplied by the Global Disease Detection and Evaluation Database through the Centers for Disease Control and Prevention (DHHS, 2010).

KEY ISSUES IN PUBLIC HEALTH SOCIAL WORK AND GLOBAL HEALTH

Despite the focus discussed in *Healthy People 2020* objectives (malaria, tuberculosis, and regional disease detection centers), a number of additional issues appear to still be paramount within the global arena, and public health social work plays a role in intervening within these areas. HIV/AIDS is one of these specific issues. According to a 2009 WHO report, nearly 33.3 million people were living with HIV, with 2.6 million people who were newly infected with HIV in 2009. The HIV/AIDS epidemic is recognized as a global threat, and funding and resources for the HIV epidemic have increased significantly since the 1990s. This epidemic, especially across sub-Saharan Africa and Asia, is predominantly concentrated and evolving among most-at-risk populations. Although there have been many successes in the HIV response over the past decade, great challenges clearly remain, especially when addressing most-at-risk populations, who are often criminalized, marginalized, and discriminated against. These groups face significant legal and social barriers to accessing HIV prevention and treatment services. Similarly, the global economic recession has also led to declining financial commitment about HIV prevention. In order to reach the Millennium Development Goal (MDG) of halting and reversing the spread of HIV by 2015 and to achieve universal access to HIV treatment, these barriers must be overcome (Le Loup, Fleury, Camargo, & Larouzé, 2010; United Nations Organization, 2010).

The U.S. President's Emergency Plan for AIDS Relief (PEPFAR; 2011) has one of the goals of integrating and coordinating HIV/AIDS programs with broader global health and development programs to maximize impact on health systems. This historic commitment and initiative of the U.S. government is not only to combat a single disease, but also to help internationally alleviate suffering from other diseases across the global health spectrum. The major focus of PEPFAR is to improve the health of women, newborns, and children, and save the greatest number of lives by supporting the countries in the world as they work to improve the health of their own people.

UNAIDS and the World Bank predict that HIV, which was responsible for 8.6% of deaths from infectious diseases in the developing world in 1990, will be responsible for 37.1% of such deaths among adults between the ages of fifteen and 59 by 2020 (World Bank, 1997). If treatment advances and other recent scientific advances give us reason for optimism, there is equally good reason for concern, as HIV/AIDS continues to stand as one of the most significant global health problems that must be confronted in the new millennium. The Global Fund to Fight HIV/AIDS, Tuberculosis, and Malaria (GFATM) was founded to increase political and financial commitments toward health and development, in the aftermath of the Millennium Declaration, and on track to implement the MDGs. This fund has mobilized over $16 billion U.S. through its partnership, and spent over $8 billion through 620 contracts in 140 countries for these three diseases (Kerouedan, 2010). The main focuses are given to accelerate and expand HIV, tuberculosis, and malaria prevention, awareness, care, and treatment-related activities in the poorest and the most affected countries worldwide. Despite the global application, a special emphasis has been placed upon Africa. The rationale is that

Africa is the continent with the highest disease burden, especially with respect to HIV/AIDS. An estimated 22.5 million people are living with HIV in sub-Saharan Africa—around two-thirds of the global total. In 2009, approximately 1.3 million people died from AIDS in sub-Saharan Africa and 1.8 million people became infected with HIV (AVERT, 2011).

The Asia Pacific region has an estimated 4.9 million people living with HIV, including 440,000 new cases and 300,000 deaths annually (UNAIDS, 2008). Over 95% of infections occur in eight countries: Cambodia, China, India, Indonesia, Myanmar, Nepal, Thailand, and Vietnam. In addition, within these countries, HIV is concentrated in the most-at-risk populations within communities, wherein HIV prevalence is often over 5% (Commission on AIDS in Asia, 2008). Although there are major challenges to ensuring universal access to HIV services in Asia, many of the barriers can be overcome if there is political will and civil society is adequately involved in the response. Human rights violations, the detention of large numbers of people (often for long periods and in poor conditions, simply for using or possessing drugs), the criminalization of HIV and of homosexuality in many countries, and stigma and discrimination continue to impede the national and global responses to the epidemic (Rao, Mboi, Phoolcharoen, Sarkar, & Carael, 2010). A concerted effort will be needed to remove these barriers by changing legislation, policies, and practices.

The global economic downturn has had a particularly devastating impact on low-income and middle-income countries and dropped millions of people below the poverty line. Thus, it will be critical to continue investing in prevention and treatment and, more broadly, in health systems in these countries, which already bear a disproportionate burden of HIV, malaria, and tuberculosis. Great progress has been made in recent years in the response to HIV and AIDS, but this progress remains fragile; a reduction in prevention efforts could jeopardize the positive results achieved and allow AIDS to gain force again (Smith, Poobalan, & Van Teijlingen, 2008). Despite these potential reductions in efforts, it is still possible to achieve, or even exceed, the health-related MDGs by 2015. The Millennium Development Goal related to the health sector also marks a major milestone for efforts aimed at achieving the MDG to "halt and reverse the spread of HIV by 2015" (United Nations, 2010). Only a few countries in Asia are on track to meet this target by 2015 (United Nations, 2010) due to a widespread failure or reluctance to properly address the local epidemiological contexts and to target the most-at-risk populations among whom the epidemic is largely concentrated, such as people who use drugs (and their partners), men who have sex with men, and sex workers (and their clients). In particular, the prevention of millions of new HIV infections dramatically reduce deaths from AIDS, and virtually eliminate transmission of HIV from mother to child in Asia—but only with targeted and expanded input from donors (United Nations, 2010).

The effects on HIV prevalence are more complex. *Prevalence* is the proportion of at-risk people who are living with a disease; successful treatment and prevention efforts of PEPFAR will have opposing near-term effects on prevalence. Connor et al. (1994) suggested that successful treatment reduces the number of newly infected infants and may also prevent new sexually acquired infections, which would decrease prevalence. By rapidly reducing the death rate in advanced infection, treatment increases the number of patients alive and living with HIV. Improving access to anti-retroviral therapy prevents AIDS-related deaths and increases prevalence. As a result, both aspects of PEPFAR—treatment and prevention—could be working without affecting HIV prevalence. So, the changes in global health and aid architecture have meant that development assistance for HIV/AIDS since the 2000s has increasingly been provided through partnerships and Global Health Initiatives (GHIs; Buse & Walt, 2000). GHIs have been successful in leveraging large amounts of new funding for HIV/AIDS. The three largest GHIs—the PEPFAR, the GFATM, and the World Bank Multi-Country AIDS Program—together provide two-thirds of all external funding for HIV/AIDS (Bennett, Boerma, & Brugha, 2006). Given that the GHIs are rapidly evolving, consistent nomenclature is difficult across countries and systems of care. Brugha (2008) defined GHIs as "a blueprint for financing, resourcing, coordinating and/or implementing disease control across several countries in more than one region of the world" (p. 74). Despite their levels of funding and influence, evidence and detailed understanding of the impact of GHIs, especially at the subnational level, is limited although this body of evidence is growing (Biesma et al., 2009; WHO Maximizing Positive Synergies, 2009).

In addition to the HIV pandemic and the importance it raises for global health issues, the GDDs are critical initiatives within the global arena for detection, intervention, surveillance, and workforce development (Taboy, Chapman, Albetkova, Kennedy, & Rayfield, 2010). These centers were developed with the goal of strengthening public health systems and building essential infrastructure in host countries and meeting the objectives outlined in the International Health Regulations of 2005 (Fidler, Low-Beer, & Sarkar, 2010; Yamin, 2005; IHR, 2005). A number of core capacities were identified by internal and external GDD stakeholders to help build a country's ability to rapidly identify and control emerging infectious diseases at the time of detection. The core capacities that the GDDs deliver include (1) response and detection of emerging infectious diseases, (2) manpower development in field epidemiology and laboratory methods, (3) preparedness and response for pandemic influenza, (4) disease detection and response with animal–human interface, (5) emergency preparedness and risk communication, and (6) laboratory systems development and improvement (CDC, 2011). These core capacities are in direct response and help promote compliance with IHR 2005, which calls for strengthened national capacity for surveillance and control; prevention, alert, and response to public emergencies; and accountability (Andrus, Aguilera, Oliva, & Aldighieri, 2010; Armstrong et al., 2010). It is hoped that using these mechanisms of the GDDs will impact the social determinants of health and reduce health inequities (Barten, Mitlin, Mulholland, Hardoy, & Stern, 2007; Bell, Taylor, & Marmot, 2010; Fox & Meier, 2009; Koh, Piotrowski, Kumanyika, & Fielding, 2011; Payne, 2006; Pfeiffer et al., 2008).

THE CORE FUNCTIONS OF PUBLIC HEALTH IN RELATION TO GLOBAL HEALTH

The core public health functions of assessment, policy development, and assurance play an important role in several aspects of global health functioning. Each of the specific core functions defines a set of essential services and competencies to carry out these functions effectively. These can also be tied to public health social work competencies. This next section outlines each of the core functions, their priorities in the global health arena, and some associated public health social work competencies.

Assessment

Public health social workers who work in global settings play a key role in surveillance, disease detection, and monitoring as well. Depending upon the setting, different areas of health status may be monitored. Infant mortality and maternal mortality rates may be monitored in some situations, and incidence rates for malaria, tuberculosis, polio, or other life-threatening diseases may be the subject of monitoring. Public health social workers will use skills related to epidemiology to help track incidence and prevalence of specific conditions. In addition, they will utilize practice and epidemiologic theories to substantiate interventions and programming designed to promote health and behavioral change. In like manner, public health social workers will use these same skills to monitor the health status of a community and to help use this information to identify community health problems and health hazards.

Evaluation skills are useful for public health social workers to help assess interventions, as well as the effectiveness, accessibility, and quality of personal and population-based health services available to people, regardless of location. These skills become essential when working in small villages in countries such as Ecuador, Nepal, Bangladesh, or Niger. Although services and resources may be available in larger centers or cities within these countries, the same access and quality may not be consistently available in villages or smaller communities. Public health social workers in these roles may have to make use of demographic data and apply primary, secondary, and tertiary strategies to address the health issues of individuals, families, and communities within these settings.

Policy Development

The arena for policy development within global health settings becomes important as public health social workers move into these settings. Health policy can range from clear language with statements that have been developed through the use of evidence to policy statements which have been developed in a vacuum with vague, unclear, or nonexistent evidence (Jurkowski, 2008). In communities where no public policy exists, public health social workers will need to assume a role to help key community stakeholders develop policies and plans that support individual and community health efforts, particularly in countries where limited health policies exist. Soliciting support from key stakeholders and enlisting the support of elders where relevant (i.e., in tribal communities, or communities where elders make key decisions) will be paramount for successful policy development to take place when working in global settings.

Within the realm of policy development, public health social workers will also need to help enforce laws and regulations that protect health and ensure safety and empower local individuals to be comfortable speaking up in support of regulations that enforce the public's safety. An example to showcase this would be developing safe driving regulations. Although speed limit and seat belt legislation may exist in a local community such as Niamey, Niger (the capital city), rarely are people stopped by legal authorizes for not wearing seat belts, and thus people do not consistently wear these devices. Public health social workers can work toward assisting the local stakeholders within these communities to enforce these policies and develop campaigns to educate the public on the benefits and risks to seat belt use.

Moreover, within the realm of policy development, public health social workers will work toward developing strategies and projects which will promote research for new insights and innovative solutions to health problems. Often, strategies and research studies that have been developed in the United States or Canada do not seem relevant, or may need adaptation in order to be executed in other countries within the global context. Resources, cultural expectations, and workforce expertise will all play a role in the technology transfer between different countries. Public health social workers will help work with facilitating this type of technology transfer and often assist in building research methodologies to replicate studies that are culturally relevant.

Some of the specific public health social work competencies which may be used in this policy development arena will include skills related to leadership and communication and skills in public health advocacy. These may include networking toward inter-multidisciplinary team building and group processes, social work community organization, and coalition building to address the issues of social and health disparities and to develop strategies for soliciting and maintaining consumer and other constituencies involved at all levels of an organization.

Assurance

The last core function assures services, a competent workforce, and the provision of strategies to inform and educate the public. Within this function, public health social workers link people to needed personal health services and assure the provision of health care when otherwise unavailable. This may include educating, informing, and empowering people about health issues. Public health social workers working with indigent families may need to educate mothers about the importance of immunizations or use of primary health care services when a child is showing signs of persistent illness.

Assurance of a competent public health and personal health care workforce becomes more critical as we move into the global health arena, where resources and person-power may be limited. Often times, the village health worker may play a key role in the detection and cursory assessment of health issues, and then refer the individual or his/her family to a local primary care center. The village workers require training and preparation in terms of skills for triage; often, public health social workers working in global settings help to identify people for these roles. GDDs also play a role in the development of a local workforce to help with the development of specific skills/competencies within local laboratories or health care settings. Public health social workers can work with these resources to help facilitate and engage the local workforce to pursue training and human resource development.

Last, public health social workers will mobilize community partnerships to identify and solve health problems when working in global settings. These partnerships may pursue public education campaigns to erase the stigma of many common public health issues and remove barriers to care that have been created through myths and taboos. This process of informing, educating, and empowering people about health issues is also a critical function of public health social workers working in global contexts.

SUMMARY

This chapter thus far has provided an overview of the description of global health, some of the key issues that are faced within the context of global health, and an agenda for the roles public health social workers can play in the global health arena. In addition, the chapter has discussed the priorities established as benchmarks in *Healthy People 2020*, and showcased how public health social workers can carry out the core functions and essential services within global health and health care settings. Despite the current developments to improve the health status of individuals within a global context, a number of new issues are emerging and will help shape an agenda for public health social workers in the future. The next segment addresses these future/emerging issues.

Emerging Issues for the Future

Promoting intervention through social determinants of health

In the future, the social determinants of health, which include genetics, lifestyle, social support environment, and health care systems, will be integrated into the spectrum of factors which affect health. This framework will be used in the future when working with the global health community and in the training process of public health social workers (Koh et al., 2011; Morris, 2011; Venkatapuram, 2010).

Building capacity

An increased emphasis will be seen on building technological expertise and capacity for workers functioning in global settings. As talent is imported, international experts will provide education and technology to help cultivate an educated workforce, and to help build local capacity.

Blending public health promotion with social work intervention

In the future, we will see an increase in the role social workers play with health promotion efforts. Public health social workers will increasingly take the lead in developing and carrying out health promotion interventions with people, especially in global settings.

Promoting mental health

Over the past two decades, the focus of global health efforts, particularly in low-income countries, has been on reducing infant and maternal mortality rates, increasing sanitation, and improving running water and the safety of environments. As the rates of mortality have decreased and living conditions have improved, some communities and national/state health policy see an increased recognition about mental health. In some countries, there has been an increase in suicide rates and thus there will be a need to address risk factors which impact suicide and the public's overall mental health. In the future, an increased level of attention will be paid to promoting mental health across the life span (Canadian Medical Association, 2010; Jenkins, Baingana, Ahmad, McDaid & Atun, 2011a, 2011b).

Building public health policy and regulations

Last, an issue for the future will be the development and inclusion of public health policies and regulations which will target the building of safe communities in industrial and residential environments. Chemical regulations will also play a critical role in the future as communities and practitioners work toward building safe environmental conditions and communities (Olowokure, Pooransingh, Tempowski, Palmer & Meredith, 2005). Increasingly, the process of building health policy and regulations will lead to health reform and healthy community initiatives (Fielding, Teusch, & Koh, 2012).

CLASSROOM EXERCISES

1. Using the database from the WHO develop a comparison chart on several countries of interest. Secure data from different points in time over a 10-year time span and plot the data on a graph.
   - Are the trends improving over time?
   - What factors can be contributing to these improvements or declines?
   - What reasons can you attribute to the changes in these trends?
   - What differences are evident from the countries selected, and what do you speculate accounts for these differences?
2. You and a team of your colleagues are charged with the task of developing a needs assessment to be submitted to the CDC Global Health Division, for the development of a GDD.
   (a) What would you include in your needs assessment?
   (b) How do these elements align themselves with the core areas of a GDD?
3. You are going to work as a Peace Corps volunteer once you complete your degrees in Public Health and Social Work. You have been told that you will be working as a public health social worker in villages in any one of the following countries: Bangladesh, India, Nepal, or Niger. The role you will take on will be in public health education/health promotion in the areas of family planning, immunizations, and/or malaria control.
   (a) What skills will you need to bring to this role?
   (b) How will you prepare for your assignment as a Peace Corps volunteer?

INTERNET RESOURCES

The World Health Organization (WHO)

(www.who.int/en/)

The WHO serves as a repository of information that is useful for countries worldwide. The WHO collects data on a number of health and social indicators, which are made available to the general public. It also provides reports on various health topics, publications on various health topics, and comprehensive information on projects and programs that it runs throughout the world. The WHO serves as the coordinating authority for health within the United Nations system. It is charged with the responsibility for providing leadership on global health matters, shaping the health research agenda, setting norms and standards, articulating evidence-based policy options, providing technical support to countries, and monitoring and assessing health trends.

The Division of the Global Disease Detection and Emergency Response; Centers for Disease Control and Prevention

(www.cdc.gov/globalhealth/gdder/)

The Division of Global Disease Detection and Emergency Response protects Americans and the global community from urgent public health threats and provides public health relief for humanitarian emergencies. It houses the GDDs and several other initiatives designed to promote the health of people in the United States from diseases brought to the United States by foreign means. It also provides infrastructure and expertise to countries within the global community.

Global Health Council

(www.globalhealth.org/Home_Page.html)

The Global Health Council serves as an advocacy organization to provide comprehensive and evidence-based information to the global community.

REFERENCES

Andrus, J., Aguilera, X., Oliva, O., & Aldighieri, S. (2010). Global health security and the international health regulations. *BMC Public Health*, *10*(Suppl. 1), 1–4.

Armstrong, K., McNabb, S., Ferland, L., Stephens, T., Muldoon, A., Fernandez, J., et al. (2010). Capacity of public health surveillance to comply with revised international health regulations, USA. *Emerging Infectious Diseases*, *16*(5), 804–808.

AVERT. (2011). *HIV and AIDS in Africa*. Retrieved from http://www.avert.org/hiv-aids-africa.htm

Barten, F., Mitlin, D., Mulholland, C., Hardoy, A., & Stern, R. (2007). Integrated approaches to address the social determinants of health for reducing health inequity. *Journal of Urban Health: Bulletin of the New York Academy of Medicine, 84*(3, Suppl.), i164-i173.

Beaglehole, R., & Bonita, R. (2010). What is global health? *Global Health Action, 3*(514), 5142-5143. doi: 10.3402/gha.v3i0.5142

Bell, R., Taylor, S., & Marmot, M. (2010). Global health governance: Commission on social determinants of health and the imperative for change. *The Journal of Law, Medicine & Ethics, 38*(3), 470-485. doi: 10.1111/j.1748-720X.2010.00506.x

Bennett, S., Boerma, J. T., & Brugha, R. (2006). Scaling up HIV/AIDS evaluation. *The Lancet, 367*(9504), 79-82.

Biesma, R., Brugha, R., Harmer, A., Walsh, A., Spicer, N., & Walt, G. (2009). The effects of global health initiatives on country health systems: A review of the evidence from HIV/AIDS control. *Health Policy Plan, 24*(4), 239-252.

Brown, T., Cueto, M., & Fee, E. (2006). The World Health Organization and the transition from "international" to "global" public health. *American Journal of Public Health, 96*(1), 62-72.

Brugha, R. (2008.) Global health initiatives and public health policy. In K. Heggenbouge & S. R. Quah (Eds.), *International encyclopedia of public health* (pp. 72-81). San Diego: Academic Press.

Buse, K., & Walt, G. (2000). Global public-private partnerships: Part I. A new development in health? *Bulletin of the World Health Organization, 78*, 549-561.

CDC. (2011). *Global Disease Detection Program: 2010 Monitoring & Evaluation Report*. Center for Global Disease Detection and Emergency Response.

CMA. (2010). Mental Disorders seek space at the global health table. *Canadian Medical Association Journal, 182*(7), E3767-E3768.

Commission on AIDS in Asia. (2008). *Redefining AIDS in Asia: Crafting an effective response*. New Delhi: Oxford University Press.

Connor, E. M., Sperling, R. S., Gelber, R., Kiselev, P., Scott, G., O'Sullivan, M. J.... Balsey, J. (1994). Reduction of maternal-infant transmission of human immunodeficiency virus type 1 with zidovudine treatment. *The New England Journal of Medicine, 331*, 1173-1180.

Fidler, D., & Gostin, L. (2006). The new international health regulations: An historic development for international law and public health. *The Journal of Law, Medicine & Ethics, 34*(1), 85-94.

Fielding, J. E., Teutsch, S., & Koh, H. (2012). Health reform and healthy people initiative. *American Journal of Public Health, 102*(1), 30-33. doi: 2105/AJPH.2011.300312

Fox, A., & Meier, B. (2009). Health as freedom: Addressing social determinants of global health inequities through the human right to development. *Bioethics, 23*(2), 112-122.

IHR. (2005). World Health Assembly. *Revision of the International Health Regulations*, WHA58.3 (May 23, 2005).

Jenkins, R., Baingana, F., Ahmad, R., McDaid, D., & Atun, R. (2011a). Mental health and the global agenda: Core conceptual issues. *Mental Health in Family Medicine, 8*(2), 69-82.

Jenkins, R., Baingana, F., Ahmad, R., McDaid, D., & Atun, R. (2011b). Social, economic, human rights and political challenges to global mental health. *Mental Health in Family Medicine, 8*(2), 87-96.

Jurkowski, E. T. (2008). *Policy and program planning for older adults: Realities and visions.* New York, NY: Springer Publishing.

Kerouedan, D. (2010). The global fund to fight HIV/AIDS, TB and malaria evaluation policy issues. *Bulletin for Social Pathology, 103*(2), 119-122.

Kickbush, I. (2006). The need for a European strategy on global health. *Scandinavian Journal of Public Health, 34,* 561-565.

Koh, H., Piotrowski, J., Kumanyika, S., & Fielding, J. (2011). Healthy people: A 2020 vision for the social determinants approach. *Health Education & Behavior, 38*(6), 551-557.

Koplan, J. P., Bond, T. C., Merson, M. H., Reddy, K. S., Rodriguez, M. H., Sewankambo, N. K., et al. (2009). Towards a common definition of global health. *Lancet, 373,* 1993-1995.

LaLonde, M. (1974). *A new perspective on the health of Canadians.* Retrieved from http://www.healthpromotionagency.org.uk/Healthpromotion/Health/section6a.htm

Le Loup, G., Fleury, S., Camargo, K., & Larouzé, B. (2010). International institutions, global health initiatives and the challenge of sustainability: Lessons from the Brazilian AIDS programme. *Tropical Medicine & International Health: 15*(1), 5-10.

Low-Beer, D., & Sarkar, S. (2010). Systematic HIV prevention in Asia: Scaling up from individual to population level impact. *Journal of AIDS, 24*(Suppl. 3), 12-19.

Macfarlane, S. B., Jacobs, M., & Kaaya, E. E. (2008). In the name of global health: Trends in academic institutions. *Journal of Public Health Policy, 29,* 383-401.

Morris, K. (2011). Healthy People 2020: Thirty years of moving towards health. *Ohio Nurses Review, 86*(3), 16-17.

Olowokure, B., Pooransingh, S., Tempowski, J., Palmer, S., & Meredith, T. (2005). Global surveillance for chemical incidents of international public health concern. *Bulletin of the World Health Organization, 83*(12), 928-934.

Payne, M. (2006). International social work research and health inequalities. *Journal of Comparative Social Welfare, 22*(2), 115-124. doi: 10.1080/17486830600836099

Pfeiffer, J., Johnson, W., Fort, M., Shakow, A., Hagopian, A., Gloyd, S., et al. (2008). Strengthening health systems in poor countries: A code of conduct for nongovernmental organizations. *American Journal of Public Health, 98*(12), 2134-2140.

Rao, P., Mboi, I., Phoolcharoen, W., Sarkar, S., & Carael, M. (2010). AIDS in Asia amid competing priorities: A review of national responses to HIV. *Journal of AIDS, 24*(3), 41-48.

Smith, W., Poobalan, A., & Van Teijlingen, E. (2008). Global themes in international public health. *Leprosy Review, 79*(2), 128-129.

Taboy, C., Chapman, W., Albetkova, A., Kennedy, S., & Rayfield, M. (2010). Integrated disease investigations and surveillance planning: A systems approach to strengthening national surveillance and detection of events of public health importance in support of the International Health Regulations. *BMC Public Health, 10*(Suppl. 1S6), 1-6. doi: 10.1186/1471-2458-10-S1-S6

UNAIDS. (2008). *Regional review of HIV and AIDS in Asia-Pacific region.* Geneva, Switzerland: UNAIDS.

United Nations. (2010). *UN. Millennium development goals.* Geneva, Switzerland: United Nations. Retrieved April 19, 2011, from http://www.un.org/millenniumgoals/

U.S. Department of Health and Human Services. (2010). *Healthy People 2020: Health objectives for the nation.* Baltimore, MD: U.S. Government Printing Office.

The U.S. President's Emergency Plan for AIDS Relief. (2011). Retrieved from http://www.pepfar.gov/documents/organization/171303.pdf

Venkatapuram, S. (2010). Global justice and the social determinants of health. *Ethics & International Affairs, 24*(2), 119-130.

WHO Maximizing Positive Synergies. (2009). An assessment of interactions between global health initiatives and country health systems. *The Lancet, 373*(9681), 2137–2169.

World Bank. (1997). *Confronting AIDS: Public priorities in a global epidemic*. New York, NY: Oxford University Press.

World Health Organization. (2009). *Global summary of the AIDS epidemic*. Retrieved from http://www.who.int/hiv/data/2009_global_summary.png

World Health Organization. (2011). *Data and statistics*. Retrieved from http://www.who.int/whosis/whostat/EN_WHS2011_Full.pdf

Yamin, A. (2005). The right to health under international law and its relevance to the United States. *American Journal of Public Health, 95*(7), 1156–1161.

CHAPTER 13

Mental Health

Mary Helen Hogue and Elaine T. Jurkowski

INTRODUCTION

*I*n his message on World Mental Health Day (Oct. 10, 2011), United Nations Secretary-General Ban Ki Moon stated, "There is no health without mental health. Mental disorders are major contributors to illness and premature death, and are responsible for 13 percent of the global disease burden. With the global economic downturn and associated austerity measures—the risks for mental ill-health are rising around the globe" (United Nations World Health Organization (UNWHO, 2011).

Mental health plays a significant role in the health and well-being of individuals and communities. This chapter will explore the definition of mental health; examine the incidence and prevalence of mental health from a national perspective; explore some of the major disorder groups; and examine major mental health concerns, such as suicide. It will also explore how public health social workers can respond to these issues using public health core functions and the public health social work standards and competencies. The chapter will conclude with interactive exercises and resources for further exploration.

WHAT IS MENTAL HEALTH?

The 1999 *Surgeon General's Report on Mental Health* (U.S. Department of Health and Human Services (DHHS), 1999, p. 4) defined *mental health* as "Successful performance of mental function, resulting in productive activities, fulfilling relationships with other people, and the ability to change and to cope with adversity." Mental health disorders are largely preventable, non-communicable diseases which include disorders such as: Anxiety, Bipolar, Eating, Depression and Suicide. These disorders are identified as the leading causes of illness and death and impact persons or any age, race, religion or income (National Adolescent Health Information Center, 2008; National Institutes of Mental Health [NIMH], 2010).

Are mental health issues preventable, or are they inherent to the individuals who are genetically predisposed to developing them? McKeowan (1971), in efforts to reshape the British health care system, addressed this question and argued that the behavior and lifestyle of the individual played a role in one's physical and mental health well-being, as do factors such as environment and genetics. Marc Lalonde, the Minister of Health in Canada (1974), built upon McKeown's theory to articulate five main criteria that undergird the health of individuals. These determinants, articulated in his health plan for Canadians (Lalonde, 1974), have been embraced by the World Health Organization (WHO) in a variety of seminal documents, and have most recently been used to help identify social determinants of health (WHO, 2005 & 2009), including economics, behavior/lifestyle, genetics, environment, and social networks. Although there is significant documentation within the literature to suggest that these factors have a significant impact on one's health, the literature summarized in various reports exploring mental health conditions, etiology, and epidemiology (DHHS, 1999; WHO, 2009) also suggests that these factors individually or in combination also contribute to one's mental health (Bahrer-Kohler, 2011; Jurkowski, 2011).

THE SCOPE OF THE PROBLEM: MENTAL HEALTH INCIDENCE AND PREVALENCE

Suicide

Suicide is a major, preventable public health problem. Over the past 45 years, suicide rates have increased by 60% worldwide (UNWHO, 2012). Suicide is among the three leading causes of death among people aged 15 to 44 in some countries, and the second leading cause of death in the 10- to 24-year-old age group; these figures do not include suicide attempts, which are up to 20 times more frequent than completed suicide. Moreover, suicide was the 10th leading cause of death in the United States, accounting for 34,598 deaths (National Institute of Mental Health (NIMH), 2012). The overall rate was 11.3 suicide deaths per 100,000 people, and an estimated 11 attempted suicides occur per every suicide death (National Alliance on Mental Illness, 2011).

Suicide is complex, with psychological, social, biological, cultural, and environmental factors involved. Every year, almost 1 million people die from suicide; a "global" mortality rate of 16 per 100,000, or one death every 40 seconds. Suicide worldwide is estimated to represent 1.8% of the total global burden of disease in 1998, and 2.4% in countries with market and former socialist economies in 2020 (WHO, 2011). Although traditionally suicide rates have been highest among the male elderly, rates among young people have been increasing to such an extent that they are now the group ranked at highest risk in at least one-third of all countries worldwide, within both the developed and developing world. Mental disorders (particularly depression and alcohol use disorders) are a major risk factor for suicide in Europe and North America. In Asian countries, impulsiveness plays a key role as a motivating factor in suicide (WHO, 2011).

A National Perspective

Each year in the United States, approximately 2 million U.S. adolescents attempt suicide, and almost 700,000 receive medical attention for their attempt (American Academy of Child and Adolescent Psychiatry, 2010). According to the Youth Risk Behavior Surveillance System (Centers for Disease Control and Prevention [CDC], 2011a), 2.6% of students reported making a suicide attempt that had to be treated by a doctor or nurse. It is estimated that each year in the United States, approximately 2,000 youth aged 10 to 19 complete suicide. In 2000, suicide was the third leading cause of death among young people aged 15 to 24, following unintentional injuries and homicides (CDC Web-based Inquiry Statistics Query and Reporting System, 2011b). In 2007, suicide was the third leading cause of death for young people aged 15 to 24 (National Adolescent Health Information Center, 2006).

Suicide is the result of many complex factors. More than 90% of youth suicide victims have at least one major psychiatric disorder, although younger adolescent suicide victims have lower rates of psychopathology than adults (Gould et al., 2003). It is important to note that while the majority of suicide victims have a history of psychiatric disorder, especially mood disorders, very few adolescents with a psychiatric disorder will go on to complete suicide.

According to the CDC (2011), the suicide rate among children aged 10 to 14 was 1.5/100,000, or 300 deaths among 19,895,072 children in this age group. The suicide rate among adolescents aged 15 to 19 was 8.2/100,000, or 1,621 deaths among 19,882,596 adolescents in this age group. The suicide rate among young people aged 20 to 24 was 12.8/100,000, or 2,373 deaths among 18,484,615 people in this age group. Of every 100,000 young people in each age group, the following number died by suicide.

- Children aged 10 to 14—0.9 per 100,000
- Adolescents aged 15 to 19—6.9 per 100,000
- Young adults aged 20 to 24—12.7 per 100,000

Gender differences in suicide were also noted among young people, whereby nearly 5 times as many male adolescents as female adolescents aged 15 to 19 died by suicide. In addition, more than 6 times as many young men as young women aged 20 to 24 died by suicide (CDC, 2011). Youth who attempt suicide are particularly difficult to treat because they often leave treatment prematurely, and no specific interventions exist that reliably reduce suicidal thinking and behavior (CDC, 2010; Copeland-Linder, Lambert, & Ialongo, 2010; Fox, Halpern, & Forsyth, 2008). Risk factors for attempted suicide by youth include depression, alcohol or other drug use disorder, physical or sexual abuse, and disruptive behavior (Kuehn, 2011; Degnan et al., 2010; Muehlenkamp, 2010; NAHIC, 2008).

The elderly (aged 65 and older) comprise 15% of the U.S. population and account for over 18% of all suicides (CDC, 2010). They account for 7% of all inpatient psychiatric services, and 9% of private psychiatric patients. It is estimated that 18% to 25% of elders need mental health care for depression, anxiety, psychosomatic disorders, adjustment to aging, and schizophrenia associated with elder suicide. Even though 17 older individuals kill themselves each day, depression is not a part of normal aging; other illnesses and medications play a role (National Center for Injury Prevention and Control, 2012). The elderly are afraid of losing their autonomy if they became dependent on help from the health services. Moreover, encounters between the elderly and providers of mental health services frequently occur in a manner that is not conducive to disclosing the risk of suicide (Kjolseth, Ekeberg, & Stelhaug, 2010).

Statistics from the NIMH (2011) suggest that older Americans are disproportionately likely to die by suicide. For example, of every 100,000 people aged 65 and older, 14.3 died by suicide in 2007. This figure is higher than the national average of 11.3 suicides per 100,000 people in the general population. Non-Hispanic White men aged 85 or older had an even higher rate, with 47 suicide deaths per 100,000 (CDC, 2011; Cole, Stevenson, & Rogers, 2009; & Karlin & Zeiss, 2010). An estimated 11 nonfatal suicide attempts occur per every suicide death. Men and the elderly are more likely to have fatal attempts than are women and youth (NIMH, 2011). Some of the risk factors with nonfatal suicide attempts by adults include depression and other mental disorders, alcohol and other substance abuse, and separation or divorce (NIMH, 2007).

Since research shows that older adults and women who die by suicide are likely to have seen a primary care provider in the year before their death, improving primary-care providers' abilities to recognize and treat risk factors may help prevent suicide (Blakemore, 2009; Snowden, Dhingra, Keyes, & Anderson, 2010). Improving outreach to men at risk is a major challenge in need of investigation. Risk factors that have been identified for this target group include at least one prior suicide attempt; a family history of mental disorder or substance abuse; a family history of suicide; family violence, including physical or sexual abuse; firearms in the home (the method used in more than one-half of all suicides); incarceration; and/or exposure to the suicidal behavior of others, such as family members, peers, or media figures (Degnan et al., 2010; Flood & Buckwalter, 2009; Karlin & Fuller, 2007; Luoma, Pearson, & Martin, 2002; Substance Abuse and Mental Health Services Administration (SAMHSA), 2009).

Obesity, Body Image, and Eating Disorders

An eating disorder is an illness that causes serious disturbances to one's everyday diet, such as eating extremely small amounts of food or severely overeating. Severe distress or concern about body weight or shape may also characterize an eating disorder. Obesity and body image are key issues in relation to eating disorders, which also impact many adolescents.

Stigma and discrimination toward obese persons are pervasive and pose numerous consequences for psychological and physical health. Despite decades of science documenting the impact of weight stigma, its public health implications are widely ignored (Wilson, 2009). Obese persons are blamed for their weight, with common perceptions that weight stigmatization is justifiable and may motivate individuals to adopt healthier behaviors. However, stigmatization of obese individuals threatens health, generates health disparities, and interferes with effective obesity intervention efforts. These findings highlight weight stigma as both a social justice issue and a priority for public health (Peul & Heuer, 2010; Hensley, Corrigan, Watson, Byrne, & Davis 2005).

Causes of obesity can include poor eating habits, overeating or bingeing, lack of exercise (e.g., couch potato kids), a family history of obesity, medical illnesses (endocrine, neurological problems), medications (steroids, and some psychiatric medications), stressful life events or changes (separations, parental divorce, abuse, or death), family and peer problems, low self-esteem or emotional problems, and/or depression (Copeland-Linder, Lambert, & Ialongo, 2010).

Disordered Eating in Adolescence

A person with an eating disorder may have started out just eating smaller or larger amounts of food, but at some point the urge to eat less or more spiraled out of control. Severe distress or concern about body weight or shape may also characterize an eating disorder. Eating disorders frequently appear during the teen years or young adulthood but may also develop during childhood or later in life (NIMH, 2011). Eating disorders frequently coexist with other illnesses, such as depression, substance abuse, or anxiety disorders.

Risks and Complications of Obesity

Physical consequences associated with obesity include an increased risk of heart disease, high blood pressure, diabetes, problems with breathing and respiratory issues, and trouble sleeping.

The problem of childhood obesity in the United States has grown considerably in recent years. Between 16% and 33% of children and adolescents are obese. Obesity is among the easiest medical conditions to recognize but one of the most difficult to treat. Unhealthy weight gain due to poor diet and lack of exercise is responsible for over 300,000 deaths each year. The annual cost to society for obesity is estimated at nearly $100 billion. Overweight children are much more likely to become overweight adults unless they adopt and maintain healthier patterns of eating and exercise. Child and adolescent obesity is also associated with increased risk of emotional problems.

The reason most obese adolescents gain back their lost pounds is that after they have reached their goal, they go back to their older maladaptive eating and exercise habits. An obese adolescent must therefore learn to eat and enjoy healthy foods in moderate amounts and to exercise regularly to maintain the desired weight. Parents of an obese child can improve their child's self-esteem by emphasizing the child's strengths and positive qualities rather than just focusing on their child's weight problem. Finally, teens with weight problems tend to have much lower self-esteem and be less popular with their peers (Hoffman, Baldwin, & Cerbone, 2003).

MAJOR DEPRESSIVE DISORDER

Major depressive disorder (MDD) is a condition characterized by a long-lasting depressed mood or marked loss of interest or pleasure (anhedonia) in all, or nearly all, activities. Children and adolescents with MDD may be irritable instead of sad. These symptoms, along with others described below, must be sufficiently severe to interfere significantly with the person's daily functioning in order for the person to be diagnosed with MDD.

MDD is a serious mental condition that profoundly affects an individual's quality of life. Unlike normal bereavement or an occasional episode of "the blues," MDD causes a lengthy period of gloom and hopelessness, and may rob the sufferer of the ability to take pleasure in activities or relationships that were previously enjoyable. In some cases, depressive episodes seem to be triggered by an obviously painful event, but MDD may also develop without a specific stressor. Research indicates that an initial episode of depression is likely to be a response to a specific stimulus, but later episodes are progressively more likely to start without a triggering event. Mental efficiency and memory are affected, causing even simple tasks to be tiring and irritating (Cuijper & Smit, 2008).

Although by some estimates there are over 400 different treatment approaches—all of which attempt to alleviate psychological distress among children and adolescents—not all mental health therapies for young people are created equal. Resources are currently being poured into evidence-based interventions, and thus researchers are constantly evaluating and comparing the effects of various treatments for a variety of mental health problems.

For reasons that are not well understood, prior to puberty MDD is about equally common in girls and boys (Hoffman et al., 2003). Adolescence is a high-risk period for MDD; while suicide may result from impulsive behavior under stress, rather than from MDD, it is noteworthy that about 14% of all teenage deaths are due to suicide (NAHIC, 2008).

Depression appears to have become a more common disorder over the past century. Epidemiologists studying the incidence of depression across time compared groups of people born between 1917 and 1936, between 1937 and 1952, and between 1953 and 1966; their results indicated that the rate of depression increased progressively from one generation to the next (Kuhn, 2009). While no single explanation for the rise in depressive disorders emerged, some researchers have suggested that the breakdown of social support networks caused by higher rates of family disruption and greater social mobility may be important contributing factors.

Eight to 20% of older adults in the community and up to 37% in primary care settings suffer from depressive symptoms. Treatment is successful, with response rates between 60% and 80%, but the response generally takes longer than that for other adults. Depression in older people is hard to disentangle from the many other disorders that affect older people, and its symptom profile is somewhat different from that in other adults.

Evidence-based practices (EBPs) are treatments that are based directly on scientific evidence that has revealed the strongest contributors and risk factors for psychological symptoms. Most EBPs have been studied in several large-scale clinical trials, involving thousands of children and/or adolescents. These trials have carefully compared the effects of EBPs with other types of psychological treatments. Dozens of multiyear studies have shown that EBPs can reduce symptoms significantly for many years following the end of psychological treatment.

The most commonly used EBP approaches for the treatment of psychological symptoms involve cognitive/behavior therapies (CBT). The efficacy of CBT has been demonstrated for a wide range of symptoms in adults, adolescents, and children.

When parents look for mental health treatment for a child or adolescent, it is common to search for a psychotherapy provider who has an open schedule, affordable fees, or is covered by a specific insurance plan. However, it is also essential that parents or guardians in search of treatment get specific information about the type of treatment that a mental health care provider will offer for their child. Not all mental health treatments for young people are equally efficacious, and parents must be educated when searching for a therapist (Kuehn, 2011).

Mental health care providers (i.e., psychotherapists, such as psychologists, social workers, and psychiatrists) may subscribe to different "schools of thought," or philosophies on how to effectively reduce psychological symptoms in young people. Some of these philosophies are based directly on scientific evidence that indicates the best routes to symptom relief, whereas other mental health care providers may offer treatment that is not based on strong scientific evidence, or for which no evidence is available to date.

Healthy People 2020 Objectives Related to Mental Health

Healthy People 2020 (DHHS, 2010) has introduced a number of objectives for our nation related to mental health. Consistent with some of the major issues people experience within the mental health arena, these include objectives related to suicide, eating disorders, treatment, employment, screening, and intervention. Some specific objectives that relate to mental health and adolescents address suicide and eating disorders and screening practices.

Screening, Referral, and Access to Services

In terms of screening to reduce the suicide rate, target baselines seek to reduce the number of people that are affected by suicide to 10.2 per 100,000 by the year 2020, and reduce the number of suicide attempts made by adolescents. In efforts to meet these goals, some additional objectives have been identified to include increasing the proportion of children with mental health problems who receive treatment, and increasing the proportion of primary care physician office visits that screen youth aged 12 to 18 for depression.

With regard for eating disorders, specifically, *Healthy People 2020* seeks to reduce the proportion of adolescents who engage in disordered eating behaviors in an attempt to control their weight. According to the most recent version of the Behavioral Risk Factor Surveillance System data (CDC, 2011), nearly 15% of the population is afflicted by eating disorders at the current time. Ideally, the target that CDC would like to see is a reduction to 10.2% of our youth population that suffer from eating disorders. Without some careful and committed interventions, reaching this goal will be difficult, thus interventions targeting this group of young adults will be important.

Access to mental health services will also be an important dimension to consider when working to address the mental health needs of our population. Screening is the first line of defense in this goal. *Healthy People 2020* seeks to increase the proportion of primary care physician office visits that screen people 12 and older for depression. According to the National Medical Care Ambulatory Care Survey (CDC, 2010), only 2.4% of the population is being screened for depression during visits to their primary care physician. Meeting the goal of 10% of the population to be screened by 2020 may seem arduous, but with efforts, this benchmark may be reached. Overall, *Healthy People 2020* would also like to reduce the number of people who suffer from depression, and see a 10% improvement in depression rates. According to the National Survey on Drug Use and Health, (SAMHSA, 2008), nearly 7.5% of the population aged 12 to 17 were diagnosed with depression, and slightly over 6% of adults identified themselves as suffering from depression.

Children and adolescents who reside in juvenile residential facilities have also been identified in *Healthy People 2020* as in need of receiving screening and treatment for mental health issues. According to the National Health Interview Survey (2008), about 75% of children who are identified with mental health concerns do not receive adequate treatment for their issues. In addition, only 64% of juvenile facilities screen for mental health issues upon admission. Within both of these areas, the *Healthy People 2020* goals identified seek to improve the use of screening and treatment by 10% by the year 2020. In addition to these goals, *Healthy People 2020* seeks to increase the proportion of primary care facilities that provide mental health treatment onsite or by paid referral.

Other *Healthy People 2020* goals include the need to increase the proportion of people with serious mental illness who are employed by 10% from 58.4% (SAMHSA, 2008) and increase the proportion of people who receive treatment for co-occurring disorders such as mental health and drug abuse by 10%. According to the National Survey on Drug Use (SAMHSA, 2008), only 3% of this population actually received treatment for their co-occurring disorders.

Public health social workers play a role in these goals through a number of standards and competencies that are exercised through public health practice at the micro, mezzo, and macro levels. The next section of this chapter explores the specific public health social work competencies and how they are intertwined with public health social work within the mental health arena.

THE CORE FUNCTIONS OF PUBLIC HEALTH AND MENTAL HEALTH AND PUBLIC HEALTH SOCIAL WORK COMPETENCIES

The core functions of public health articulate a series of essential services framed under the three core functions of assessment, policy development, and assurance within the field of mental health. This section examines each of the three core functions, 10 essential services, and public health social work competencies that play a role within each of the core functions.

Assessment

1. *Monitor health status to identify community health problems*. Public health social workers working in the area of mental health assess the individual, place, and environment in efforts to address the impact conditions may have on individuals, families, and communities. In addition, community assessment is conducted to carry out needs assessments in a variety of situations. For example, following Hurricane Katrina, and the 2011 tsunami in Japan, public health social workers were available to assist victims with the traumatic events, including loss of families, homes, and communities. An overall assessment of the community situation also led to efforts to provide debriefing to communities and people within the communities. Public health social workers also assess the impact of need for individuals, families, groups, and communities, following catastrophic events such as shootings, or massive community injury. Follow-up and debriefing with the community in Arizona following the shooting rampage in a parking lot that took the lives of many and seriously injured U.S. Representative Gabrielle Giffords is another example of community assessment.

2. *Diagnose and investigate health problems and health hazards in the community*. Public health social workers utilize their assessment skills to identify, investigate, and address health hazards in various ways. The counting of mental health disorders to identify incidence and prevalence is a skill carried out by public health social workers in their role as an investigator of health problems within a given community. Collaborative investigation with medical examiners can identify environmental conditions that may be of concern, as well as situations where individuals may be at risk of suicide. The evaluation and investigation of nuisance complaints is also within the purview of public health social workers working in mental health situations.

3. *Evaluate effectiveness, accessibility, and quality of personal and population-based health services*. Public health social workers

working in the arena of mental health carry out a variety of tasks that examine the mental health outcomes of service delivery systems. Most state mental health divisions or departments have reporting procedures based on outcomes and diagnoses, which can then be used to help identify the need for additional services. Public health social workers also contribute to our understanding of the incidence and prevalence of psychiatric disorders through data management and can examine the effectiveness of interventions through performance-plan monitoring. Needs assessments are also easily carried out through the use of data and performance monitoring.

Policy Development

1. *Develop policies and plans that support individual and community health efforts*. Public health social workers play key roles in policy development, and utilize a variety of skills and competencies to support individuals and facilitate community health efforts. In many states, communities, or counties, a mental health board provides oversight of and regulatory mandates for mental health services. In some instances, like in the state of Illinois, county boards have regulatory oversight for mandated mental health services, and public health social workers play a pivotal role in overseeing that these services are carried out. Public hearings may address proposed changes to state legislation impacting the provision and delivery of mental health services. Grants are sometime given to community-based agencies to provide services to people with severe and persistent mental illness. Often, the monitoring and performance planning activities are supervised and managed by public health social workers.

2. *Enforce laws and regulations that protect health and ensure safety*. Under the guise of professional licensure and regulation, public health social workers have worked together to establish public health social work competencies, which govern their practice across all fields, including mental health. In addition, each state has its own rules concerning safety for its citizens and protection from those who are a danger to themselves and others. Public health social workers are often consulted to weigh in on which changes to the existing legislation will affect both the consumers and the people in the general community. Public health social workers often find cases of people who may have diagnoses of a severe and persistent mental illness as they go about their work in the enforcement of state/county/local health-related rules and ordinances.

3. *Conduct research to determine new insights and innovative solutions to health problems*. The practice of conducting health needs

assessments, especially in an effort to identify the health needs of a population, are carried out by public health social workers. In addition to needs assessments, the practice of surveying consumers to identify if they were satisfied with services and practices also falls under this essential function. Competencies used to carry out these functions include the ability to utilize leadership and skills to take initiative toward orchestrating data collection and analysis and dissemination.

Assurance

1. *Link people to needed personal health services and assure the provision of health care when otherwise unavailable.* This essential function calls public health social workers to practice the act of referral and to collaborate with other programs and services in an effort to assure a total care plan for the individual/family and community. Three specific areas where referrals are often made across helping professions occurs within the Maternal and Child Health programs, the Women and Infant Children programs, and critical access hospitals. Cases of women who suffer from post partum depression are often identified by public health social workers, who refer these women on for more intensive screening, intervention, and treatment. Critical access hospitals and emergency rooms can often be the first line of intervention in many cases, especially in remote and rural communities.

2. *Assure a competent public health and personal health care workforce.* The assurance of a competent public health workforce is a key factor in the process of building capacity and developing needs assessments and planning interventions of mental health issues within the community. Public health social workers often survey mental health practitioners, case aides, and agencies that serve individuals with mental illness to identify needed training areas for professional development and continuing education courses. In like manner, the same public health social workers will participate in regional committees, such as regional bio emergency councils, to help identify training needs and training topics for community, and professional members.

3. *Inform, educate, and empower people about mental health issues.* Public health social workers inform and educate the public about mental health issues in a variety of ways. Community education efforts are carried out annually to educate people about the signs and symptoms of depression. These efforts include public awareness through the local school systems and through the use of community public media campaigns. Another example of community health education and health promotion efforts include media campaigns that

have taken place to educate people on the signs and symptoms, detection of, and intervention for various types of dementia. Public health social workers have engaged in local community and grassroots efforts by using public health education through the media and other community presentations. Examples of these interventions include weekly newspaper articles about mental health topics that are written in regional newspapers, such as the "Mind and Body" column published in *The Southern Illinoisan*. Each week, public health social workers take turns writing on specific mental health topics to increase awareness of diagnostic information and potential interventions as a way to reach the community.

Health fairs are also strategies to provide information to the general public on mental health topics. Information fairs that target senior citizens or older adults also provide similar information are strategies that public health social workers use to educate the public. In addition, public health social workers can participate in senior fairs, and provide handouts on topics of interest to older adults. Working within the school system, public health social workers also carry out educational efforts by educating the general public on mental health topics such as eating disorders, bullying, and self-esteem.

4. *Mobilize community partnerships to identify and solve health problems*. Public health social workers work tirelessly with community partnerships in various fields to develop coalitions and collaborations in efforts to build resources and address community issues that improve the mental vitality and well-being of communities' residents. Across the nation we see coalitions for addressing the mental health needs of children, people affected by domestic violence, and older adults and grandparents raising grandchildren. Community partnerships including membership from a variety of factions include academia, faith-based communities, education, recreation, industry, law enforcement, county attorneys, community-betterment groups, disability rights groups, and housing authorities. A specific example of such a coalition includes the Coalition for Mental Health and Aging, operated nationwide, with state chapter affiliates.

SUMMARY

This chapter has reviewed a number of issues affecting the mental health status of individuals and communities. Notably, screening and assessment for mental health disorders, access to care, and timely intervention are a few strategies identified. Eating disorders and suicide risk factors were also addressed in the chapter. *Healthy People 2020* objectives related to mental health were also explored. Last, an exploration of how the core public health functions and public health social work standards and competencies are interwoven into the work of public health social workers with respect to mental health were explored. Despite the issues discussed, a host of other issues for the future remain and require some discussion. The next segment will address emerging issues for the future.

EMERGING ISSUES/ISSUES FOR THE FUTURE

This chapter has explored a series of issues that impact mental health for individuals and communities. Issues that will affect the field in the future include mental health and older adults, children's mental health, telemedicine options for rural and difficult-to-reach population groups (Crilly, Keefe, & Volpe, 2011), screening and assessment strategies, and interdisciplinary collaboration.

Mental health and older adult needs

Traditionally, disorders in older adults that relate to psychopathology have been neglected and often perceived as a part of the aging process. Issues such as depression and anxiety, which can be commonly found in older adults, are often misdiagnosed as simply medical issues. The increasing numbers of baby boomers will put ongoing pressure on mental health programs to address the screening and education needs of older adults.

Children's mental health

Evidence suggests that children struggle with various mental health issues. Programs and services will be needed as professionals and parents become more aware of how children have distinct but specialized psychiatric needs. *Healthy People 2020* calls for the need to address children's access to mental health screenings through primary care physicians and through juvenile detention centers. As the incidence of mental health disorders in children increases, the need to address children's mental health issues in the future will be critical (Joe & Bryant, 2007).

Telemedicine options

Increasingly, rural and smaller communities will not have access to psychiatric specialties; thus, the need for other strategies to provide diagnosis and treatment will be necessary. Telemedicine, the ability to provide interactive health care utilizing modern technology and telecommunications, will provide options for small and rural communities to provide assessment and treatment for difficult–to-reach populations in the future (Crilly, Keefe, & Volpe, 2011).

Gatekeeper functions

Gatekeepers are trained professionals or service workers who naturally engage with older adults and other citizens in the community, such as the water meter reader, or postal workers. In the future, these individuals will be critical in communities to help detect and recognize people who could easily become isolated in the community, such as older adults.

Depression screening

Screening for depression can be an effective way of locating cases of people who could be at risk for suicide or chronic episodes of depression. In an effort to reduce the current level of depression by 10% (as defined by *Healthy People 2020*), screening will become an integral clinical practice. In the future, we can expect that resources will be built into primary care practices to provide screening for depression through the use of a social worker who will visit with the patient, prior to the visit with the primary care practitioner. In the future, we can also anticipate major efforts to provide depression screening through community events, on college campuses, and in high schools. Hand in hand with screening efforts, we can expect that we will see an increase in educational resources about depression that target groups and interventions tailored for different cohorts across the life span (i.e., teens, college-aged people, young adults, middle-aged adults, and older adults).

Interdisciplinary practice with other specialties to provide integrated services

Shrinking resources, financial and economic limitations and competition for resources will force mental health and other professionals to work in concert with each other through multi-disciplinary and inter-disciplinary collaboration. This will include professionals such as substance abuse help providers, aging service providers, adult protective services, elder abuse investigators, and child welfare and child protective service workers along with public health social workers.

CLASSROOM EXERCISES

Activity #1

Consider the following case scenarios: You are part of a campus-wide committee that has been appointed to develop a series of community interventions (on campus and within the local high schools) for Mental Health Month.

What would you do to address the issues described, and how would you integrate the *Healthy People 2020* objectives, core functions (assessment, policy development, and assurance), and public health social work competencies?

1. Suzie's mother died a year ago, but Suzie just cannot seem to "move on." Suzie is still having a hard time sleeping at night and concentrating in school. Last week, I even caught Suzie crying in the school washroom. Some people have seen her take some pills (depression).
2. Brandon has recently graduated from high school and will be attending a local university this year. Brandon was always exercising and working out in high school. He now spends a lot of time weight training at the gym. He has been putting on a lot of muscle lately, and he is always talking about working out and getting bigger. Brandon takes supplements, drinks protein shakes, and has started using creatine (an amino acid). When I am talking to Brandon he almost sounds as if he wants to become the next Superman. I am really worried about Brandon because he gets agitated and angry very easily (muscle dysmorphia).
3. Jenny and Sam are best friends. They have played volleyball together since Grade 7. Sam has noticed that every winter Jenny withdraws from her friends and always seems sad. Every winter, Sam thinks that it is her fault ... that she has done something to Jenny to upset her. Once spring arrives, Jenny slowly returns to her "normal" self (seasonal affective disorder).
4. Chris is constantly worried about catching colds. In fact, he washes his hands about 20 times a day. When asked, Chris says that he cannot afford to be sick, and then goes into a lecture about how many germs there are around at any given time. Sometimes Chris washes his hands so much that they bleed (obsessive–compulsive disorder).
5. Hailey's parents were divorced when she was 6. Since then, she has been spending every second weekend with her father. She is now 16, in high school and does not want to go to her father's house every second weekend anymore. Instead, she wants to work and spend more time with her school friends. Her father lives in another part of the city, which is quite a distance from where she lives. When Hailey is at his house there is not much to do. Her father smokes, which bothers her, but she realizes that he is lonely and needs her help to do household chores (stress).

Activity #2

How would you develop an action plan for a Depression Screen Day within your community? Using essential services defined by the core functions, develop a plan and timeline to meet this goal.

Activity #3

You call to visit Mr. E, a 68-year-old man with a long history of psychosis. When you arrive to visit him, you are met by his neighbor, who comes to tell you that Mr. E has been pacing up and down in the street in a very agitated state and talking to himself. The neighbor does not know where Mr. E is now but is very worried about him. During the course of the conversation, you discover that there are several more older adults living in the community high-rise building with behaviors that seem to be abnormal.

What kinds of screening, intervention, and educational strategies can be implemented in this high-rise building?

How would you develop an action plan to meet these needs as a public health social worker?

INTERNET RESOURCES

National Alliance for the Mentally Ill

(www.nami.org)

This website provides information to consumers to help them adapt, cope, or adjust to the impact of a mental illness. It provides helpful information about how to adjust to the stigma of mental illness, locate helpful resources, connect to legislative action, and find additional sources of support.

National Institute of Mental Health

(www.nimh.nih.gov)

This website, established by the federal government's National Institute of Mental Health, provides a plethora of resources and related topics to mental health. Its scientific division provides information and statistics on mental health topics, funding alerts, legislative action, and fact sheets on a range of mental health topics. Various health topics are also showcased on the website, as are educational resources. Some specific modules have also been developed which address topics of interest related to mental health.

National Mental Health Association

(www.nmha.org)

The National Mental Health Association is an advocacy-based group that works to advance the needs within the field of mental health. It provides advocacy and publishes policy statements in various areas, including system transformation as well as issues on rights and privacy, service use, children, criminal justice, and procedures.

American Psychiatric Association

(www.psych.org)

The American Psychiatric Association is known for the development of the *Diagnostic and Statistical Manual of Mental Disorders*. The American Psychiatric Association was founded in 1844, and is currently the largest organization focused on psychiatric concerns. It represents over 36,000 psychiatrists in the United States and worldwide. The organization works toward the assurance of humane care and the effective treatment of people with mental disorders.

American Psychological Association

(www.apa.org)

This group serves as a scientific and professional organization that represents the field of psychology in the United States. The organization, which is based in Washington, DC, boasts of more than 154,000 members, and works toward fulfilling the mission of advancing communication and dissemination of psychological knowledge to benefit society and improve the lives of people. The website provides an overview of current research, educational forums, and materials to educate psychologists and the general public.

National Mental Health Information Center (for the) Substance Abuse and Mental Health Services Administration

(www.mentalhealth.samhsa.org)

This website provides information about pertinent interventions and treatments for various mental disorders. It provides a range of resources, including evidence-based treatments and interventions that have been identified to have been proven to be clinically effective.

REFERENCES

American Academy of Child and Adolescent Psychiatry. (2010). *Tips for clinical practice*. Retrieved from http://www.aacap.org/

Bahrer-Kohler, S. (2011). *Social determinants of mental health*. Hauppauge, NY: Nova Publishers.

Blakemore, S. (2009). Age discrimination hinders access to quality services. *Mental Health Practice, 12*(9), 8–9.

Bloom, B., Cohen, R. A., & Freeman, G. (2009). Summary health statistics for U.S. children: National health interview survey, 2008. *National Center for Health Statistics. Vital Health Stat 10*(244). http://www.cdc.gov/nchs/data/series/sr_10/sr10_244.pdf

Centers for Disease Control and Prevention. (2006). *National adolescent health information*. Fact sheet. Retrieved from www.cdc.gov/HealthyYouth/Injury

Centers for Disease Control and Prevention. (2011a). *Behavioral risk factor surveillance system*. Retrieved from http://apps.nccd.cdc.gov/youthonline/App/Default.aspx?SID=HS

Centers for Disease Control and Prevention. (2011b). Suicide Prevention: Youth Suicide. Web-based Injury Statistics Query and Reporting System. Retrieved October 2011, from http://www.cdc.gov/injury/wisqars/index.html

Cole, E., Stevenson, M., & Rogers, B. (2009). The influence of cultural beliefs on self-reported mental health status and mental health service utilization in an ethnically diverse sample of older adults. *Journal of Feminist Policy Theory, 21*, 1–17.

Copeland-Linder, N., Lambert, S., & Ialongo, N. (2010). Community violence, protective factors, and adolescent mental health: A profile analysis. *Journal of Clinical Child & Adolescent Psychology, 39*(2), 176–186.

Crilly, J. F., Keefe, R. H., & Volpe, F. (2011). Use of electronic technologies to promote community and personal health for individuals unconnected to healthcare systems. *American Journal of Public Health, 101*(7), 1163–1167.

Cuijpers, P., & Smit, F. (2008). Has the time come for broad-scale dissemination for prevention of depressive disorders? *Acta Psychiatrica Scandinavica*, 419–420. doi:10.1111/j.1600-0447.2008.01294.x

Degnan, K. A., Almas, A. N., & Fox, N. A. (2010). Temperament and the environment in the etiology of childhood anxiety. *Journal of Child Psychology and Psychiatry, 51*(4), 497–517.

Flood, M., & Buckwalter, K. (2009). Recommendations for mental health care of older adults: Part 2—An overview of dementia, delirium, and substance abuse. *Journal of Gerontological Nursing, 35*(2), 35–47.

Fox, J. K., Halpern, L. F., & Forsyth, J. P. (2008). Mental health checkups for children and adolescents: A means to identify, prevent, and minimize suffering associated with anxiety and mood disorders. *Clinical Psychology: Science & Practice, 15*(3), 182–211.

Gould, M., Greenberg, T., Velting, D., & Shaffer, D. (2003). Youth suicide risk and preventive interventions: A review of the past 10 years. *Journal of the American Academy of Child and Adolescent, 42*(4), 386–405.

Hensley, M., Corrigan, P., Watson, A., Byrne, P., & Davis, K. (2005). Mental illness stigma: Problem of public health or social justice? *Social Work, 50*, 363–368.

Hoffman, J., Baldwin, S., & Cerbone, F. (2003). Onset of major depressive disorder among adolescents. *Journal of the American Academy of Child Adolescent Psychiatry, 47*(2), 217–224.

Joe, S., & Bryant, H. (2007). Evidence-based suicide prevention screening in schools. *Children & Schools, 29*(4), 219–227.

Jurkowski, E. T. (2011). Psychosocial determinants of mental health. In S. Bahrer-Kohler (Ed.), *Social determinants of mental health* (pp. 19–36). Hauppauge, NY: Nova Publishers..

Karlin, B., & Fuller, J. (2007). Meeting the mental health needs of older adults: Implications for primary care practice. *Geriatrics, 62*(1), 26.

Karlin, B. E., & Zeiss, A. M. (2010). Transforming mental health care for older veterans in the veterans health Administration. *Generations, 34*(2), 74–83.

Kuehn, B. (2011). New guidance for clinicians on avoiding mental health problems in young people. *Journal of the American Medical Association, 305*(15), 1525–1526.

Kjolseth, I., Ekeberg, O., & Steihaug, S. (2010). Suicides in later life. *Curr Psychiatry Rep. 2011 June, 13*(3), 234–241. doi:10.1007/s11920-011-0193-3.

LaLonde, M. (1974). *A new perspective on the health of Canadians: A working document.* Ottawa, Ontario: Government of Canada.

Luoma, J., Pearson, J., & Martin, C. (2002). Contact with mental health and primary care prior to suicide: A review of the evidence. *American Journal of Psychiatry, 159,* 909–916.

McKeowan, T. (1971). *A historical appraisal of the medical task, from "Medical History and Medical Care."* Oxford, UK: Oxford University Press.

Muehlenkamp, J., Walsh, B., & McDade, M. (2010). Preventing non-suicidal self-injury in adolescents: The signs of self-injury program. *Journal of Youth & Adolescence, 39*(3), 306–314.

National Adolescent Health Information Center. (2006). Fact Sheet on Suicide: Adolescents & Young Adults. San Francisco, CA: Author, University of California, San Francisco. http://nahic.ucsf.edu/downloads/Suicide.pdf

National Adolescent Health Information Center (2008). Fact Sheet on Demographics: Adolescents and Youth. Retrieved from http://nahic.ucsf.edu/downloads/Demographics08.pdf

National Alliance on Mental Illness. (2011). *Eating Disorders.* Retrieved from http://www.nami.org/

National Center for Injury Prevention and Control (2012). Centers for Disease Control and Prevention, National Center for Injury Prevention and Control. Web-based Injury Statistics Query and Reporting System (WISQARS) [online]. Available January 31, 2012 from http://www.cdc.gov/ncipc/wisqars and http://www.nimh.nih.gov/health/publications/older-adults-depression-and-suicide-facts-fact-sheet/index.shtml

National Health Interview Survey: Data review (2008). http://www.cdc.gov/nchs/nhis/nhis_2008_data_release.htm

National Institute of Mental Health (2010). Teens who recover from hard to treat depression still at-risk for relapse. Retrieved from: http://www.nimh.nih.gov/science-news/2010/teens-who-recover-from-hard-to-treat-depression-still-at-risk-for-relapse.shtml

National Institute of Mental Health. (2011). *Spotlight on Eating Disorders.* Retrieved from http://www.nimh.nih.gov/health/publications/eating-disorders/complete-index.shtml

National Institute of Mental Health (NIHM, 2012). Suicide in America. National Institute of Mental Health. Office of Science Policy, Planning and Communications Science Writing, Press and Dissemination Branch

Peul, R., & Heuer, C. (2010). Obesity stigma: Important considerations for public health. *American Journal of Public Health, 100*(6), 1019–1028.

Practice Standards Development Committee. (2005). *Public health social work standards and competencies.* Columbus, OH: Ohio Department of Health. Retrieved March 5, 2012, from http://oce.sph.unc.edu/cetac/phswcompetencies_May05.pdf

Snowden, M., Dhingra, S., Keyes, C., & Anderson, L. (2010). Changes in mental well-being in the transition to late life: Findings from MIDUS I and II. *American Journal of Public Health*, *100*(12), 2385–2388.

Substance Abuse and Mental Health Services Administration (SAMHSA). (2008). National Survey on Drug Use and Health: National findings. http://oas.samhsa.gov/nsduh/2k8nsduh/2k8Results.cfm

Substance Abuse and Mental Health Services Administration (SAMHSA). (2009). Results from the 2008 National Survey on Drug Use and Health: National Findings (Office of Applied Studies, NSDUH Series H-36, HHS Publication No. SMA 09-4434), Rockville, MD. http://www.kap.samhsa.gov/products/manuals/tips/pdf/TIP50.pdf

United Nations World Health Organization. (2011). Investing in Mental Health . *UN World News Center, Oct. 10, 2011.* Retrieved from http://www.un.org/apps/news/story.asp?NewsID=39981&Cr=health&Cr1

United Nations World Health Organization. (2012). *Depression: A Global Crisis.* Retrieved from www.who.int/mental_health/en/

United States Department of Health and Human Services (1999). *The Surgeon General's report on mental health.* Washington, DC: U.S.: Government Printing Office.

United States Department of Health and Human Services. (2010). Depression: A Global Crisis. *Healthy People 2020.* Retrieved from http://www.healthypeople.gov/2020/about/default.aspx .

Wilson, M. (2009). Achieving a better balance. *Mental Health Practice*, *12*(9), 13.

PART IV

Selected Settings

*P*ublic health social workers will often work within geographic-specific communities such as rural towns, urban neighborhoods, and military bases. While working in these communities, they work to help residents assess the communities' needs, plan an approach to address those needs, and evaluate the approach used.

In this section, the chapters focus on public health social work practice in each of these communities. Chapter 14 focuses on the unique challenges public health social workers face practicing in rural areas. Some of the challenges include lack of formal resources, limited funding, and the "aging" of rural communities. To address these challenges, the federal government has developed policies and charged existing funding sources to provide support for research that identifies some of the unique needs inherent in rural public health social work practice.

Chapter 15 addresses neighborhoods and health, with a primary focus on urban neighborhoods. The author discusses the distinction between the built and social environments of various neighborhoods and some of the successful intervention efforts that have helped ameliorate the negative effects of living in neighborhoods that have negative health outcomes. Building on Chapters 14 and 15, Chapter 16 considers efforts public health social workers can engage in to empower the community to do its own research that assesses neighborhood problems, develops an intervention to eliminate those problems, and evaluates the intervention. The author provides helpful examples of interventions she has developed and evaluated.

The final chapter in this section addresses public health social work in the uniformed services. The author discusses some of the federal initiatives to involve social workers, the types of interventions needed to work with returning veterans, and the differences in practicing in the various branches of the military.

As you read the chapters in this section, consider other types of communities that are not geographic specific, but are rather communities of interest. Examples include the lesbian/gay/bisexual/transgender community, the community of breast cancer survivors, the Hispanic community, or any other community whose members are not clustered within an area but are widely distributed that needs our assistance as public health social workers. How would you reach out to these communities, help them to identify problems, develop a plan of action, and evaluate their intervention efforts? Consider the federal, state, and local policies in place that help or hinder access to services. What advocacy efforts could you engage in that would help to enhance access to services or perhaps develop additional services to meet the needs you have identified?

CHAPTER 14

Rural Health and Mental Health

Jeanne Saunders and Edward Saunders

INTRODUCTION

*P*ublic health social work practice in rural communities offers both rewards and challenges. This chapter explores the unique aspects of rural social work practice—as it can be distinguished from practice in urban communities. This chapter will provide public health social workers with (1) an understanding of definitions of "rurality" and "rural health," (2) an appreciation of the health and mental health disparities between rural and urban residents, (3) an understanding of the barriers to health and preventive health in rural communities, (4) an appreciation of research challenges within rural communities, (5) an appreciation of evolving practice strategies by public health social workers in rural communities, and (6) an understanding of the application of public health core functions and public health social workers competencies to rural practice.

WHAT IS *RURAL,* AND WHAT IS *RURAL HEALTH*?

There are a number of challenges to discuss "rural health" because the definition of "rural" varies among government officials, policymakers, and researchers. The U.S. Census Bureau defines rural as "open country and settlements with fewer than 2,500 residents"; this describes about 80% of the land mass of the United States (Economic Research Service, 2009). According to this definition, about 20% of the U.S. population (~50 million Americans) resides in rural areas. Economic Research Service researchers, working for the U.S. Department of Agriculture to examine the economics of food, farming, and natural resources in rural America, use the terms "metro" and "nonmetro" to distinguish urban from rural areas. These researchers identify *counties* in each state to identify metro and nonmetro areas for their research purposes. Using those definitions, approximately 25% of the U.S. population resides in rural, nonmetro, areas

(Economic Research Service, 2009). From a health perspective, urban or metro areas are easily identified as those with large populations and multiple services. Rural areas, by contrast, are those with much smaller communities and many fewer services.

While rural areas are often addressed as though they are homogeneous, they have unique characteristics based on their geographic location, historic and current racial/ethnic and cultural composition, population density, and economic base (Rainer, 2010). Rural areas are more economically diverse than urban areas. For example, a larger proportion of rural residents are engaged in manufacturing compared to urban residents. Rural areas are increasingly becoming more culturally diverse as immigrant populations move into them. These characteristics contribute to a local culture that influences the daily lives and the service needs in a given area.

As Davenport and Davenport (2008) pointed out, the diversity within rural communities refutes the prevalent myth of one rural America. Human needs, including health and mental health care, differ significantly as in, for example, between residents of a rural retirement community and a mining community (especially a boom town with many young families). Similarly, the needs of a rural university town with many educated affluent persons would vary from those of an impoverished rural community in the Mississippi Delta. Understanding such differences is vital for good social and health care policy and necessary for public health social workers' practice.

Another unique difference among rural areas is the variance in their proximity and access to larger urban areas for health services. A rural area that has ready access to a major highway has better access to services provided in an urban area, making it less isolated or "less rural" (Dye, Willoughby, & Battisto, 2011). Therefore, among rural areas, there is considerable variation that influences access to health, mental health, and related supportive services.

Demographic trends in the United States suggest that rural areas are increasingly becoming "older" as younger persons and families move to urban/suburban areas for employment and educational opportunities (Kaufman, Scogin, Burgio, Morthland, & Ford, 2007). Elders in rural areas have traditionally chosen to stay in their home or local community. Elders are more likely to have different health needs and require different services (because of chronic health problems) when compared to the needs of younger families living in the same area. This changing demographic provides challenges to the limited health providers and facilities available to rural residents.

Practitioners and researchers have long identified the unique health and mental health challenges faced by rural residents and providers (Smalley et al., 2010). The federal government recognized these needs by establishing the Office of Rural Health Policy and the National Rural Health Advisory

Committee within the Health Resources and Services Administration (HRSA) in 1987. These offices have provided support for research to identify rural health issues and policy development for their resolution (Ricketts, 1999). Yet, challenges related to geography; rural infrastructure; federal, state, and local policies; and limited funding all contribute to ongoing problems of access to health and mental health care in rural America.

Health disparities and access to health and mental health care services in rural or remote areas are not unique to the United States. Other nations that have a similar geographic space and population distribution experience many of the same challenges. For example, Australia and Canada (two countries similar to the United States) have given equal attention to rural health issues in their efforts to ensure that rural residents receive comparable health and mental health care as their urban counterparts. Recognizing the need for increased health promotion; reducing barriers related to transportation; the limited size, scope, and availability of services; and recruiting and retaining health professionals in rural areas are common issues (Humphreys, 2009).

CHANGING DEFINITIONS OF HEALTH AND HEALTH DISPARITY

Early definitions of health service access largely focused on access to primary health and acute care services. Today, health is defined more broadly to include holistic and preventative care, care for chronic conditions and mental health; and care to support individuals, families, communities, and health care providers to manage all aspects of health (Wakerman, 2009).

By virtue of their training, public health social workers are especially aware of the social determinants of health. In particular, the socioeconomic circumstances—the places where people live and work—strongly influence health and contributes to health disparities.

Healthy People 2020 defined a health disparity as a

> Particular type of health difference that is closely linked with social, economic, and/or environmental disadvantage. Health disparities adversely affect groups of people who have systematically experienced greater obstacles to health based on their racial or ethnic group; religion; socioeconomic status; gender; age; mental health; cognitive, sensory, or physical disability; sexual orientation or gender identity; geographic location; or other characteristics historically linked to discrimination or exclusion. (U.S. Department of Health and Human Services, 2010)

In the following section, disparities associated with *geographic location* are described, with attention given to both health and mental health conditions.

HEALTH AND MENTAL HEALTH DISPARITIES BETWEEN RURAL AND URBAN RESIDENTS IN THE UNITED STATES

Rural areas of the United States have a distinct set of health and mental health problems. According to the Economic Research Service/U.S. Department of Agriculture (Jones, Parker, Ahearn, Mishra, & Variyam, 2009), rural residents in the United States have higher rates of age-adjusted mortality, disability, and chronic disease than urban residents. Rural residents are also more likely to be older, less likely to be from a minority group (if they are farmers), have lower incomes and education levels and are also more likely to smoke, to be obese, and to be physically inactive compared to urban residents (Eberhardt & Pamuk, 2004). Rural areas also have a higher incidence of infant mortality and preterm infants than urban areas (Baldwin et al., 2009). Health disparities previously documented between racial and ethnic groups compared to Whites (Keefe, 2010) add to the complexity of the disparities found by geographic location for those populations.

Injuries associated with rural occupations (farming, mining, lumbering) are of particular concern in rural areas, not only because of their higher incidence but also because of the higher per capita trauma death rates and the limited resources available to treat them. Delayed discovery of injuries, long transportation times, rudimentary training of prehospital personnel, fewer available physicians, and less experience with trauma patients all lead to poorer prognoses for patients injured in rural than in urban settings (*Encyclopedia of Public Health*, 2011).

In addition, health problems are unique to certain rural areas. Farming communities, for example, have a higher prevalence of zoonotic diseases (those transmitted between animals and humans), insecticide and pesticide poisoning, farm machinery accidents, and farmers' lung disease. By comparison, rural areas in West Virginia have health problems such as black lung disease, which is unique to coal miners (*Encyclopedia of Public Health*, 2011). All warrant the attention of public health social workers.

The prevalence of HIV/AIDS and sexually transmitted diseases is growing in rural America and requires increasing attention from public health social workers.

> In contrast to the early 1980s, the twenty-five US counties with the highest rates of increase in HIV infection during the 1990s were mostly rural counties with an average population of 73,000. The expansion of the AIDS epidemic to rural areas is worrisome because rural communities have fewer adequate health care facilities and services than urban areas, particularly for the care of such a complex and multifaceted disease as AIDS. (*Encyclopedia of Public Health*, 2011, p. 2)

HIV/AIDS is also one example of a health condition that carries a social stigma that further limits rural residents' access to needed care.

Disparities in mental health between rural and urban residents have been documented. While some have found that the difference in prevalence is small, but significant, the impact of those problems is greater for residents in rural areas that have limited access to, and availability of, services and a greater stigma attached to mental health care (HRSA, 2005). Epidemiological studies have documented higher levels of depression, substance abuse (and co-occurring disorders), domestic violence, incest, and child abuse among rural residents compared to urban residents (Hutchison & Blakely, 2003).

An estimated 34% to 41% of patients in primary care in rural areas have a diagnosable mental health disorder (Sears, Evans, & Kuper, 2003). Suicide, especially among adolescents, is more prevalent among rural residents (Eckert, Kutek, Dunn, Air, & Goldney, 2010; Gamm, Stone, & Pittman, 2003). However, despite the differences in prevalence and recognized greater impact of poor mental health, rural residents receive less mental health care than urban residents (Hauenstein et al., 2007). The adjusted odds of receiving mental health care in urban areas are 47% higher than in rural areas; the adjusted odds of receiving specialized mental health care are 72% higher in urban areas than in rural areas.

Lenardson, Ziller, Lambert, Race, and Yousefian (2010) reported that there is a small but significant difference in the prevalence of mental health problems between rural and urban children, with a higher prevalence among rural children. Rural parents report that they are able to access some services for their child, often in a school setting, but are unlikely to access all of the services their child needs and spend a significantly greater amount of time trying to access and coordinate services for their child compared to urban parents.

The common perception of adolescent problems and the interventions used to treat them are based on urban models, which often results in the perception that problems are not present among rural youth because of the different demographics (Myers, 2010). For example, in urban areas, issues of alcohol and drug use and gang violence are often believed to be problems among African American or other minority youth. However, in rural areas White youth typically have a higher prevalence of tobacco and alcohol use compared to African American or other minority youth. Moreover, rural youth, compared to urban youth, have higher rates of depression and substance use, including alcohol, tobacco, methamphetamines, inhalants, marijuana, and cocaine (Substance Abuse and Mental Health Services Administration, 2001).

BARRIERS TO HEALTH AND HEALTH PREVENTION IN RURAL COMMUNITIES

Rural residents face more challenges and barriers associated with accessing appropriate, timely, and cost-effective care than urban residents. Access to health care can be understood as comprising three factors: (1) physical access; (2) financial access; and (3) psychological access (Mohatt, 2000).

Poor physical access is generally understood as the difficulty that rural residents experience in obtaining health or mental health services due to geographic distance and the absence of services within their communities. Rural communities suffer from a shortage of health care providers. Approximately 60% of rural White Americans and 75% of rural minority Americans live in Health Professions Shortage Areas (Probst et al., 2002). Only about 10% of physicians in America practice in rural areas despite the fact that approximately one-fourth of the U.S. population lives in these areas (Gamm, Castillo, & Pittman, 2003). As a result, critical service delivery functions may go understaffed, employees are overworked, and there are fewer health care and long-term care facilities in rural communities. Rural health care facilities that do exist are less likely than urban facilities to be "state of the art" (Dye et al., 2011).

Similarly, availability of mental health services in rural America is limited by mental health professional shortages (Gamm, Stone et al., 2003); more than 85% of Mental Health Professional Shortage Areas are in rural regions (Bird, Dempsey, & Hartley, 2001). These practitioner shortages are largely associated with an inability of rural communities to recruit and retain mental health professionals because of lower salaries; limited social/cultural opportunities; and increased risk of ethical dilemmas, primarily dual relationships, in rural practice (Smalley et al., 2010).

Transportation is a key barrier that limits physical access to all services in rural areas. Because there are very few, if any, alternatives to owning a personal vehicle, rural residents totally rely on their vehicle and assume that roads are maintained and accessible at all times of the year. When the vehicle breaks down, there is not enough money for gas, or roads are not passable, access to health and mental health services is impossible (Dye et al., 2011). Transportation problems can result, for example, in a pregnant woman who does not routinely obtain quality prenatal care, a child with a chronic illness who misses appointments with a specialist to evaluate one's treatment progress, or an elderly person who is not able to refill a prescription that controls one's diabetes. Rural residents also experience longer response times by emergency medical services, and transport time to urban health settings at times of an emergency are considerably longer than for urban residents (Rawlinson & Crews, 2003).

Just as important as access to health and mental health care for acute and chronic conditions are the opportunities for prevention of health and mental

health problems. Health-promotion activities and smoking cessation programs are often limited in rural areas due to cost, population density, and
available professionals. Opportunities for exercise that would decrease
stress and obesity—and the attendant social interaction that reduces isolation and promotes mental health—that might be accessed at a local gym
or park in an urban area are often nonexistent or inconsistently available
in rural areas (Kaiser & Baumann, 2010). The inadequacies of programs
make it difficult to maintain an exercise routine. Rural women, in particular,
often feel it is unsafe to take walks on deserted roads and have few resources
for child care that allows them to maintain a routine. Other strategies for
better health, such as access to fresh fruits and vegetables, can be compromised in some communities by the reluctance of grocery stores to stock
these items because of a limited number of customers and the need to
contain costs.

Poor financial access, according to Mohatt (2000), is related to poverty as
well as the level and sources of funding on a larger community-wide scale. In
2009, 16.6% of rural residents, compared to 13.9% of urban residents, were
living in poverty (U.S. Census Bureau, 2009). Because of higher rates of
poverty in rural America, a greater proportion of rural residents, when compared to their urban counterparts, will often choose against costly health
and/or mental health care in favor of more basic needs for food, shelter,
and other necessities. Overall, rural households are more likely than urban
households to report that health care costs limit their medical care (Jones
et al., 2009).

There is a strong relationship between poverty and physical and mental
health and physical impairments over the life span (Wickrama, Kway, Lorenz,
Conger, & Surjadi, 2010). This is especially concerning given that approximately 22% of America's rural children live in poverty (O'Hare, 2009). Part
of the relationship between poverty and health/mental health impairment
is accounted for by material deprivation (e.g., lack of quantity and quality
of food). Psychological and social experiences associated with poverty also
contribute to health/mental health impairment in rural residents and
include physical illness and depression.

Access to health care in rural areas is often limited because a small population base does not allow for the economy of scale possible in urban areas. It
is often difficult to recruit and retain a health care workforce in rural areas
when urban centers are able to offer higher pay, access to up-to-date equipment and facilities, and a large network of providers (Humphreys, Wakerman, & Wells, 2006). While poverty is a factor that limits access to health
care at the individual level across urban and rural settings, it is exacerbated
at the rural level because rural areas also experience poverty that limits
the ability to provide services. Older rural residents with limited incomes
are especially at risk for less quality health care, particularly mental health

care, because of the additional mobility and isolation challenges they experience (Kaufman et al., 2007).

The number of health care facilities and providers are more limited in rural areas, resulting in rural residents needing to seek services in urban areas. Costs incurred from traveling these distances are not covered by Medicare, Medicaid, or private insurance—resulting in rural residents paying a higher out-of-pocket cost. Alternative forms of transportation between rural and urban areas are not typically available or are limited to a small number of destinations (Smalley et al., 2010). Collectively, these issues result in health and mental health care for rural residents that is often inefficient and expensive.

The lack of health insurance is another serious factor influencing access to health care among impoverished rural residents. Rural residents are more likely than urban residents to be uninsured (Bolin & Gamm, 2003), which often results in greater likelihood that they will not seek preventive health care or obtain needed tests and prescriptions. When self-employed rural residents—notably farmers—face economic problems, they often sacrifice their health insurance and are less likely to seek care until the problems become serious. Among all farm-operated households, 14% did not have health insurance during 2007 (Jones et al., 2009). Similarly, small rural businesses often do not provide health insurance to their employees due to the cost of a small group policy, contributing to a lack of access to health and mental health care among rural residents when compared to urban residents.

By "psychological access," Mohatt (2000) referred to the consumer traits that interfere with or facilitate health and/or mental health service utilization. Previous narrow definitions of "access" to health care have been expanded because regardless of whether or not there is a primary health care provider available in one's community, an individual may not seek care for other reasons. Race/ethnicity, education, age, "rural culture," perceptions of confidentiality, and stigma associated with some health and mental health diseases are among the factors that also determine whether or not an individual seeks care (Kaufman et al., 2007).

A rural, impoverished farmer, for example, may not have access to health care information (poor health literacy), have limited access to nutritious foods, and might smoke because "everyone in town smokes." Because of limited health literacy, he might not recognize some indicators of health problems and thus not know to seek medical care. It is possible that he recognizes a health problem, but because he was raised in a "stoic" rural culture he might be less inclined to seek medical care in the belief that he can "tough it out." This individual might also believe that the health care provider will not understand his situation because the provider is of a different race or ethnicity, has a different sexual orientation, or is "too young." In any case, this farmer is unlikely to seek out care unless a serious health crisis occurs.

Perceived stigma related to a health or mental health condition is another factor that influences access to health and mental health care in rural areas (Gorman et al., 2007; Rainer, 2010). Anonymity and privacy are much harder to maintain in a small, tight-knit community, and the fear of being identified as having a mental illness, for example, keeps some rural residents from seeking the help they need (Gorman et al., 2007). Stigma toward mental health services has been shown to have an inverse relationship with population size; the smaller the community, the larger the stigma (Hoyt, Conger, Valde, & Weihs, 1997).

For some racial/ethnic groups and indigenous populations (i.e., American Indian and Alaska Natives), health and mental health care and access to services are further jeopardized by a dearth of culturally appropriate services; many services, in fact, are provided using an urban model and do not integrate cultural and spiritual beliefs important to rural residents. Issues of past and current oppression, racism and discrimination, and little regard for effective indigenous practices in service provision and funding decisions create major barriers to health and mental health care for indigenous populations (Goodkind et al., 2010).

CHALLENGES IN CONDUCTING RURAL-BASED RESEARCH

To date, the vast majority of research on rural health care has provided descriptive data on perceptions of access to care. Although these data are important, it is equally important to study effective rural models of health care delivery to build our knowledge of evidence-based practice in rural communities (Wakerman, 2009). Service delivery models must be evaluated, as must clinical information systems, use of consumer input, and levels of community engagement. It is not practical to develop a service delivery system that is dependent on one key person or the beneficence of one community, which cannot be replicated in other areas. Information on how the system adapts and changes over time with the changing context is also useful information.

In many respects, conducting research in rural areas is not unlike conducting research in urban areas. However, conducting culturally competent research is perhaps most important (Goodkind et al., 2010; Kaufman et al., 2007). Understanding the cultural context of a given community or group within a community is necessary if a researcher is to receive the dual support of community leaders and potential participants. To produce the most valid research, a researcher needs to understand community beliefs and values, cultural practices, widely held religious or spiritual beliefs, stigma that might be attached to participating in a research study (e.g., an admission of having a mental health problem), and possible resistance to "outsiders" who are not part of the community or population group being studied.

Researchers also need to be mindful of the potential for additional costs when conducting research in rural areas (Kaufman et al., 2007). If researchers are not embedded in the community, costs for transportation and those related to travel time, communication, and the time needed to become "accepted" into the community must all be calculated into the cost of the research study. Given the short deadlines sometimes connected to grant funding, these issues need to be addressed prior to application for funds.

Because there is no clear definition of "rural culture," future research is needed to understand how the intersection of individuals in their unique rural communities (i.e., culture) makes a difference in their health (Hartley, 2004). Wakerman (2006) argued that there is an ongoing need to ensure that research is used for policy development so that the health and mental needs of rural residents are better understood among urban-centric policymakers.

EVOLVING SOCIAL WORK PRACTICE STRATEGIES IN RURAL COMMUNITIES

Given the many challenges of providing adequate, culturally appropriate, and cost-effective health and mental health care to rural residents, public health social workers continually explore "new and improved" strategies for providing services. Increasingly, computer technology is being used in rural communities to improve access to care and the quality of care available to rural residents. This section provides two examples of the use of new technologies over the past decade: mental health screenings and telemedicine (inclusive of telepsychiatry).

Given the limited number of providers of health and mental health services in rural areas, it is important to identify, through early screening processes, individuals who require follow-up care. Screening for depression by primary care physicians is a good example. Farrell et al. (2009) describe the use of brief computer screening completed by patients awaiting their primary care visit. Based on the instant feedback from the screening tool, primary care providers can readily identify individuals who will need further mental health screening and intervention.

Telemedicine is believed to be one of the most promising strategies to increase access to physical and mental health care for rural residents and their providers; however, it is not without challenges (Rainer, 2010; Spaulding, Cain, & Sonnenschein, 2011). Telemedicine connects patients in one area with providers in another area (via computer), thus eliminating the need for costly travel by patients in rural counties to urban health care centers. Telemedicine is theoretically available in any location that has access to a computer. Mental health clients can now receive screening and/ or counseling from a practitioner hundreds of miles away via a computer connection. Similarly, physicians, nurses, and other health providers (e.g., occupational therapists, physical therapists) in a rural office can now consult with health specialists in large urban health centers. However, barriers in using telemedicine include the discomfort that some clients feel in "talking to a computer screen," and a lack of infrastructure needed to facilitate these interactions. For example, health and mental health professionals often require the medical records of rural patients for whom a consultation is needed. However, because developing and maintaining electronic medical records is both time consuming and expensive, many rural providers do not use electronic medical files. A lack of electronic medical records consequently limits the exchange of medical information necessary for telemedicine.

The poor quality of computer networks in remote rural areas of America is also a concern; slow, dial-up connections make the transmission of data, voice, and video slow and cumbersome, if not impossible. Even when these technical problems can be overcome, special medical tests are often needed by consulting physicians to make an accurate diagnosis. Unfortunately, in too many cases, rural medical facilities are not able to conduct these tests because they lack costly, specialized equipment or adequately trained personnel.

Public health social workers should advocate for increased federal funds for rural health and mental health care and use these funds to develop more creative strategies to care for rural residents. Using their advocacy skills, public health social workers can encourage more health and mental health professionals to move to rural areas and promote increased training for existing professionals (Johnson, Brems, Warner, & Roberts, 2006). State and federal funding have been used successfully in the past, for example, to recruit health and mental health professionals to rural areas, to facilitate the supervision of rural-based physician assistants by physicians in urban areas, and to improve facilities and technology in rural communities.

CORE PUBLIC HEALTH FUNCTIONS AND COMPETENCIES IN RURAL PRACTICE

Public health social workers practicing in rural communities across the United States use their micro, mezzo, and macro practice skills to carry out the three core public health functions of assessment, policy development, and assurance (Institute of Medicine, 1988). The continuing assessment of health and mental health status of rural residents to identify community health problems is a critical role that public health social workers play within their practice settings.

As these professionals investigate the specific health problems and health hazards facing rural residents, they can promote policy development that will support improved health and mental health services for the population. Policy improvement must focus on improved financial access to health and mental health services in impoverished rural communities. Public health social workers use their knowledge of research methods and statistics to investigate physical and mental health issues within the community. This research contributes to new insights and innovative solutions to health problems within their rural service areas. Continuing research into problems of access is necessary to improve health outcomes for rural residents.

In meeting the *assurance* function of public health, public health social workers use their micro-level skills to link rural residents to needed health and mental health services. Public health social workers must reach out to the most vulnerable of populations in rural America: the impoverished, the elderly, children, and persons with disabilities. Public health social workers must inform and educate rural residents about health issues. Finally, public health social workers use their community-organizing skills to mobilize community partnerships to identify and solve health problems unique to their communities. Public health social workers use their networking skills to build capacity within the physical and mental health infrastructures of rural America to better serve vulnerable rural residents.

Because of the core competencies attained as part of their professional training (Public Health Social Work Standards and Competencies, 2005), public health social workers have the knowledge, skills, values, and ethics to carry out the essential core public health functions in rural practice. Public health social workers can better address the health and mental health needs of rural residents by using their knowledge of social epidemiology, population-based health promotion and empowerment, life span perspective, planned change, protective and risk factors within population groups, and characteristics of health systems. Of particular importance is the cultural competence that public health social workers bring to their practice settings. Cultural competence is especially important in rural communities. Social workers possess professional knowledge of the strengths, needs, values, and practices of diverse cultural, ethnic, and socioeconomic groups. This knowledge is necessary to understand how various factors influence a group's access to care and how to develop more culturally responsive systems of care for them.

Using their methodological and analytic skills, public health social workers are prepared to engage in research that documents health and mental health needs within the community and help to evaluate strategies designed to address those needs. By collecting and interpreting data from vital statistics, censuses, surveys, service utilization, and other relevant community-based data, public health social workers can identify the most vulnerable and underserved populations in a community and the gaps in services (or access) that exist within their rural community.

Public health social workers have a wealth of leadership and communication skills to bring to their rural practice settings. Using their management and planning skills, public health social workers can effectively work to improve systems of physical and mental health care in rural communities. Workers can use their cultural competence to promote "best practice" prevention and intervention strategies to eliminate social inequity and health disparities within vulnerable minority populations.

Public health social workers' knowledge and skills in policy development and advocacy are critical to resolve systemic problems of access to care among rural residents. Coalition building and agenda setting to address the gaps in the physical and mental health systems in rural communities are essential. As workers mobilize support for policy changes, they communicate the effects of current barriers to care and identify policy options to remove these barriers.

Through the combination of knowledge, skills, values, and ethics they possess, public health social workers can enhance the health and mental health of rural Americans. Many public health social workers have found that the rewards of working in such close-knit communities and a sense of "making a difference" in these communities far outweigh the challenges they face in their rural practice.

QUESTIONS FOR DISCUSSION

1. Assume you are a public health social worker engaged in a "community empowerment effort" in rural Mississippi. What strategies would you use to help this community accomplish its stated goal of "including a public health Maternal and Child Health program in the new community center" being built in town?

2. Assume a public health nurse has asked you to intervene with a young Native American teen mother in rural South Dakota who refuses to have her newborn vaccinated because the mother says it is against tribal custom. Given your culturally competent clinical skills training, how would you intervene?

3. Assume you are on the "search committee" for the next director of the local mental health agency in a rural Iowa county. What questions do you want to pose to the job applicants, and what answers will you be looking for to determine if they are the "best fit" for the rural Iowa county in which you practice?

4. From among the many access-related barriers identified in this chapter to rural health/mental health services, what do you consider *the most serious barrier*, and how would you go about eliminating that barrier?

CASE STUDY

Tom (aged 38) and Cheryl (aged 34) reside in a rural community in Wyoming. Tom and Cheryl met when they were both working in Cheyenne. After getting married, they moved to this small community about 100 miles away when a new small business opened there. They believed that this rural area was perfect to raise their future family because it was away from the urban congestion of Cheyenne. Additionally, Tom's mother lived only 20 miles away. Their new employer offered higher incomes compared to their previous employer, but because the business employed only eight persons it did not provide health insurance. Tom and Cheryl believed that they could save enough from their extra income to purchase a family health insurance plan in the future. At the time, both were in excellent health.

Two years after moving to this rural community, Tom and Cheryl had twin boys, who were born prematurely at 32 weeks. Cheryl had received minimal prenatal care because the closest physician was approximately 45 minutes away and she lost a half day at work to attend each appointment. After realizing that she would be having twins, Cheryl tried to make more of her prenatal visits. They planned to have the babies at the hospital 45 minutes away. However, when Cheryl went into premature labor, her physician told her she would need to get to the hospital in Cheyenne (2 hours away), which was the closest hospital with a neonatal intensive care unit (NICU). Cheryl spent a week in the hospital before the babies were born. Both boys needed care in the NICU for 6 weeks. The doctors explained to the parents that the boys would need to receive follow-up care to monitor health concerns typical of premature infants. While Tom and Cheryl were thrilled with the birth of the boys, they quickly became overwhelmed with the health care costs associated with the birth and future follow-up care.

Tom talked with the county public health social worker about his concerns of not having a way to pay the medical bills and ensuring that the boys got the follow-up care they needed. He had been missing work while Cheryl and the boys were hospitalized. They had gone from two incomes to no income for the past 2 months. Tom also shared with the social worker that he was responsible for caring for his 60-year-old mother, who was living alone and showing signs of increasing dementia. Initially, the couple thought that his mother might help care for the babies, but it now appeared she might need as much care as the babies need.

INTERNET RESOURCES

National Rural Health Association

(www.ruralhealthweb.org/)

Rural Health Research and Policy Center

(www.ruralhealthresearch.org/)

Office of Rural Health Policy

(www.hrsa.gov/ruralhealth/)

Rural Social Work Caucus

(ruralsocialwork.org)

National Rural Health Resource Center

(ruralcenter.org/)

REFERENCES

Baldwin, L., Grossman, D. C., Murowchick, E., Larson, E. H., Hollow, W. G., Sugarman, J. R., et al. (2009). Trends in perinatal and infant health disparities between rural American Indians and Alaska Natives and rural whites. *American Journal of Public Health*, *99*(4), 638–646.

Bird, D. C., Dempsey, P., & Hartley, D. (2001). *Addressing mental health workforce needs in underserved rural areas: Accomplishments and challenges*. Portland, ME: Maine Rural Health Research Center.

Bolin, J., & Gamm, L. (2003). Access to quality health services in rural areas—Insurance. In L. Gamm, L. Hutchins, B. Dabney, & A. Dorsey (Eds.), *Rural Healthy People 2010: A companion document to Healthy People 2010* (Vol. 1, pp. 19–24). College Station: Texas A&M University System Health Science.

Davenport, J. A., & Davenport, J. (2008). Rural practice. In T. Mizrahi & L. Davis (Eds.), *Encyclopedia of social work.* New York: Oxford University Press.

Dye, C. J., Willoughby, D. F., & Battisto, D. G. (2011). Advice from rural elders: What it takes to age in place. *Educational Gerontology, 37,* 74–93.

Eberhardt, M. S., & Pamuk, E. R. (2004). The importance of place of residence: Examining health in rural and nonrural areas. *American Journal of Public Health, 94,* 1682–1686.

Eckert, K. A., Kutek, S. M., Dunn, K. I., Air, T. M., & Goldney, R. D. (2010). Changes in depression-related mental health literacy in young men from rural and urban South Australia. *Australian Journal of Rural Health, 18,* 153–158.

Economic Research Service. (2009). *Rural population and migration*. Retrieved from www.ers.usda.gov/Briefing/Population

Encyclopedia of Public Health. (2011). *Rural public health*. Retrieved from http://www.enotes.com/public-health-encyclopedia/rural-public-health

Farrell, S. P., Mahone, I. H., Zerull, L. M., Guerlain, S, Akan, D., Hauenstein, E., et al. (2009). Electronic screening for mental health in rural primary care: Implementation. *Issues in Mental Health Nursing, 30*, 165-173.

Gamm, L., Castillo, G., & Pittman, S. (2003). Access to quality health services in rural areas—Primary care. In L. Gamm, L. Hutchins, B. Dabney, & A. Dorsey (Eds.), *Rural Healthy People 2010: A companion document to Healthy People 2010* (Vol. 1, pp. 45-51). College Station: Texas A&M University System Health Science Center, School of Rural Public Health.

Gamm, L., Stone, S., & Pittman, S. (2003). Mental health and mental disorders—A rural challenge. In L. Gamm, L. Hutchins, B. Dabney, & A. Dorsey (Eds.), *Rural Healthy People 2010: A companion document to Healthy People 2010* (Vol. 1, pp. 165-170). College Station: Texas A&M University System Health Science Center, School of Rural Public Health.

Goodkind, J. R., Ross-Toldo, K., John, S., Hall, J. L., Ross, L., Freeland, L., et al. (2010). Promoting health and restoring trust: Policy recommendations for improving behavioral health care for American Indian/Alaska Native adolescents. *American Journal of Community Psychology, 46*, 386-394.

Gorman, D., Buikstra, E., Hegney, D., Pearce, S., Rogers-Clark, C., Weir, J., et al. (2007). Rural men and mental health: Their experiences and how they managed. *International Journal of Mental Health Nursing, 16*, 298-306.

Hartley, D. (2004). Rural health disparities, population health and rural culture. *American Journal of Public Health, 94*(10), 1675-1678.

Hauenstein, E. J., Petterson, S., Rovnyak, V., Merwin, E., Heise, B., & Wagner, D. (2007). Rurality and mental health treatment. *Administration and Policy in Mental Health and Mental Health Services Research, 34*, 255-267.

Health Resources and Services Administration. (2005). *Mental health and rural America: 1994 − 2005*. Rockville, MD: Author.

Hoyt, D. R., Conger, R. D., Valde, J. G., & Weihs, K. (1997). Psychological distress and health seeking in rural America. *American Journal of Community Psychology, 25*(4), 449-470.

Humphreys, J. S. (2009). Key considerations in delivering appropriate and accessible health care for rural and remote populations: Discussant overview. *Australian Journal of Health, 17*, 34-38.

Humphreys, J. S., Wakerman, J., & Wells, R. (2006). What do we mean by sustainable rural health services? Implications for rural health research. *Australian Journal of Rural Health, 14*, 33-35.

Hutchison, L., & Blakely, C. (2003). Substance abuse—Trends in rural areas. In L. Gamm, L. Hutchins, B. Dabney, & A. Dorsey (Eds.), *Rural Healthy People 2010: A companion document to Healthy People 2010* (Vol. 1, pp. 223-226). College Station: Texas A&M University System Health Science Center, School of Rural Public Health.

Institute of Medicine. (1988). *The future of public health*. Washington, DC: National Academies Press.

Johnson, M. E., Brems, C., Warner, T. D., & Roberts, L. W. (2006). Rural–urban health care provider disparities in Alaska and New Mexico. *Administration and Policy in Mental Health Services Research, 33*(4), 504-507.

Jones, C. A., Parker, T. S., Ahearn, M., Mishra, A. K., & Variyam, J. N. (2009 August). *Health status and health care access of farm and rural populations* (Publication No. EIB-57). Washington, DC: U.S. Department of Agriculture.

Kaiser, B. L., & Baumann, L. C. (2010). Perspectives on healthy behaviors among low-income Latino and non-Latino adults in two rural counties. *Public Health Nursing, 27*(6), 528–536.

Kaufman, A. V., Scogin, F. R., Burgio, L. D., Morthland, M. P., & Ford, B. K. (2007). Providing mental health services to older people living in rural communities. *Journal of Gerontological Social Work, 48*(3/4), 349–365.

Keefe, R. H. (2010). Health disparities: A primer for public health social workers. *Social Work in Public Health, 25*, 237–257.

Lenardson, J. D., Ziller, E. C., Lambert, D., Race, M. M., & Yousefian, A. (2010, October). *Access to mental health services and family impact of rural children with mental health problems*. Maine Rural Health Research Center, Working Paper #45.

Mohatt, D. F. (2000). Access to mental health services in frontier America. *Journal of the Washington Academy of Sciences, 86*, 35–47.

Myers, L. L. (2010). Health risk behaviors among adolescents in the rural South: A comparison of race, gender, and age. *Journal of Human Behavior in the Social Environment, 20*, 1024–1037.

O'Hare, W. P. (2009). *The forgotten fifth: Child poverty in rural America*. Durham, NH: Carsey Institute, University of New Hampshire.

Probst, J., Samuels, M., Jespersen, K., Willert, K., Swann, R., & McDuffie, J. (2002). *Minorities in rural America: An overview of population characteristics*. Columbia, SC: South Carolina Rural Health Research Center, University of South Carolina.

Public Health Social Work Standards and Competencies. (2005). Columbus: Ohio Department of Health.

Rainer, J. (2010). The road much less travelled: Treating rural and isolated clients. *Journal of Clinical Psychology: In Session, 66*(5), 475–478.

Rawlinson, C., & Crews, P. (2003). Access to quality health services in rural areas—Emergency medical services. In L. Gamm, L. Hutchins, B. Dabney, & A. Dorsey (Eds.), *Rural Healthy People 2010: A companion document to Healthy People 2010* (Vol. 1, pp. 77–81). College Station: Texas A&M University System Health Science Center, School of Rural Public Health.

Ricketts, T. C. (Ed.). (1999). *Rural health in the United States*. New York: Oxford University Press.

Sears, S. F., Evans, G. D., & Kuper, B. D. (2003). Rural social services systems as behavioral health delivery systems. In B. H. Stamm (Ed.), *Rural behavioral health care: An interdisciplinary guide* (pp. 109–120). Washington, DC: American Psychological Association.

Smalley, K. B., Yancey, C. T., Warren, J. C., Naufel, K., Ryan, R., & Pugh, J. L. (2010). Rural mental health and psychological treatment, a review for practitioners. *Journal of Clinical Psychology: In Session, 66*(5), 479–489.

Spaulding, R., Cain, S., & Sonnenschein, K. (2011). Urban telepsychiatry: Uncommon service for a common need. *Child and Adolescent Psychiatric Clinics of North America, 20*(1). Retrieved from http://www.mdconsult.com/das/article/body/250534209-4/jorg=journal&source=&sp=23783914&sid=1162911360/N/776027/1.html?issn=1056-4993.

Substance Abuse and Mental Health Services Administration. (2001). *Summary of findings from the 2001 National Household Survey on Drug Abuse.* Rockville, MD: Office of Applied Studies.

U.S. Census Bureau. (2009). *American Community Survey.* Retrieved from www.census.gov.

U.S. Department of Health and Human Services. (2010). *Healthy People 2020* (Office of Disease Prevention and Health Promotion Publication No. B0132) Washington, DC: U.S. Government Printing Office.

Wakerman, J. (2009). Innovative rural and remote primary health care models: What do we know and what are the research priorities? *Australian Journal of Rural Health, 17,* 21-26.

Wickrama, K. A. S., Kway, K. H., Lorenz, F. O., Conger, R. D., & Surjadi, F. F. (2010). Dynamics of family economic hardship and the progression of health problems of husbands and wives during the middle years: A perspective from rural mid-west. *Journal of Aging and Health, 22*(8), 1132-1157.

CHAPTER 15

Neighborhoods and Health

Robert H. Keefe

INTRODUCTION

*P*ublic health social workers have been at the forefront of promoting neighborhood health for nearly 100 years. Regardless of whether we work in urban or rural areas, as public health social workers we help bring about change that improves the health and well-being of neighborhood residents. As public health social workers, we use our micro-, mezzo-, and macro-level practice skills to work with neighborhood residents to start Neighborhood Watch programs, provide access to no-cost influenza vaccines, and work with recreational services to start after-school programs.

Neighborhoods are living systems that continue to grow and change and meet many of its residents' needs. As a result, neighborhoods have a significant effect on the quality of schools, health care services, and available job opportunities (Moore, Diez Roux, Evenson, McGinn, & Brines, 2008; Ross & Mirowsky, 2008). In well-functioning neighborhoods, the residents know each other, can access services, and feel safe in and outside their homes.

However, many neighborhoods that require our help are very dysfunctional: Crime rates are high, health outcomes are poor, and neighborhood cohesion is low. Escaping the dysfunctional, poverty-stricken neighborhoods is challenging, because the neighborhoods typically lack employment opportunities and the necessary services that lead to upward mobility. There may be fewer community members who have sufficient resources to help neighbors achieve a higher standard of living (Bayer & McMillan, 2005; Cubbin, Pedgron, Egerter, & Braveman, 2008). Moreover, problems such as redlining and other forms of housing discrimination restrict many people from moving into neighborhoods that have better health outcomes and offer more opportunity (Cubbin et al., 2008; Lane et al., 2008).

In this chapter we will explore many of the factors that lead to poor health in neighborhoods and what we as public health social workers can do to alleviate negative health outcomes.

CORE FUNCTIONS OF PUBLIC HEALTH AND NEIGHBORHOODS

The core functions of public health include assessment, policy development, and assurance. The National Institutes of Health consider each of these areas as crucial to reaching the objectives set forth in the U.S. Department of Health and Human Services' (DHHS) *Healthy People 2020*. To help neighborhoods become higher functioning and reach their goals, public health social workers must conduct thorough assessments to help structure effective interventions that in turn effect policy development and assure the public of safe and effective health care.

ASSESSMENT

The causes of poor neighborhood health are extremely varied. In order to conduct a thorough assessment of the causes, public health social workers use their critical thinking and observation skills. Prior research informs us that living in poor neighborhoods exposes individuals to stressors that lead to chronic illnesses such as cardiovascular diseases (Cox, Boyle, Davey, Feng, & Morris, 2007; Diez Roux et al., 2001; Stafford & Marmot, 2003; Stimpson, Ju, Raji, & Eschbach, 2007), and diabetes (Krishnan, Cozier, Rosenberg, & Palmer, 2010), and to negative child health outcomes (Kim, 2008; Lane et al., 2008; Msall, Avery, Msall, & Hogan, 2007; Pickett & Pearl, 2001; Riva, Gauvin, & Barnett, 2007; Sellstrom & Bremberg, 2006). Low-income neighborhoods also pose other risk factors such as poverty, crime victimization, and housing instability (Lindberg et al., 2010). Housing instability contributes to adverse health outcomes, including increased asthma, tuberculosis, developmental delays, and school failure (Buckner, 2008). Homes adjacent to major highways often expose residents to pollutants and other toxins that affect pulmonary and cardiac health (Brugge, Durant, & Rioux, 2007; Houston, Wu, Ang, & Winer, 2004). A neighborhood's socioeconomic conditions affect whether its residents have healthy diets (Lee & Cubbin, 2002), smoke (Chuang, Cubbin, Ahn, & Winkleby, 2005), and practice safer reproductive behaviors (Lane et al., 2004).

To help us address these problems, we can separate neighborhood assessment into two broad domains: the built environment and the social environment (Diez Roux & Mair, 2009). The built environment includes land-use and transportation patterns; street designs; and other features, such as parks and recreational facilities. The social environment includes the social connection and familiarity among neighbors, the presence of social norms, and the levels of safety and violence (Diez Roux & Mair, 2009). Many diseases are associated with the built environment (Coburn, 2004; Malizia, 2006; Northridge, Sclar, & Biswas, 2003) and include asthma and other pulmonary problems. Other diseases are more often associated with the social environment, such as sexually transmitted diseases (Lane et al., 2004). The built and social environments work together to give rise to other illnesses, such as mental illness (Stafford & Marmot, 2003), obesity (Cecil-Karb & Grogan-Kaylor, 2009), and diabetes (Northridge et al., 2003).

Once we have thoroughly observed the built and social environments, we must learn who the key members in the neighborhood are and where people turn for guidance. In many neighborhoods, merchants, religious leaders, and perhaps gang leaders wield the most influence. Other available sources of information include county-level public health data (such as electronic birth certificate, Medicaid, and Healthy Start enrollments and drug and alcohol arrest records), key-informant interviews and census tract data. (Census tracts are small areas within counties that consist of 2,500 to 8,000 residents [U.S. Census Bureau, 2000].)

Public health social workers use other tools to help them with their assessments. One is the *systematic social observation approach*. Using this approach, a public health social worker drives or walks throughout a neighborhood looking for built and social environmental features of neighborhoods that cannot be obtained by using surveys or public-access data. This approach is helpful to public health social workers, who may wish to videotape social activities (e.g., neighborhood residents watching a Little League baseball game) and physical features (e.g., graffiti or abandoned cars) to create an index of physical and social order or disorder. A second approach is *space–time analysis*. This approach considers where a group resides and the location of its daily activities (e.g., traveling to work, bicycling through parks, or running along pedestrian trails). A third approach comprises *surveys and questionnaires,* which can be used to gather information from a large number of individuals to measure attitudes on key variables of interest (e.g., perceptions of safety during certain time periods of the day or the quality of neighborhood services). A fourth approach includes *Geographic Information System* (GIS) and *spatial analysis techniques,* which allow for the examination of space in a much more detailed manner (Rushton, 2003). GIS has been used in conjunction with a variety of databases to construct measures of neighborhood density and accessibility of resources such as corner markets (Lane et al., 2008), as well as measures of features of the built environment related to the design, road networks, and land-use patterns (Handy, Boarnet, Ewing, & Killingsworth, 2002). Each of these approaches is then used to examine health outcomes for a specific group within the neighborhood, such as diabetes in the elderly, accessible buildings for people with disabilities, and food sources for women with high-risk pregnancies (Diez-Roux, 2007).

POLICY DEVELOPMENT

Public health social workers often encounter resistance from city officials when advocating for policy change and grant-funding organizations when seeking funds for neighborhood improvement. Some of the obstacles that have hindered the improvement of neighborhood conditions include competition for scarce resources (e.g., should funding be provided for after-school programs or for senior citizens centers), the lack of agreement on individual versus public responsibility for self-improvement (e.g., the argument that poverty and poor neighborhoods are caused by individual failings rather than by social conditions), the political support for groups that have less clout than other groups (e.g., providing funding for neighborhood cleanup in areas that have high rates of vandalism without assurance that future vandalism will not occur), and the limited research on evidence-based solutions to community problems (e.g., isolating which variables seem to predict adoption of health lifestyle behaviors, such as walking in particular neighborhoods) (Heymann & Fischer, 2003).

One example of a successful project based on federal housing policy that can help neighborhoods with secure housing or help neighbors move to better neighborhoods is The Housing Choice Voucher Program (often referred to as "Section 8"). Section 8 assists very-low-income families, older people, and people with disabilities to access safe and sanitary housing at reduced rental costs (U.S. Department of Housing and Urban Development, 2009a). Program participants can use the vouchers in any neighborhood with available housing units that meet the U.S. Housing and Urban Development's health and safety standards.

Section 8 policy allows state and local housing agencies flexibility in determining income-eligibility limits. The amount a voucher pays toward housing costs is based on a payment standard set by the local housing agency and can range from 90% to 110% of the area's fair market rent; the actual cost for rent and utilities for the particular housing unit; and the household's annual adjusted income, which factors in information such as the number of children in a household, child care costs, and disability status (Center on Budget and Policy Priorities, 2008). In general, the program aims for households to contribute 30% of their income toward the housing costs.

Although the program has been effective in many ways, only one in every four households eligible for the program receives federal housing assistance

(Center on Budget and Policy Priorities, 2008). Additional federal and state funding is required to reach the actual number of people needing Section 8 housing. Public health social workers can work with neighborhood groups to develop letter-writing and voter-registry campaigns that will put pressure on legislators to endorse the expansion of the Section 8 program.

ASSURANCE

Public health social workers do much to assure neighborhood health. On an individual (or micro-practice) level, public health social workers encourage individual clients to exercise, stop smoking, and eat healthier foods. On a neighborhood (or mezzo-practice) level, public health social workers encourage the development of after-school programs, social connection among neighbors, and community gardens (Berkman, 1995; House, Landis, & Umberson, 1988; Kawachi, Kennedy, Lochner, & Prothrow-Stith, 1997; Litt et al., 2011). On the national (or macro-practice) level, public health social workers use their skills to assist in the development of various interventions (Sable, Schild, & Hipp, 2012).

One public health issue affecting many inner cities is childhood lead poisoning. We have known for many years that living in areas with broken windows and dilapidated housing can be indicative of high crime, poverty, and poor health care (Cohen et al., 2000). Despite the 1978 federal law that outlawed the use of lead-based paint, many inner-city homes contain old paint that, when chipped or peeled away, leaves behind lead residue. Lead is also found in the soil surrounding houses with exteriors that have peeling lead-based paint (Schilling & Bain, 1988) and in lead-tainted water from corroded lead solder in old copper pipes (American Academy of Pediatrics, 2005). Many new mothers who, as children, ate lead-based paint chips have lead poisoning. These new mothers later passed the lead poisoning on to their newborn infants during pregnancy and in breast milk after delivery.

One project that helped assure neighborhood health was aimed at lead-based paint removal from dilapidated homes (Lane et al., 2008) and healthy food options available at corner markets (Lane et al., 2008). This project used county-level census data to study the long-term effects of lead poisoning in run-down housing on maternal and child health outcomes and GIS mapping and systematic observation to generate a map of corner markets and record sales of merchandise at the corner markets (Lane et al., 2008). The results indicate that increased blood-lead levels were associated with increased tobacco and alcohol use, teen pregnancy, and school dropout rates. Additionally, the data revealed that store owners sold limited healthy foods but were doing a thriving business selling tobacco, alcohol, and drug paraphernalia. The mothers in the census tracts that had elevated rates of lead poisoning and low birth weight infants often had negative health outcomes due to limited food options.

The researchers later provided the data to neighborhood groups and agencies to develop tutoring programs that encouraged students to stay in school, neighborhood education services to advise residents how to safely clean up chipped and peeling paint, and advocacy training to help residents petition corner store owners to stock healthy foods. Since that time, the city has procured funding from the U.S. Department of Housing and Urban Development for lead abatement and is developing policies requiring landlords to follow specific guidelines to assure that all rental properties are free of lead paint.

HEALTH DISPARITIES

The DHHS launched its Racial and Ethnic Health Disparities Initiative, which focused on key health areas, including infant mortality, diabetes, cardiovascular disease, cancer screening and management, HIV/AIDS, and child and adult immunizations (Bullard, Warren, & Johnson, 2001). The relationship between these areas and the built and social environments has been closely documented (Lane et al., 2008).

For instance, the limited access to healthy food options in many poverty-stricken inner-city neighborhoods helps explain the diabetes epidemic facing much of the United States. Many inner-city neighborhoods have been referred to as "food deserts" (Wrigley, Warm, & Margetts, 2003) in which residents have very limited access to high-quality food, enjoy fewer options in the variety of foods available to them, and pay higher prices for groceries (Bolen & Hecht, 2003). Limited access to supermarkets is strongly associated with greater body mass index (BMI; Wang, Cubbin, Ahn, & Winkleby, 2008), heart disease, and diabetes (Johnson, Bazargan, & Cherpitel, 2001), whereas physical activity and better neighborhood food environments are associated with significantly lower BMI (Mujahid et al., 2008), as are lower prices of fruits and vegetables (Sturm & Datar, 2008). Inner city neighborhoods are disproportionately composed of African Americans and Hispanics, who have significantly greater adverse outcomes for each of the key areas than Whites.

Moreover, inner-city neighborhoods are often inhabited by low-income individuals who have limited health insurance or providers available to them. Consequently, they tend to have worse health outcomes and die at younger ages (Lane et al., 2004).

PUBLIC HEALTH SOCIAL WORK PRACTICE

Public health social workers have worked for many years to improve neighborhood health. The settlement houses of the 1900s focused on meeting the health and social service needs of poor families. The New Deal Era of the 1930s focused on "slum clearance." The Great Society initiatives of the 1960s led to a variety of social programs that attempted to eliminate inner-city poverty. The 1990s brought forward projects such as "comprehensive community initiatives" and empowerment zones that were designed to improve neighborhoods.

Despite these efforts, however, neighborhood problems persist. Public health social worker standards help to address these ongoing problems.

Standard: Identify, Measure, Assess, and Monitor Social Problems Affecting Health Status

Funding organizations have policies in force that require programs to identify, measure, assess, and monitor their progress in alleviating the problems that affect neighborhoods. As public health social workers, we use our research, intervention, and epidemiologic skills to help programs continue to improve neighborhood health and receive future funding. Many of the neighborhood programs described above have effected change, but none has provided a consistent roadmap that can be applied to all neighborhoods. Consequently, we are forced to rely on untested methods in our work with neighborhoods. Therefore, it is of vital importance that we contribute to the knowledge base on neighborhoods and health by testing various intervention methods, identifying problems, assessing the impact of our interventions, measuring the intervention progress, and monitoring our success. Finally, we need to make available to public health social workers in other areas our best practices that have been shown to have an effect on reducing neighborhood health problems.

Standard: Provide Quality Services Within a Cultural, Community, and Family Context

Various methods can be used to provide services. Bringing people into the process of relieving neighborhood health problems helps assure that the approach will be culturally valid. Grassroots organizing is one approach public health social workers can use to reach many individuals in a culturally relevant manner. Often, grassroots-organizing efforts come about by citizens who are dissatisfied with efforts made by city officials who have not accurately assessed the need for services or the methods by which the services should be provided (Bullard et al., 2001; Keefe, Lane, & Swarts, 2006). In such cases, public health social workers engaged in grassroots organizing used a bottom-up leadership approach by helping neighborhood groups organize.

Well-known examples of grassroots organizing techniques include women living with breast cancer, gay men living with HIV, and people who use intravenous drugs. Members from each group educated themselves on the dynamics of their own health issues and the unfair and unjust legal practices that kept them from receiving current treatment. By organizing themselves, they formed strong coalitions so as to gain political control over issues such as the expanded use of alternative and complementary medicines for the treatment of breast cancer; the shortened length of time for the approval of new and effective drugs to treat people living with HIV; and the increased use of bleaching kits and development of needle-exchange programs to prevent the spread of HIV, hepatitis C, and dermatitis among intravenous drug users. Over time, survival rates increased as the rates of death for people with breast cancer and with HIV decreased and the services have become more relevant. The Centers for Disease Control and Prevention now requires HIV service organizations to have people living with HIV be actively involved with the operations of the service organization.

These grassroots efforts started where the communities were first understanding their community members' issues, setting specific goals, formulating an intervention plan, and evaluating success.

Standard: Develop Primary Prevention Strategies That Promote Health and Well-Being

The emphasis in public health over the past few decades has been to develop and implement effective health promotion strategies by primary prevention approaches to reduce the burden of disease in populations. Primary prevention strives to put a stop to the occurrence of illness or injury before it occurs. As such, primary preventions are less costly than other secondary and tertiary approaches and help preserve good health and longevity. Some frequent examples of primary prevention efforts in inner-city neighborhoods include yearly influenza immunizations and prostate cancer screenings. More recent examples are gathering support for mobile screening vans to provide mammography and HIV screenings; and school health programs to help prevent the spread of head lice, teen pregnancy, and school violence.

CLASSROOM EXERCISES

Case Scenario 1: "The Riverfront" neighborhood

Haverville is a large, urban area located in a northeastern state. At the last census, the population of Haverville was 390,200. The population was 70% White, 12.5% African American, 12.5% Hispanic, 3% Native American, and 2% other. Like many northeastern cities, Haverville has seen much change in the recent years. Many middle-class families have left the city for the suburbs, along with many of the resources, including health and recreational facilities, supermarkets, and small-business owners, leaving lower-income individuals to fend for themselves. In the recent years Haverville's inner city has also declined. Crime rates have risen, as has the incidence of various health problems, including cardiovascular disease, diabetes, obesity, and HIV.

In your role as a master of social work intern, your field educator has required you to conduct an assessment, plan an intervention, and propose an evaluation method for an area of Haverville known as "the Riverfront neighborhood," which is located in the inner city along a large river that goes through the downtown and empties into the ocean an hour's drive away. In order for you to accomplish this large task you must answer the following:

1. How would you go about finding the key people in the neighborhood who have influence?
2. What assessment methods would you use?
3. How would you gain support from various individuals so as to conduct your assessment and later intervene effectively?
4. What policies in your state are in place that would affect your intervention methods if Haverville were located in your state?
5. How would you assure the citizens that they have the influence to address their neighborhood needs once your project is finished?
6. How would you go about addressing concerns from others that the residents of "the Riverfront" simply need to "pick themselves up by their bootstraps?"

Case Scenario 2: Stephenstown

Stephenstown is a small town of 2,300 people located in a midwestern state. The residents of Stephenstown go back many generations and take pride in the close-knit ties in their community. Recently, you read in the town newspaper that a large corporation informed the people of the town that they wanted to purchase open land located just outside the town limits to be used as a waste site. The company has informed the state legislature that none of the material to be left at the site is hazardous, the material will be stored in appropriate waste bins, and no environmental harm will come to the area.

You brought this matter to your field educator at a local neighborhood center, who was likewise disturbed by the newspaper article and encouraged you to look into the matter further and to organize a grassroots effort to stop the corporation from coming to Stephenstown.

In order to go about starting such an effort, discuss how you would do the following:

1. Mobilize key people of interest.
2. Look up legislation that may help you keep the corporation from moving in.
3. Get the word out that you plan to have a community meeting and where you would host the meeting.
4. Plan an intervention effort such as picketing, petitioning the town manager/mayor, and other legislators to keep the company away.
5. Come up with benchmarks to monitor your progress toward keeping the company from coming to the Stephenstown area.

KEY ISSUES

There are many key issues we face in public health social work. Selecting from among them is a difficult task. We must focus first and foremost on understanding what we need to do to foster good neighborhood health. Some of these issues focus on the built environment, including safe neighborhoods with affordable housing, markets that sell healthy food, and schools that provide a rigorous curriculum that will help young people with life options. Others focus on the social environment, including community participation in decision making and interaction among neighbors.

As we move forward in our work as public health social workers involved in neighborhood health, there will continue to be many obstacles to face. Among them are the ongoing problems of neighborhood violence, school dropout, dilapidated housing, and chronic illnesses. We will be forced to intervene with fewer financial and in-kind resources.

In order to do all that we need to do to be effective, we must be culturally sensitive and aware of the values of various neighborhood groups, work to promote the dignity and self-worth of the people living in the neighborhoods, recognize the talents and resources within each neighborhood, acknowledge the neighborhood's right to exercise its own self-determination, strengthen and expand the social networks in various neighborhoods, and strengthen neighborhoods to work with various community-based organizations (Aronson, Lovelace, Hatch, & Whitehead, 2005).

INTERNET RESOURCES

There are many websites available to help public health social workers in their work with various neighborhoods. Below is a list of some of the more commonly used ones.

The Urban Institute

(www.urban.org/publications/410819.html)

Neighborhood Watch

(https://entp.hud.gov/sfnw/public/)

Promise Neighborhoods

(http://promiseneighborhoods.org/policies/school-based-health-centers-sbhcs/)

National Association of Community Health Centers

(www.nachc.org/)

U.S. Housing and Urban Development

(http://portal.hud.gov/portal/page/portal/HUD)

REFERENCES

American Academy of Pediatrics Committee on Environmental Health. (2005). Lead exposure in children: Prevention, detection, and management. *Pediatrics, 116*(4), 1036–1046.

Aronson, R. E., Lovelace, K., Hatch, J. W., & Whitehead, T. L. (2005). Strengthening communities and the roles of individuals in community life. In B. Levy & V. Sidel (Eds.), *Social injustice and public health.* New York: Oxford University Press.

Bayer, P., & McMillan, R. (2005). *Racial sorting and neighborhood quality.* National Bureau of Economic Research Working Paper No. W11813. Retrieved July 15, 2011, from http://www.nber.org/papers/w11813

Berkman, L. (1995). The role of social relations in health promotion. *Psychosomatic Medicine, 57,* 245–254.

Bolen, E., & Hecht, K. (2003). *Neighborhood groceries: New access to healthy food in low-income communities*. San Francisco: California Food Policy Advocates.

Brugge, D., Durant, J. L., & Rioux, C. (2007). Near-highway pollutant in motor vehicle exhaust: A review of epidemiologic evidence of cardiac and pulmonary health risks. *Environmental Health, 6,* 23.

Buckner, J. C. (2008). Understanding the impact of homelessness on children: Challenges and future research directions. *American Behavioral Scientist, 51*(6), 721-736.

Bullard, R. D., Warren, R. C., & Johnson, G. S. (2001). The quest for environmental justice. In R. L. Braithwaite, & S. E. Taylor (Eds.), *Health issues in the Black community* (2nd ed.). San Francisco: Jossey-Bass Publishers.

Cecil-Karb, R., & Grogan-Kaylor, A. (2009). Childhood body mass index in community context: Neighborhood safety, television viewing, and growth trajectories of BMI. *Health & Social Work, 34,* 169-177.

Center on Budget and Policy Priorities. (2008). *Introduction to the housing voucher program*. Washington, DC: Center on Budget and Policy Priorities.

Chuang, Y. C., Cubbin, C., Ahn, D., & Winkleby, M. A. (2005). Effects of neighborhood socioeconomic status and convenience store concentration on individual-level smoking. *Journal of Epidemiology and Community Health, 59,* 568-573.

Coburn, J. (2004). Confronting the challenges in reconnecting urban planning and public health. *American Journal of Public Health, 94,* 541-546.

Cohen, D., Spear, S., Scribner, R., Kissinger, P., Mason, K., & Wildgen, J. (2000). "Broken window" and the risk of gonorrhea. *American Journal of Public Health, 90*(2), 230-236.

Cox, M., Boyle, P. J., Davey, P. G., Feng, Z., & Morris, A. D. (2007). Locality deprivation and type 2 diabetes incidence: A local test of relative inequalities. *Social Science and Medicine, 65,* 1953-1964.

Cubbin, C., Pedgron, V., Egerter, S., & Braveman, P. (2008). *Where we live matters for our health: Neighborhoods and health*. Issues Brief 3: Neighborhoods and health. Robert Wood Johnson Foundation. Retrieved July 21, 2011, from http://www.rwjf.org/files/research/commissionneighborhood102008.pdf

Diez-Roux, A. V. (2007). Neighborhoods and health: Where are we and where do we go from here? *Revue d'Epidemiologie et de Sante Publique, 55*(1), 13-21.

Diez Roux, A. V., & Mair, C. (2009). Neighborhoods and health. *Annals of the New York Academy of Sciences, 1186,* 125-145.

Diez Roux, A. V., Merkin, S., Arnett, D., Chambless, L., Massing, M., Nieto, F. J., et al. (2001). Neighborhood of residence and incidence of coronary heart disease. *New England Journal of Medicine, 345*(2), 99-106.

Handy, S. L., Boarnet, M. G., Ewing, R., & Killingsworth, R. E. (2002). How the built environment affects physical activity: Views from urban planning. *American Journal of Preventive Medicine, 23*(2, Suppl.), 64-73.

Heymann, J., & Fischer, A. (2003). Neighborhoods, health research, and its relevance to public policy. In I. Kawachi, & L. F. Berkman (Eds.), *Neighborhoods and health*. New York: Oxford University Press.

House, J., Landis, K. R. & Umberson, D. (1988). Social relationships and health. *Science, 84,* 541-545. Retrieved July 17, 2011, from http://www.npc.umich.edu/publications/policy_briefs/brief20/policy_brief_20_web.pdf

Houston, D., Wu, J., Ang, P., & Winer, A. (2004). Structural disparities of urban traffic in Southern California: Implications for vehicle-related air pollution exposure in minority and high poverty neighborhoods. *Journal of Urban Affairs, 26*(5), 565–592.

Johnson, S. H., Bazargan, M., & Cherpitel, C. J. (2001). Alcohol, tobacco, and drug use and the onset of type 2 diabetes among inner-city minority patients. *The Journal of the American Board of Family Practice, 14*, 430–436.

Kawachi, I., Kennedy, B. P., Lochner, K., & Prothrow-Stith, D. (1997). Social capital, income inequality, and mortality. *American Journal of Public Health, 87*, 1491–1498.

Keefe, R. H., Lane, S. D., & Swarts, H. J. (2006). From the bottom up: Tracing the impact of four health-based social movements on health and social policies. *Journal of Health & Social Policy, 21*(3), 55–69.

Kim, D. (2008). Blues from the neighborhood? Neighborhood characteristics and depression. *Epidemiologic Reviews, 30*, 101–117.

Krishnan, S., Cozier, Y. C., Rosenberg, L., & Palmer, J. R. (2010). Socioeconomic status and incidence of type 2 diabetes: Results from the Black Women's Health Study. *American Journal of Epidemiology, 171*(5), 564–570.

Lane, S. D., Keefe, R. H., Rubinstein, R., Levandowski, B. A., Webster, N., Cibula, D. A., et al. (2008). Structural violence, urban retail food markets, and low birth weight. *Health & Place, 14*, 415–423.

Lane, S. D., Rubinstein, R. A., Keefe, R. H., Webster, N., Cibula, D. A., Rosenthal, A., et al. (2004). Structural violence and racial disparity in HIV transmission. *Journal of Healthcare for the Poor and Underserved, 15*, 319–335.

Lane, S. D., Webster, N. J., Levandowski, B. A., Rubinstein, R. A., Keefe, R. H., Wojtowycz, M. A., et al. (2008). Environmental injustice: Childhood lead poisoning, teen pregnancy, and tobacco. *Journal of Adolescent Health, 42*, 43–49.

Lee, R. E., & Cubbin, C. (2002). Neighborhood context and youth cardiovascular health behaviors. *American Journal of Public Health, 92*(3), 428–436.

Lindberg, R. A., Shenassa, E. D., Acevedo-Garcia, D., Popkin, S. J., Villaveces, A., & Morley, R. L. (2010). Housing interventions at the neighborhood level and health: A review of the evidence. *Journal of Public Health Management Practice, 16*(5, Suppl. E), S42–S52.

Litt, J. S., Soobader, M. J., Turbin, M. S., Hale, J. W., Buchenau, M., & Marshall, J. A. (2011). The influence of social involvement, neighborhood aesthetics, and community garden participation on fruit and vegetable consumption. *American Journal of Public Health, 101*(8), 1466–1473.

Malizia, E. E. (2006). Planning and public health: Research options for an emerging field. *Journal of Planning, Education, and Research, 25*, 428–432.

Moore, L. V., Diez Roux, A. V., Evenson, K. R., McGinn, A. P., & Brines, S. J. (2008). Availability of recreational resources in minority and low socioeconomic strain areas. *American Journal of Preventive Medicine, 34*(1), 16–22.

Msall, M. E., Avery, R. C., Msall, E. R., & Hogan, D. P. (2007). Distressed neighborhoods and child disability rates: Analyses of 157,000 school-age children. *Developmental Medicine, & Child Neurology, 49*, 814–817.

Mujahid, M. S., Diez Roux, A. V., Shen, M., Gowda, D., Sanchez, B., Shea, S., et al. (2008). Relation between neighborhood environments and obesity in the multi-ethnic study of artherosclerosis. *American Journal of Epidemiology, 167*, 1349–1357.

Northridge, M. E., Sclar, E. D., & Biswas, P. (2003). Sorting out the connections between the built environment and health: A conceptual framework for navigating pathways and planning healthy cities. *Journal of Urban Health, 80,* 556-568.

Pickett, K. E., & Pearl, M. (2001). Multilevel analyses of neighbourhood socioeconomic context and health out-comes: A critical review. *Journal of Epidemiology and Community Health, 55,* 111-122.

Riva, M., Gauvin, L., & Barnett, T. A. (2007). Toward the next generation of research into small area effects on health: A synthesis of multilevel investigations published since July 1998. *Journal of Epidemiology and Community Health, 61,* 853-861.

Ross, C. E., & Mirowsky, J. (2008). Neighborhood socioeconomic status and health: Context and composition. *City and Community, 7,* 163-177.

Rushton, G. (2003). Public health, GIS, and spatial analytic tools. *Annual Review of Public Health, 24,* 43-56.

Sable, M. R., Schild, D. R., & Hipp, J. A. (2012). Public health social work. In S. Gehlert, & T. Browne (Eds.), *Handbook of health social work* (2nd ed). Hoboken, NJ: John Wiley & Sons.

Schilling, R. J., & Bain, R. P. (1988). Prediction of children's blood lead levels on the basis of household-specific soil lead levels. *American Journal of Epidemiology, 128,* 197-205.

Sellstrom, E., & Bremberg, S. (2006). The significance of neighbourhood context to child and adolescent health and well-being: A systematic review of multilevel studies. *Scandinavian Journal of Public Health, 34,* 544-554.

Stafford, M., & Marmot, M. (2003). Neighbourhood deprivation and health: Does it affect us all equally? *International Journal of Epidemiology, 32*(3), 357-366.

Stimpson, J. P., Ju, H., Raji, M. A., & Eschbach, K. (2007). Neighborhood deprivation and health risk behaviors in NHANES III. *American Journal of Health Behavior, 31*(2), 215-222.

Sturm, R., & Datar, A. (2008). Food prices and weight gain during elementary school: 5-year update. *Public Health, 122,* 1140-1143.

U.S. Bureau of the Census. (2000). *Geographic areas reference manual.* Washington, DC: U.S. Government Printing Office.

U.S. Department of Housing and Urban Development. (2009). *Housing choice vouchers fact sheet.* Washington, DC: Author.

Wang, M. C., Cubbin, C., Ahn, D., & Winkleby, M. A. (2008). Changes in neighbourhood food store environment, food behaviour and body mass index, 1981-1990. *Public Health Nutrition, 11,* 963-970.

Wrigley, N., Warm, D., & Margetts, B. (2003). Deprivation, diet, and food-retail access: Findings from the Leeds "food deserts" study. *Environment and Planning A, 35*(91), 151-188.

CHAPTER 16

Improving Local Health and Development Through Community-Based Participatory Research

Michele A. Kelley

INTRODUCTION

S ocial work has a rich history of working with vulnerable populations in various contexts (Lundy, 2004). One context in which social work has made significant contributions is in the area of community organization. While working in communities, social workers help empower residents to deploy resistance strategies and bring about change that enhances communities (Minkler & Wallerstein, 2005). Social workers also use the principles of community-based participatory research (CBPR) to bring about change that enhances the lives of community residents.

CBPR, also referred to as *antioppressive* (or *emancipatory*) *research* (Strier, 2007), is a method of participatory and action inquiry that fosters local community development and sustainable community change to improve the health and well-being of community residents. CBPR is rooted in many disciplines and traditions, and is especially suited to address health inequalities at the local level. Change is guided by a strategic-inquiry process that uses citizen engagement and empowerment strategies to investigate and document causes of health problems, including inequities in access to health care, and to develop and implement locally tailored, evidence-informed solutions to these problems (Wallerstein & Duran, 2006).

Good health is determined by many factors, including household size, neighborhood composition, and broader social policies (Frieden, 2010; Marmot, 2005). While macro-level determinants (such as poverty) need to be addressed through large-scale policy changes, it is in the smaller, local settings, such as in schools and faith-based organizations, that adaptation to policy change needs to take place (Fried et al., 2010; Trickett, 2009).

The release of *Healthy People 2020* stresses that persistent and pervasive health inequities are rampant in low-income and minority populations (Office of Disease Prevention and Health Promotion, U.S. D.H.H.S., 2011). Public health authorities stress the importance of achieving the goals and objectives, particularly those focused on chronic disease, in areas where poor and minority groups bear the greatest disease burden (Currie, 2011). Unlike previous editions of *Healthy People*, the *Healthy People 2020* objectives call for addressing social determinants of health by focusing from individual health status to larger service-delivery systems and environmental and policy factors (Johnson, 2011). Public health social workers can play a valuable role as collaborators in local change by bringing resources to local efforts and by engaging in culturally sensitive and community-building methods such as CBPR.

This chapter will briefly review the conceptual underpinnings of CBPR, consider its role in addressing health inequities as a change strategy, provide case vignettes from the author's work (including community perspectives on collaboration), and conclude with a discussion of lessons learned thus far. The broader objective is to encourage a thoughtful debate and consideration of the merits of CBPR as a resource for sustained, culturally sensitive change toward community health improvement and, ultimately, toward a vision for a more just society where the right to living conditions that foster optimal health is possible for all citizens.

BACKGROUND

Conceptual Foundation of CBPR

CBPR is defined as "a collaborative approach to research that equitably involves, for example, community members, organizational representatives, and researchers in all aspects of the research process" (Israel, Schulz, Parker, & Becker, 1998, p. 177). The Ottawa Charter, a fundamental document in public health worldwide, states that "health promotion works through concrete and effective community action in setting priorities, making decisions, planning strategies, and implementing them to achieve better health. At the heart of this process is the empowerment of communities—their ownership and control of their own endeavors and destinies" (World Health Organization, 1986, p. 2). The Ottawa Charter recognizes the importance of improving human health, broadly defined (i.e., well-being) as well as changing conditions that impact health. These dual outcomes are also recognized in applying CBPR principles to address community health.

Israel, Schulz, Parker, and Becker (2001 p. 184) identified what they referred to as *key principles* of CBPR: (1) recognizes community as a unit of identity; (2) builds on strengths and resources within the community; (3) facilitates collaborative, equitable involvement of all partners in all phases of the research; (4) integrates knowledge and action for mutual benefit of all partners; (5) promotes a co-learning and empowering process that attends to social inequalities; (6) involves a cyclical and iterative process; (7) addresses health from both positive and ecological perspectives; (8) disseminates findings and knowledge gained to all partners; and (9) involves a long-term commitment by all partners.

A key idea is to address local resources that can support healthy living, including social norms, social and organizational networks, local infrastructure and the built environment, and local policies. Thus, whole community—and, at times, broader regional development—is undertaken. Additionally, building community capacity (Goodman et al., 1998) to respond to health threats and foster healthy living is recognized as part of the process and outcome of CBPR (Wallerstein & Duran, 2010). What differentiates CBPR from other forms of community organization and action is that it is a systematic inquiry process, with a foundation of scientific research principles that use culturally rooted and participatory paradigms such as social constructivism (Splitter, 2009) and qualitative and mixed methods research (Creswell, 2009) to foster what critical theorist Jurgen Habermas referred to as *emancipatory knowledge* (Habermas, 1984 as cited in Ewert, 1991).

CBPR and Its Significance in Public Health

CBPR is related to the core public health function of assessment: Diagnose and investigate health problems and health hazards in the community. This transformative method is also related to the following essential public health services: (1) mobilize community partnerships and action to identify and solve health problems; (2) diagnose and investigate health problems and health hazards in the community; and (3) inform, educate, and empower people about health issues (Centers for Disease Control and Prevention, 2011).

Moreover, the following core competencies for public health social workers in particular, relate to social work inquiry and CBPR: (1) integration of professional values and principles of ethics within community and organizational practice settings; (2) the ethical conduct in program management, research, and data collection and storage; (3) partnerships with public health and social services communities and constituencies to foster community empowerment, reciprocal learning, and involvement in design, implementation, and research aspects of public health and social systems;

and (4) utilization of social work standards and principles in the resolution of ethical dilemmas (Association of State and Territorial Public Health Social Workers, 2005).

An emerging science of CBPR suggests that this method has the potential to advance the goals of practice and research in several ways by: (1) addressing privilege in cross-cultural research and practice, leading to insights from insider knowledge, or "emic," perspectives, and a shared commitment to the research objectives; (2) incorporating cultural assets and everyday meaning into practices (ecological validity), thereby increasing appeal and possibly effectiveness through increased response rates; (3) communicating and measuring (e.g., interpretive equivalency of assessment and survey tools) that are culturally sensitive and likely more effective; (4) deriving a more complete and locally relevant understanding of research outcomes; (5) building skills and capacity that lead to adoption and sustainability of program components in a local setting; (6) enhancing the researcher's and community partners' knowledge and skill sets for pursuing locally relevant research agendas; and (7) helping community members attain health and social benefits from participation as a social protective factor (Chavez, Duran, Baker, Avila, & Wallerstein, 2008; Leung, Yen, & Minkler, 2004; Minkler, 2004, 2005; Trickett & Espino, 2004).

While several benefits of CBPR were outlined above, it is the ultimate change-oriented outcomes that are of particular interest. Wallerstein and Duran (2010) presented a model of dynamic changes processes in CBPR, where outcomes are characterized as (1) system and capacity changes in both research-partner organizations (e.g., universities, health departments) as well as in communities (including policy, cultural sensitivity and revitalization, and empowerment) and (2) health changes, which include health behaviors, social norms, knowledge, and, ultimately, health status indicators (e.g., well-being, morbidity, and mortality; Wallerstein & Duran, 2010).

Challenges in Conducting CBPR and Public Health Adoption

There are several obstacles and challenges to both researchers and community partners that need to be discussed in advance and throughout the duration of the partnership and specific project. Some of these challenges are suggested in the model presented above. Certainly, historical factors that inform how the project is perceived from the beginning, and the perceived trustworthiness of the principal investigator and research team, as well as the perceived capacity of the community partners to adhere to research protocols, are paramount. Then there are the delicate issues related to research "fidelity," when a local context may dictate flexibility or change in the research design, which suggests attention to relational dynamics in terms of how university and community members communicate and negotiate inevitable issues. Obviously, there are issues with the capacity of funding agencies and with the researcher's home institution if the scope of work needs to be changed to adapt to local conditions. However, if indicated changes are made in collaboration with mutual learning and understanding, the research will be more acceptable and locally relevant, and such changes could enhance validity of the project (Ka'opua, Park, Ward, & Braun, 2011).

Another issue to be considered are changes in researcher and community partner roles as the research progresses from one stage to another (e.g., data analysis and dissemination). During various phases of the research process, CBPR can fall short as resources, including time, become limited. Lack of adequate resources to support collaboration, especially for community members who do not have time that can be allowed just for research, and sustained follow-up and "sweat equity" on the part of researchers once the research objectives or contract have been satisfied, are critical issues that any one project may not be able to address.

Addressing power issues is a constant concern and not fully appreciated in CBPR. The material and fiscal resources of academic and governmental public health agency research teams, no matter how modest, outweigh those of local organizations whose missions and limited resources are directed at solving community problems and often exclude formal research (Minkler, 2004). In addition to these challenges, other relational concerns matter in the CBPR paradigm. Wallerstein and Duran (2006) suggested that the notion of *cultural humility* is more useful than the more widely used (but seemingly misunderstood) term *cultural competency.* Cultural humility is "a lifelong commitment to self-evaluation and self-critique" (Tervalon & Murray-Garcia, 1998, p. 117) to redress power imbalances and "develop and maintain mutually respectful and dynamic partnerships with communities" (Tervalon & Murray-Garcia, 1998, p. 118). In line with these considerations of power issues, Chavez and colleagues (2008) offered an excellent discussion of racism, oppression, and culture in collaborative research with a framework that is very helpful to the novice researcher. Therefore, researcher commitments over the long haul in the absence of funding and working to build community capacity and foster health equity are of paramount importance.

Burdine, McLeroy, Blakely, Wendel, and Felix (2010) reminded us that to engage in CBPR fully is to engage in community health development, which they liken to Rothman's locality development model (Cnaan & Rothman, 2001). However, the good stewardship exhibited by social work researchers who follow this model more closely risk doing so in the face of their own organizational constraints, as many higher education institutions and even local health agencies adopt more entrepreneurial organizational cultures and reward systems (Olssen & Peters, 2005).

APPLYING CBPR PRINCIPLES AND PROCESSES WITH YOUTH TO ADDRESS COMMUNITY HEALTH & WELL-BEING

In this section, three vignettes are presented that illustrate how CBPR principles and processes were applied across collaborative projects to improve the well-being of adolescents and young adults. In the particular community where the projects took place, there was a deep commitment and involvement of "indigenous" Puerto Rican leadership who were children during the mid-20th century migration to Chicago (Perez, 2004). These leaders were committed to building capacity, including young leadership, to improve the health and well-being of residents. Each of the three cases involved the author, students, other public health colleagues and, most important, a key community partner organization or consortia (from the same urban Latino community) in the research process. These applied practice and research cases were approved by a university institutional review board, to assure adherence to ethical research conduct.

1. ***Jóvenes Sin Fronteras: Latino Youth Take Action for Social Justice & Well-Being*** (Kelley, Benson, Estrella, & Lugardo, 2009)
   Objective: To capture the experiences of late adolescents and young adults in a culturally tailored, youth-driven after-school collective using arts and media for taking action to improve their community.
   Researcher role: The researcher supported university student involvement in the project as young collaborators striving for cultural humility. The principal investigator/student university team discussed the project outcomes with community youth, conducted observations, interviewed youth, performed member-checking of results with youth (a validity check; Morse, Barrett, Mayan, Olson, & Spiers, 2002), and co-presented with youth to elders at community events. At project completion, the researcher responded to a community request to assist with writing a grant to expand the program to a new community venue for youth-driven health promotion to prevent underage drinking. Funding was awarded to the community, and the researcher donated her time for this new project. One of the participating university students went on to work on a funded community-health initiative upon completing her academic program.
   Youth reflection from the data: "Liberation of seeing other young people like them—Puerto Ricans and Latinos—be able to articulate ideas, be able to put together concepts—that may be things that they know, but don't know that words exist for those things, like gentrification, or people putting up condos, or yuppies moving in. And that it's just not your average analysis of what that's about and what you can do."

"Because of racism and displacement, our neighborhoods are depicted as slums . . .[critiquing the status quo] so the way you change things is putting lights on the streets . . .. displacement."

Community leader reflection on project and research collaboration: "There are certain partners that you know you have a more genuine or more intimate relationship with that you may be able to discuss certain things."

"Our idea has always been to create alternatives and not necessarily have the same outlook as some of the city programs would, where they're really looking for who to blame in the sense of these young people that are behaving badly or being criminalized or some of those things that I think we all know about. But more importantly is what we can create. And so a lot of our intervention in the way that we work is really kind of a participatory process, and so in that way young people that are actually affected by the problem are the people that are finding the solutions to the problems."

2. *Community Youth Participatory Democracy Campaign*

Objective: To describe the impact on Latino youth participants of a culturally tailored youth arts and media campaign, to enhance social capital and engage youth and community members in an intergenerational dialogue to address community issues pertaining to residential stability, health, and quality of life.

Researcher role: The researcher provided unfunded technical assistance on program evaluation and held group debriefing interviews with youth. She presented key results of dialogue sessions to youth and adult leaders for making improvements and expanding programs addressing local health-promotion topics. She then used selected findings in community grant applications to expand the program. Later, the researcher presented a model for community-wide dissemination in terms of "culminating events" and tracked attendees' feedback at that event. Additionally, she held individual sessions with nascent youth leaders to assist them in tracking program participants and in keeping progress notes for project reports. Together with the community partner organization, concepts for enhancing the program and for sustainability were developed.

Youth reflection from the data: "It has changed my mind . . . how young people can communicate, and seeing what other people think outside the community; all the negativity on people's mind about the community. Through participatory democracy, I'm able to do something, it's important because of awareness."

"I don't know what I want to do in the future, but doing something like this—it opens doors to the future." "I'm not thinking the worst about people. You can interview people, you learn people are human beings, they have their own stories. Something that changed within me—I forgot where people come from."

Community leader reflection on project and research collaboration: "It's an organizational outlook that takes into account the unjust balance of power, the health disparities, as well as the policies and practices of those in the universities or governmental organizations that tend to be funders and how we can try to implement them in a way that not only is there sustained intervention but the sustained intervention for us is also a matter of reducing the health disparities or health inequities and I think bring forth a message of social justice in whatever program we're in."

"There is an indigenous reservoir of resources [in this community] that often we don't validate in the academic world or even in most foundations."

"So I think that in many ways we also impact on those [academic] organizations that we work with and transform them in some respects."

3. *A Latino Community Responds to the HIV/AIDS Crisis: The Role of Social Capital* (Kelley, Concha, Molina, & Delgado, 2007)

Objective: To capture the locally relevant meaning of *social capital* as a community resource that is deployed to address a critical health threat.

Researcher role: The researcher was funded for traditional aspects of the research project, including a percentage of her time. The community received a subcontract. The researcher conducted interviews and engaged community members in research methods such that one member pursued and completed her master's degree in the researcher's department. Additionally, she conducted continuous "member checking" throughout the project, delivered co-presentations with community members at national public health meetings, and supplemented project funding with self-pay for a community member to participate in a national public health conference so that the community was represented in the dissemination of the findings. She then provided data to community partners to use for future local public health grants and later, after project termination. She linked the community agency with academic public health resources for the community to plan a conference on best practices to prevent HIV/AIDS. She regularly attends community fundraising events, such as for local celebrations/commemorations of World AIDS Day and an annual AIDS walk to benefit the community prevention programs. She involves students in practical and technical assistance on an ongoing basis with the organization.

Youth reflection from the data: "The community knows that [agency name] has been here for a long time, and they know the faces [of] the workers."

"We know what social capital is, it's how we get so much done here with no money."

"And for instance in the parade . . . we're going to have the gay flag and . . . we've always invited other Latino gay organizations to be a part of it."

"I guess we just, you know, we know that as Puerto Ricans we're strong but as Puerto Ricans and Mexicans we're stronger."

Community leader reflection on project and research collaboration: "A good CBO [community-based organization], . . . just like a good scientific undertaking, must ultimately be premised on some social reality that people are articulating."

"It's like Columbus discovered America. America was always here and occupied by people who knew how to survive. We have always understood social capital before the academy named it."

"I believe universities and research institutions exist to basically be able to systematize the knowledge that they draw from the people that they are supposed to be studying."

Community Engagement and Ripple Effects From CBPR Projects

In addition to the researcher (author) roles in the projects described above, the author found it necessary and desirable to learn as much as possible about the origins and history of the community if she were to be in a lasting relationship, which is one of the tenets of Israel et al.'s (2001) nine principles described above. Therefore, she traveled to Puerto Rico to co-present with community members at international and more locally focused conferences addressing topics on community health and culture, stayed with members of kin networks from the Chicago community, visited key historical sites in Puerto Rico of interest to the local community, and read historical and ethnographic accounts of migration to Chicago (Near Northwest Neighborhood Network, 2005; Perez, 2004).

The earliest project, initiated over a decade ago and developed from a local public health collaborative to improve maternal and child health (Peacock et al., 2001), resulted in an alliance with a "cultural broker" (Ferré, Jones, Norris & Rowley, 2010), whose family befriended her and introduced her to the community with a walking ethnographic tour, where she was introduced to several key programs and leaders. So while the researcher (author) was developing more of an appreciation of the community and, in Bordieu's terms, more *cultural capital* (Kang & Glassman, 2010) to work with the community, the community itself was becoming more interested and competent in accessing and applying public health knowledge and skills to their tremendous health challenges, which were facilitated by collaboration with a key urban institute's community assessment findings (Shah & Whitman, 2010).

Therefore, the author began to be called upon as a liaison with the university to engage in strategic plans that resulted in (1) community input into the development of a baccalaureate degree in public health in the state's only urban research-intensive public university; (2) the development of core courses in a community college located in the community; (3) a "pipeline program" for high school students to prepare for entrance into college and receive intensive field experiences using community public health programs and tutorials for strengthening academic skills; (4) codevelopment of the community's first high school public health course, which also focused on social justice and community assets as overarching themes.

Items (3) and (4) above were informed by the author's role as providing technical assistance and mentoring to a teacher, and were driven by the community. At the same time, the author was assisting the community in developing a multisector coalition (Kelley, 2007) that focused on resources for youth. A formal structure with a funded executive director (a former student of the author's) was in place to address community health issues and apply for funding for initiatives. The author was not the sole academic helping the community. Other researchers who were acting as allies (Wallerstein & Duran, 2006) were from other area institutions. One researcher in particular took a lead role in identifying community health issues and in writing grants. Most of the time, however, the author was the only person from her department or institution who was engaged in this work until recently, when the community's success with health and educational initiatives became more widely known and celebrated, including when the coalition won the outstanding community development strategy of the year (Ballesteros, 2011).

Graduate students and alumni from the university were involved in all of these developments, and two in particular took lead roles. The author is currently collaborating with the community leadership in organizing several local elementary and high schools within the boundaries of the greater community toward a vision of a *community of wellness* for youth. This community-driven concept by a well-respected lifelong community member and professor considers the whole community as a campus, where schools and youth are connected to assets in the local ecology and where public health knowledge and skills training, including personal health and social skills, will be made available in a culturally tailored curriculum and in after-school experiences. This initiative will help to assure a healthier and engaged young citizenry that will shape the health and vitality of the community in the future.

DISCUSSION: SUMMARY OF LESSONS LEARNED

The Centrality of Community Building

Excerpts from the rich narratives in the three vignettes above show a high degree of community awareness and capacity for reflection among the younger and older community members. This is at least in part due to the Freirean philosophy of education and action, which is rooted in local culture and lived experience (Chalmers & Bramadat, 1996), and is embraced by the community in all its work. Intergenerational and multisector leadership through community building are viewed as essential to the community's health (Harpham, 2009). Additionally, the community has made an effort to stabilize itself from the threat of gentrification (Perez, 2004) and grow an educated class of young talent who now will have the opportunity to obtain public health education in high school, community college, and in an undergraduate program, which would also be a strong foundation for graduate social work education.

Partnerships with academic or professional outside partners are considered strategic and purposeful in a larger vision of community development that supports healthy living (Robinson, 2005a). Community members are able to critique the nature of the partnerships, exercise control over the production of knowledge, and take ownership of critical health issues (Chavez et al., 2008; Wallerstein & Duran, 2006). The synergy described in the section above could not happen without sustained effort over a number of years, with collective reflection and discussion within the health coalition, and without cooperation from the university, city agencies, and others in the academy. Most importantly, what drove all of these innovations was vision from the community, and then being willing to put "sweat equity" into a collaborative effort because community building for health requires sustained momentum over time and transcends efforts of time-limited categorical health grants. However, to bear witness to the unfolding of a community's capacity for health action is one of the most rewarding and ethical things that one can engage in. Changes in community capacity can outlast the particulars of partnerships and form a foundation for the future.

It Is All About Relationships and Commitment

The idea of community partners strategically engaging White allies and managing these alliances demonstrates a high degree of local leadership development. Another concept that the community used to describe these allies is the *organic intellectual*. Tickle (2001) cited and elaborated upon Becker's description of the organic intellectual as:

> Constantly interacting with society, struggling to change minds, engaged in the evolution of knowledge, raising issues in the public domain and defending decent standards of social well-being, freedoms and justice. This is a distinction between "those who simply represent the information that they were trained to pass along and those who are innovative, daring and public in their re-presentation of their own personal interaction with the world." (Becker, 1996 as cited in Tickle (2001, p. 161)

Thomas, Quinn, Butler, Fryer, and Garza (2011) described the importance of researchers engaging with their communities of interest:

> CBPR is a valuable tool, [but] it is only one means of community engagement. Community engagement is essential to fully understand and grapple with the impact of the ordinariness of racism on community members' lives, to expand our understanding of race and racism as well as the intersectionality of other factors such as gender on their lives, and to engage community members fully as partners in action. (p. 410)

The ideas advanced by Wallerstein et al. (2008) regarding the capacity and readiness of the researcher and community partner, as well as their historical relationship and successes as key starting points that inform future success, are relevant here.

CBPR as an Intervention With Ethical and Power Issues

One thing that is difficult to present in traditional journals is the process behind collaborative research, such as the researcher's accommodation to the community norms and life world (Wicks & Reason, 2009). In articulating ethical issues and responsibilities of White researchers in communities of color, Helms and colleagues (2005) cautioned that, "given their research omnipotence and the pervasiveness of Whiteness, there are many opportunities for white researchers to do harm to ALANA (African American, Latino/a, Asian American and Native American) and immigrant individuals and communities without necessarily intending to do so" (p. 300). Effective CBPR partnerships can potentially reduce the likelihood of harm occurring to communities during the research process. This harm could, for example, include the researcher unknowingly misrepresenting aspects of culture or history or omitting important cultural assets that could frame issues and solutions or perhaps more commonly, failure to deploy local assets and resources in ways that build capacity (Labonte, Bell, Chad, & Laverack, 2002) and community self-efficacy (Sampson, Morenoff, & Earls,

1999) and sustainability. Additionally, an effective partnership could also facilitate cultural renewal (Wallerstein et al., 2008) and have a special identity-based appeal to the community of interest, possibly enhancing the uptake of the intervention and long-term community change.

CONCLUSION

Strier (2007) offered a definition of antioppressive social work research that encompasses the goal of "the systemic study of oppression and the development of knowledge that supports people's actions to achieve freedom from oppression" (p. 4). Public health social workers—like other public health practitioner–scientists—are embracing CBPR in their efforts to address health inequities. In so doing, they are building on a rich tradition of community building and antioppressive or emancipatory practices. Such practices are also in concert with the notion of whole community development to improve and sustain health (Robinson, 2005b), but only when power and representation issues are acknowledged and addressed, which of course are continual challenges throughout the collaborative process.

Institutional, investigator, and community supports are needed for collaborative research over time to ensure the capacities for this approach are developed among a new generation of social workers, community leaders, and professionals. Renewing efforts in the profession to teach macro-level practice and community organization, participatory and action research, and emancipatory ways of engaging with socially marginalized communities (Jordan, 2004) are key to building effective and evidence-informed CBPR approaches for addressing health inequities in the future. These practices would advance several of the public health social work core competencies, especially those related to community development and collaborative research. More evidence is needed across various community contexts to understand the conditions under which CBPR "works" best, for which outcomes and for what populations and health issues. Social workers should contribute to the science of CBPR by following Trickett's (1991) advice to *make what happens a heuristic for theory* and conduct process and outcome evaluations of CBPR projects.

LEARNING ACTIVITIES

1. Look at websites of local foundations and determine the extent to which they promote and fund collaborative inquiry between organizations such as health departments or local consortia/coalitions and specific target communities and neighborhoods. What issues are being funded and what criteria are applied to capture the nature of

the collaboration or partnership? How is community development or sustainability addressed?

2. Review area universities for community-based research or community collaborative inquiry activities. Is there a portal or protocol for local organizations or community leaders to contact the university and discuss potential applied research or programmatic interests? What issues are being funded, and where are the community partners located? What types of community-based organizations are involved in these collaborations? How is community development or sustainability addressed?

3. Investigate your state or local "Ready by 21" initiative for adolescents and young adults and determine to what extent, if any, youth are involved in community inquiry and change, action research, and/or community-based participatory research (these are all variations of youth collaborations). See www.readyby21.org/. You may also want to review your state or local after school consortia or programming as well.

INTERNET RESOURCES

Community-Based Public Health Caucus

(www.sph.umich.edu/cbphcaucus/)

Community–Campus Partnerships for Health

(http://depts.washington.edu/ccph/index.html)

Community Tool Box

(http://ctb.ku.edu/en/default.aspx)

Kellogg Health Scholars Program

(www.kellogghealthscholars.org/about/community.cfm)

National Institutes of Health, Office of Behavioral and Social Sciences Research

(http://obssr.od.nih.gov/scientific_areas/methodology/community_ba sed_participatory_research/index.aspx)

REFERENCES

Association of State and Territorial Public Health Social Workers. (2005). *Public health social work standards and competencies*. Columbus: Ohio Department of Health.

Ballesteros, J. (2011). *Greater Humboldt Park community of wellness.* Retrieved May 28, 2011, from http://www.ghpcommunityofwellness.org/

Burdine, J. N., McLeroy, K., Blakely, C., Wendel, M. L., & Felix, M. R. J. (2010). Community-based participatory research and community health development. *The Journal of Primary Prevention, 31*(1), 1-7.

Centers for Disease Control and Prevention. (2011). *10 essential public health services.* Retrieved September 5, 2011, from http://www.cdc.gov/nphpsp/essentialServices. html

Chalmers, K. I., & Bramadat, I. J. (1996). Community development: Theoretical and practical issues for community health nursing in Canada. *Journal of Advanced Nursing, 24*(4), 719-726.

Chavez, V., Duran, B., Baker, Q. E., Avila, M. M., & Wallerstein, N. (2008). The dance of race and privilege in community based participatory research. In M. Minkler & N. Wallerstein (Eds.), *Community based participatory research for health: From process to outcomes* (2nd ed., pp. 81-97). San Francisco, CA: Jossey-Bass.

Cnaan, R. A., & Rothman, J. (2001). Locality development and the building of community. In J. Rothman, J. L. Erlich, & J. E. Tropman (Eds.), *Strategies of community intervention* (pp. 251-277). Itasca, IL: F.E. Peacock.

Creswell, J. W. (2009). *Research design: Qualitative, quantitative, and mixed methods approaches* (3rd ed.). Thousand Oaks, CA: Sage Publications, Inc.

Currie, D. (2011). IoM report: Some Healthy People goals need immediate attention. *The Nation's Health, 41*(4), 8.

Ewert, G. D. (1991). Habermas and education: A comprehensive overview of the influence of habermas in educational literature. *Review of Educational Research, 61*(3), 345-378.

Ferré, C. D., Jones, L., Norris, K. C., & Rowley, D. L. (2010). The Healthy African American Families (HAAF) project: From community-based participatory research to community-partnered participatory research. *Ethnicity & Disease, 20*(1, Suppl. 2), S21-S28.

Fried, L. P., Bentley, M. E., Buekens, P., Burke, D. S., Frenk, J. J., Klag, M. J., et al. (2010). Global health is public health. *The Lancet, 375*(9714), 535-537.

Frieden, T. R. (2010). A framework for public health action: The health impact pyramid. *American Journal of Public Health, 100*(4), 590-595.

Goodman, R. M., Speers, M. A., McLeroy, K., Fawcett, S., Kegler, M., Parker, E., ... Wallerstein, N. (1998). Identifying and defining the dimensions of community capacity to provide a basis for measurement. *Health Education & Behavior, 25*(3), 258-278.

Habermas, J. (1984). *The theory of communicative action.* Boston, MA: Beacon Press.

Harpham, T. (2009). Urban health in developing countries: What do we know and where do we go? *Health & Place, 15*(1), 107-116.

Helms, J. E., Jernigan, M., & Maschier, J. (2005). The meaning of race in psychology and how to change it. *American Psychologist, 60*(1), 27-36.

Israel, B. A., Schulz, A. J., Parker, E. A., & Becker, A. B. (1998). Review of community-based research: Assessing partnership approaches to improve public health. *Annual Review of Public Health, 19*(1), 173-202.

Israel, B. A., Schulz, A. J., Parker, E. P., & Becker, A. B. (2001). Community-based participatory research: Policy recommendations for promoting a partnership approach in health research. *Education for Health, 14*(2), 182-197.

Johnson, T. D. (2011). Healthy People 2020 sets new health targets for nation. *Nations Health, 40*(10).

Jordan, B. (2004). Emancipatory social work? opportunity or oxymoron. *British Journal of Social Work, 34*(1), 5-19.

Kang, M. J., & Glassman, M. (2010). Moral action as social capital, moral thought as cultural capital. *Journal of Moral Education, 39*(1), 21-36.

Ka'opua, L. S. I., Park, S. H., Ward, M. E., & Braun, K. L. (2011). Testing the feasibility of a culturally tailored breast cancer screening intervention with native Hawaiian women in rural churches. *Health & Social Work, 36*(1), 55-65.

Kelley, M. A. (2007, Summer/Fall). Building "Comunidad de bienestar" in Puerto Rican Chicago: Community culture, development and health. *ACOSA Update*, pp. 3-14. Retrieved from http://www.acosa.org/

Kelley, M. A., Benson, M., Estrella, M., & Lugardo, J. (2009). *Jóvenes sin fronteras: Latino youth take action for social justice & well-being* (Working Paper Series GCP-09-01). Chicago: University of Illinois at Chicago Great Cities Institute. Retrieved from http://www.uic.edu/cuppa/gci/

Kelley, M. A., Concha, J., Molina, A., & Delgado, J. (2007). *A Puerto Rican community responds to the HIV/AIDS crisis: The role of social and cultural capital* (Working Paper Series ed.). Chicago, IL: University of Illinois at Chicago Great Cities Institute. Retrieved from http://www.uic.edu/cuppa/gci/

Labonte, R., Bell, W. G., Chad, K., & Laverack, G. (2002). Community capacity building: A parallel track for health promotion programs (commentary). *Canadian Journal of Public Health, 93*(3), 181-182.

Leung, M. W., Yen, I. H., & Minkler, M. (2004). Community based participatory research: A promising approach for increasing epidemiology's relevance in the 21st century. *International Journal of Epidemiology, 33*(3), 499-506.

Lundy, C. (2004). *Social work and social justice: A structural approach to practice.* Toronto, Ontario, Canada: University of Toronto Press.

Marmot, M. (2005). Social determinants of health inequalities. *The Lancet, 365*(9464), 1099-1104.

Minkler, M. (2004). Ethical challenges for the "outside" researcher in community-based participatory research. *Health Education & Behavior, 31*(6), 684.

Minkler, M. (2005). Community-based research partnerships: Challenges and opportunities. *Journal of Urban Health, 82*(2), ii3-ii12.

Minkler, M., & Wallerstein, N. (2005). Improving health through community organization and community building. In M. Minkler (Ed.), *Community organizing and community building for health* (2nd ed., pp. 26-50). New Brunswick, NJ: Rutgers University Press.

Morse, J. M., Barrett, M., Mayan, M., Olson, K., & Spiers, J. (2002). Verification strategies for establishing reliability and validity in qualitative research. *International Journal of Qualitative Methods, 1*(2), 13-22.

Near Northwest Neighborhood Network. (2005). *Near Northwest Neighborhood Network/Humboldt Park empowerment partnership.* Retrieved May 14, 2006, from http://www.nnnn.org/

Office of Disease Prevention and Health Promotion (2011). *Healthy People 2020.* Retrieved May 27, 2012 from http://healthypeople.gov/2020/.

Olssen, M., & Peters, M. A. (2005). Neoliberalism, higher education and the knowledge economy: From the free market to knowledge capitalism. *Journal of Education Policy, 20*(3), 313–345.

Peacock, N. R., Kelley, M. A., Carpenter, C., Davis, M., Burnett, G., Chavez, N., et al. (2001). Pregnancy discovery and acceptance among low-income primiparous women: A multicultural exploration. *Maternal and Child Health Journal, 5*(2), 109–118.

Perez, G. M. (2004). *The Near Northwest side story: Migration, displacement, and Puerto Rican families.* Berkeley: University of California Press.

Robinson, R. G. (2005). Community development model for public health applications: Overview of a model to eliminate population disparities. *Health Promotion Practice, 6*(3), 338.

Sampson, R. J., Morenoff, J. D., & Earls, F. (1999). Beyond social capital: Spatial dynamics of collective efficacy for children. *American Sociological Review, 64*(5), 633–660.

Shah, A. M., & Whitman, S. (2010). Sinai's improving community health survey: Methodology and key findings. In S. Whitman, A. M. Shah, & M. Benjamins (Eds.), *Urban health: Combating disparities with local data* (pp. 31–68). New York, NY: Oxford University Press.

Splitter, L. J. (2009). Authenticity and constructivism in education. *Studies in Philosophy and Education, 28*(2), 135–151.

Strier, R. (2007). Anti-oppressive research in social work: A preliminary definition. *British Journal of Social Work, 37*(5), 857–871.

Tervalon, M., & Murray-Garcia, J. (1998). Cultural humility versus cultural competence: A critical distinction in defining physician training outcomes in multicultural education. *Journal of Health Care for the Poor and Underserved, 9*(2), 117–125.

Thomas, S. B., Quinn, S. C., Butler, J., Fryer, C. S., & Garza, M. A. (2011). Toward a fourth generation of disparities research to achieve health equity. *Annual Review of Public Health, 32*, 399–416.

Tickle, L. (2001). The organic intellectual educator. *Cambridge Journal of Education, 31*(2), 159–178.

Trickett, E. J. (1991). Paradigms and the research report: Making what actually happens a heuristic for theory. *American Journal of Community Psychology, 19*(3), 365–370.

Trickett, E. J. (2009). Multilevel community-based culturally situated interventions and community impact: An ecological perspective. *American Journal of Community Psychology, 43*(3), 257–266.

Trickett, E. J., & Espino, S. L. (2004). Collaboration and social inquiry: Multiple meanings of a construct and its role in creating useful and valid knowledge. *American Journal of Community Psychology, 34*(1–2), 1–69.

Wallerstein, N. B., & Duran, B. (2006). Using community-based participatory research to address health disparities. *Health Promotion Practice, 7*(3), 312–323.

Wallerstein, N., & Duran, B. (2010). Community-based participatory research contributions to intervention research: The intersection of science and practice to improve health equity. *American Journal of Public Health, 100*(S1), S40–S46.

Wallerstein, N., Oetzel, J., Duran, B., Tafoya, G., Belone, L., & Rae, R. (2008). What predicts outcomes in CBPR. In M. Minkler & N. Wallerstein (Eds.), *Community-based participatory research for health: From process to outcomes.* (2nd ed., pp. 371–392). San Francisco, CA: Jossey-Bass.

Wenger, E. C., & Snyder, W. M. (2000). Communities of practice: The organizational frontier. *Harvard Business Review, 78*(1), 139–146.

Wicks, P. G., & Reason, P. (2009). Initiating action research: Challenges and paradoxes of opening communicative space. *Action Research, 7*(3), 243–262.

World Health Organization. (1986). *Ottawa charter for health promotion*. Paper presented at the First International Conference on Health Promotion, Ottawa, Ontario, Canada.

CHAPTER 17

Public Health Social Work in the Uniformed Services

Gary Lounsberry

INTRODUCTION

*M**ilitary social work* is the term often applied to the field of social work practice in the U.S. military services. The existence of this field of practice has not been well known and is just now gaining recognition in the social work profession as the demand for trained professionals to deal with the needs of service members and their families, as the result of extended and multiple battlefield deployments, grows.

The most recent comprehensive book on social work in the military was published in 1999, prior to the wars in Iraq and Afghanistan (Daley, 1999). Articles have appeared in journals, such as *Military Medicine,* published by the services and professional associations of military personnel, but are not generally read by social work professionals outside of the military services. Much of the recent literature deals with aftercare for veterans who are no longer on active duty and are now under the care of the U.S. Department of Veterans Affairs (VA; Kelly, Howe-Barksdale, & Gitelson, 2011). The bulk of the literature focuses on clinical treatment and aftercare. Military social work is moving toward prevention, early intervention, and community-based care, but little published literature has explicitly investigated public health social work concepts and competencies applied to military personnel.

In addition to a general lack of understanding of the role of social work in the U.S. military, there is limited contemporary knowledge among the general public of the range of American uniformed services, their distinctions, and responsibilities. The terms *armed services, military services,* and *uniformed services* are often used interchangeably in the popular media. Within the services, and at times in federal regulations, distinctions are made: Armed services are the services in military combat, including the U.S. Air Force, U.S. Army, U.S. Navy, U.S. Marine Corps, and, at times, the U.S. Coast Guard; also included when activated for foreign combat are the various National Guard and Reserve units. Uniformed services include all of the above with the addition of the Commissioned Corps of the U.S. Public Health Service (USPHS) and the National Oceanic and Atmospheric Administration. While the VA is one of the primary federal employers of professional social workers, the VA is separate from the uniformed services, does not employ commissioned personnel, and serves veterans who have been honorably discharged from active duty. The Council on Social Work Education (2010) has defined military social work as including all of the above federal organizations.

All of the uniformed services employ both commissioned and civilian social workers in the entire gamut of public health social work practice (Savinsky, Illingworth & DuLaney, 2009). Each service has the responsibility to perform the three core public health functions for their service members and the service families living on service property. It is difficult to determine the exact number of people with social work degrees currently in the services because many of the billets occupied by social workers are not formally defined as social work positions. Social workers are performing everything from more traditional social work roles to front-line combat. A *billet*—a service description of position responsibilities—with public health social work in the description is most likely to be found in the USPHS, but even in the USPHS social workers are in billets that do not mention social work in their job description duties.

In 2011, there were about 8,000 civilian, contract, enlisted, and commissioned social workers in the uniformed services. Each of the uniformed services has about 150–225 commissioned social work officers. The VA has 13,179 social work positions, the Department of Defense has 3,858, and the Department of Health and Human Services (which includes the USPHS) has 2,716 (Making the Difference, 2011).

Each of the services has its own history of the utilization of social workers in its service and somewhat different contemporary roles. However, as a result of the unique stresses of repeated tours of duty in the Iraq and Afghanistan conflicts, there is growing interservice collaboration, coordination, and consolidations, including interservice assignments, particularly in health care and family support. The current military strategy of a "total force deployment" heavily utilizes the Reserve and National Guard troops for extended and multiple deployments. With the regular active-duty troop reductions after 1973, there are not enough regular active-duty service members to staff extended combat operations.

Reserve and Guard members originate from throughout the nation, are not usually residing on a military base, and may be spread over a wide geographic area. This dispersion may reduce access to the many support programs available on base. There is recognition among military social workers that public health competencies are needed to provide prevention and early intervention strategies for Reserve and Guard units to reduce posttraumatic stress disorder (PTSD) and other stress-related physical and emotional disorders among service personnel and their families.

The military population includes a cross-section of America, with somewhat larger percentages of younger, healthier, and male enlistees. However, women constitute a growing percentage of active-duty personnel and serve in 90% of the available billets (Knox & Price, 2011. The majority of active-duty personnel are parents who live on military installations. Military installations are small cities with many similarities to their civilian counterparts. The difference is that they are entirely under military command and everyone, including families, is expected to support the service mission. The installation command has responsibility for all public health, education, family services, police, court, and other civic functions. All of the public health issues of an American community are present in a military community, with the addition of the special circumstances presented by combat missions, including extended separations, and a military authority structure.

HEALTHY PEOPLE 2020 OBJECTIVES

Healthy People 2020 objectives apply to the military community just as they do to a civilian population, with some objectives having a special importance because of the unique experiences of service personnel.

Global Health objectives are a special concern because a high percentage of military personnel serve outside the United States in extremely adverse and hazardous environments. In addition to combat, service personnel are exposed to poor sanitation, environmental pollutants, close living environments, and local populations with untreated contagious diseases, among other exposures. With today's combat operations, service personnel may experience multiple deployments with subsequent returns stateside with the possibility of transmitting a disease.

Mental Health and Mental Disorders objectives identify veterans who have experienced trauma as a population of special concern. PTSD, brain injury, suicide, substance abuse, and other mental disorders all occur at higher rates among veterans and those on active duty following traumatic experiences. These documented outcomes have been a major factor in the increased role of social work in the military services.

Substance Abuse objectives identify military personnel and their families as an emerging issue in substance abuse because of the strain military deployment places on families, with subsequent family disintegration and substance abuse. Military social workers work extensively in military substance abuse programs and family services.

Preparedness objectives include responses to disease outbreaks, natural disasters, and terrorist attacks. The military is called upon to respond in all of these situations. The military is trained to respond quickly and is often the first responder. Military social workers are part of the rapid response teams and take a lead in coordinating and training civilian counterparts.

Social Determinants objectives consider the social and economic variables in health. Military personnel bring with them the social and economic variables and risk factors of their home communities. Enlisted personnel tend to come from lower income groups with an overrepresentation of rural backgrounds. Given that being a commissioned officer requires a college degree, officers tend to have somewhat better economic and educational backgrounds while still having geographic overrepresentation. Within the military community, there is a conscious effort to provide a healthy community environment and the opportunities to address prior social disadvantages. Opportunities for education, training, and advancement abound; often, making a choice from myriad opportunities is more of a problem than a lack of opportunity. It has been often observed that the contemporary military is the most merit-based sector of American society.

Access to Health Services becomes more of an issue once the service member leaves active duty. While on active duty, service members and their dependents have access to free, comprehensive health care provided by the military. Military health care uses a public health model emphasizing prevention and early intervention that ensures the service member will be fit for duty. An issue in active-duty access to health care has been access to mental health care because the services have had difficulty recruiting enough mental health professionals to meet service demands. There is a major recruitment effort now underway to meet this challenge.

If service members leave military service prior to the earliest retirement of 20 years of service, they no longer have access to the military service health care system. Veterans who retire from the service with at least 20 years of service have lifetime health insurance coverage through the TRICARE program and may also use the health services of the nearest military installation. There are some co-pays and cost-share required under the TRICARE program. Honorably discharged veterans have access to the VA health care system. Access at the VA can be an issue because veterans with combat-related disabilities and health problems have priority. The VA is experiencing such a demand from high-priority veterans of the Middle Eastern conflicts that lower priority veterans may experience long waits for service. The VA, too, has had difficulty recruiting sufficient mental health professionals to treat veterans with mental health and substance abuse problems.

PUBLIC HEALTH SOCIAL WORK CORE COMPETENCIES

Military life is organized by levels of group membership. The readiness and fitness of the total force and all its constituent subdivisions are continually being assessed and responses being evaluated. Military social workers must be familiar with epidemiology, be able to interpret demographic information, be able to construct hypotheses based on population data, and be able to operate at the macro level. Social workers are frequently called upon to analyze patterns in service personnel experiences, health outcomes, and environmental conditions and then design macro-level interventions to prevent or reduce negative consequences. Some military social workers have full-time research duties investigating service-wide issues.

Military social workers were among the first to recognize and inform senior leadership about the added stress of repeated deployment on service personnel and their families. The ability to document the increased incidence of stress-related disorders among service personnel as well as family members led to broadening the scope of mental health and support services for the entire military family.

Leadership and communication skills are expected in all military officers. Military social workers are frequently called upon to provide briefings and reports to all levels of command on issues affecting all levels of the services, especially on issues of diversity, culture, social relations, connections to civilian communities, and family dynamics. Social workers provide training and educational sessions for commissioned and enlisted personnel and their families on a wide range of topics, including adjusting to transitions into and out of military life.

Military social workers will be found at all organizational levels, from being the sole mental professional deployed with a forward combat unit to being in command of a major clinical services unit. At all levels, the social work officers are responsible for the management of their functions, which may include the management of large budgets, staff, program planning, and policy implementation.

While social work in each of the services developed along somewhat different paths, today social workers in all of the services have a wide range of duties and responsibilities that require public health social work competencies.

U.S. AIR FORCE

The U.S. Air Force became a separate military service in 1947 when it was formed out of the former Army Air Corps (Jenkins, 1999). Social work has been part of the Air Force since its formation. All active-duty social workers belong to the Air Force Medical Service and, since 1967, have been commissioned as medical officers in the Biomedical Science Corps. Social workers may be assigned to other divisions but remain Air Force Medical Service personnel (Tarpley, 1999). Active duty, commissioned social work officers number about 210 to 225. There are several hundred contracted civilian social workers in the family advocacy services (www.usmilitary.about.com).

In the early years, Air Force social workers were almost exclusively assigned to the mental health services. Over the years, their scope of practice has expanded to embrace a more public health model of preventive services in Family Advocacy programs, the integrated delivery system, and community building programs. Today, social work officers are assigned to a wide range of duties, from direct practice to research. Air Force social workers serve in command positions and are deployed to forward combat units for early intervention and other duties.

AIR NATIONAL GUARD

Air National Guard units become part of the Air Force when activated for combat. When not on combat duty, Guard units are on standby for possible domestic crises such as natural disasters and rescue missions. Historically, Guard units were part-time duty based near the service members' homes, and Guardsmen held other full-time jobs. In the current military strategy, Guardsmen face multiple deployments with long separations from the families. Guard units include social workers in multiple roles, some as social work officers, others in a wide range of command positions, including flight officers. When activated, Guard units have access to the entire array of active-duty services and benefits. When on standby, at times access to services may be an issue. Both commissioned and civilian social workers are working on this problem through the Family Advocacy and other programs.

U.S. ARMY

Army social work evolved out of the service of Red Cross social workers at Army hospitals and field units. The first Red Cross social worker was assigned on September 1, 1918, to the Plattsburgh, NY, Army General Hospital (Harris, 1999). The Red Cross social work presence continued to grow through World Wars I and II. Between 1942 and 1945, about 1,000 Red Cross social workers were assigned to Army hospitals in the United States and abroad (National Association of Social Workers, 1965).

In 1942, six enlisted men who were professionally trained social workers were assigned to the Army Mental Hygiene Consultation Service. The commissioning of social work officers was authorized in 1945. Army social work officers were concentrated in the Mental Hygiene service until 1951, when the Red Cross withdrew its social workers from Army hospitals and the Army formed the Army Medical Social Work program. In 1957, Army social workers began to serve in the military stockades, or prisons. By the 1960s, there was a major shift in the demographics of Army installations, with the majority of service members having families with the accompanying range of family problems. In response, the Army formed the Army Community Service and assigned 42 social work officers and 19 enlisted social work specialists to develop a community-based, preventive, and early intervention family program (Harris, 1999). The Army is now increasing the recruitment of social workers and has developed training affiliations with schools of social work as well as initiated training programs with the Army to meet the demand for social work officers.

ARMY NATIONAL GUARD

When not called up for active duty with the regular Army, the National Guard is under the authority of the governor of the home state. The governor may mobilize the Guard for disaster assistance, search and rescue, and civil disturbances. There are specialty units among the Guard, such as medical units that include social work officers and a family support program that may also include social workers in the state office who work with volunteer support groups of Guard family members.

U.S. COAST GUARD

The Coast Guard has undergone many administration relocations in its history. Today, the Coast Guard is located in the Department of Homeland Security. The Coast Guard relies on the Commissioned Corps of the USPHS and civilian contractors to provide health services to its members. USPHS social work officers are detailed to the Coast Guard and Coast Guard personnel utilize services at any nearby installations of the other services.

U.S. NAVY

The U.S. Navy appointed its first social work commissioned officer in 1980 assigned to the Medical Service Corps (Mahoney, 2009). In 2009, there were 24 active-duty officers, four reserve officers, 750 civilians, and 400 contract social workers. The Navy is currently expanding its social work force and has launched a major recruitment effort. Navy social workers serve in medical retreatment facilities, major military treatment centers, and Fleet and Family Support Centers throughout the world. In addition to service members and their families, Navy social workers provide clinical and community services to international civilian populations during humanitarian missions from U.S. Navy hospital ships like the USNS Mercy.

U.S. MARINE CORPS

The Marine Corps is the land force of the U.S. Navy, and their health services are provided by naval officers who may also be assigned to the Marine Corps. Social work services are provided by naval officers or civilian contract social workers. Officers assigned to the Marine Corps practice in a wide range of settings, including being embedded with forward combat units.

U.S. PUBLIC HEALTH SERVICE

The Commissioned Corps of the USPHS is among the oldest, but least known or understood, of the American uniformed services. The USPHS dates to 1798, when it was formed to operate the U.S. Marine Hospitals and Quarantine Service in every American port city. Health care and screening for infectious diseases was provided for everyone arriving by ship, including merchant marine and immigrants. USPHS officers wear naval-style uniforms, use Navy rank, and are often confused with Navy officers (Wittman & Kissel, 1979).

The USPHS is under the command of the Surgeon General of the United States. USPHS social work officers serve in a wide range of organizations and roles. The National Institutes of Health, Centers for Disease Control and Prevention, U.S. Department of Health and Human Services Bureau of Primary Care, the Indian Health Service, Federal Bureau of Prisons, U.S. Coast Guard, Department of Homeland Security Immigration and Customs Enforcement (ICE), U.S. embassies, state health departments, and other military services are all served by USPHS social work officers.

In 1921, the first civilian social worker was employed by USPHS at the Ellis Island, NY, U.S. Marine Hospital to serve immigrant families and merchant seamen. During World War II, the Marine Hospitals and Clinics added programs for the treatment of tuberculosis and narcotic addictions. These new programs resulted in the addition of more social workers in these programs. In 1949, USPHS appointed the first social work commissioned officer. By December 2010, there were 177 commissioned social work officers in the USPHS (Social Work Professional Advisory Group, 2010). While USPHS social work officers are the most likely of military social workers to have the term "public health social work" appear in their billet description, these officers hold many command, research, and policy billets that do not even mention social work.

USPHS social work officers serve uniformed service personnel in a variety of venues. They provide services to fellow USPHS service members and their families at USPHS direct-care facilities and provide macro-level leadership in a range of USPHS divisions. USPHS social work officers are detailed to the Coast Guard, Army, Navy, and Marine Corps to provide services to these sister organizations. USPHS officers also serve veterans who are also clients of other federal programs, such as the Indian Health Service, ICE, and the Bureau of Prisons.

VETERAN'S ADMINISTRATION

The VA is the largest federal employer of social workers with over 13,000 positions (Making the Difference, 2011). The VA is an independent agency, separate from the Department of Defense, and all of its social workers are civilians—although many are veterans with prior military experience. VA services are available to all honorably discharged veterans and include a wide range of educational, financial, and supportive benefits in addition to health care. Prior to 2001, VA services were focused on the aging population of veterans from the World Wars, Korea, and Vietnam with chronic health problems. With the advent of the wars in Iraq and Afghanistan, the VA has had to adapt and restructure to address the needs of younger veterans with major traumatic injuries, PTSD, high unemployment, young families, and many reentry-to-civilian-life problems.

The VA Social Work department was established on June 16, 1926, with 14 clinical social workers placed in VA psychiatric hospitals and 22 in VA regional offices. Today, social workers are in every VA facility and program (VA Social Work, 2011). The VA is affiliated with 180 schools of social work and provides 900 social work internships a year (VA Office of Academic Affairs, 2010).

Historically, the VA has been an institution-based system, with many facilities at some distance from the beneficiary population. The emphasis was on secondary and tertiary care, often with long periods of VA residential care. Since the Vietnam War, there has been a move toward community-based, primary care. This change has accelerated under the demands of returnees from the wars in Iraq and Afghanistan (Flynn & Hassan, 2010). There is also a new stress on coordination of service and client records with the military services to reduce the problems of transfer from active duty to veteran's care. VA social workers have major responsibilities in ensuring continuity of care in this community-based model.

UNIFORMED SERVICES SOCIAL WORKERS

The oldest regular meeting of all the military social workers is held in conjunction with the annual meeting of AMSUS (American Military Surgeons of the United States). The Uniformed Services Social Workers (USSW) includes social workers from all the uniformed services and the VA (AMSUS, 2011).

CURRENT TRENDS

Topics at Military Social Work Professional Meetings

A review of the USSW agenda for the November 8, 2011, professional meeting presents the current trends and themes in military social work (USSW, 2011). All the themes have a public health social work focus. Topics for the meeting include each of the services presenting a session on "Community: Purpose/possibility," "Beyond choking under pressure: New global resilience paradigms," "Review of several research-based military and veteran marriage and family relationship resilience interventions delivered via interactive technology," "Mental fitness and resiliency training," "Resiliency in Air Force couples following deployment," and "When they return from Afghanistan: The needs of the wounded."

In summary, there are five workshops on community approaches, five sessions on promoting resilience, five sessions on treating and early intervention with PTSD, three on reintegration following deployment, one on supportive care for survivors of military sexual trauma, one on identification and early intervention with veterans at risk for becoming homeless, and one regarding identification and early intervention with people in custody of ICE.

Family and Community Services

All the services, including the Reserves and National Guard, are expanding family support services. These include services for military children in public schools.

Resilience

A major theoretical framework for research and programming is the concept of resilience. Research and intervention models are framed around the concept of building resilience among service personnel and their families prior, during, and following deployment (Wheeler & Bragin, 2007).

Reintegration

As the deadlines approach for withdrawing troops from Iraq and Afghanistan, the focus is beginning to shift toward the issues of reintegrating service personnel and their families into noncombat and civilian life. As personnel leave active duty, services will move to the VA and civilian providers. Work will be needed to make this an integrated transition without the major gaps in service experienced in prior wars.

Lack of Trained Social Workers Entering the Military

The Army and Navy have developed social work training programs in conjunction with schools of social work because they are not able to recruit enough social workers to fill their service needs. Other schools of social work have identified military social work as a specialty track. The services are for the first time actively advertising to recruit both commissioned and civilian social workers.

The emphasis on collaboration and conjoint services among the uniformed services is likely to continue.

ISSUES FOR THE FUTURE

The eventual end to the conflict in Iraq and Afghanistan will likely present challenges to military social work. An abrupt withdrawal and discharge of troops would result in major adjustment problems and a potential break in continuity of services. Reentry into civilian life of large numbers of veterans in the current economy would present a host of social and economic issues (Simmons & Rycraft, 2010). However the current conflicts end, there will be large numbers of former service personnel with long-term physical, mental, employment, and social challenges that will require decades of care through the VA and other programs.

When there is an end to the present hostilities, there are likely to be pressures on the Department of Defense to reduce expenses. An area the Department of Defense is studying is the merger of many health services, which would likely include many areas of military social work. The 2011 closure of the historic Walter Reed Army Medical Center and move of the new Walter Reed to the Bethesda Naval Medical Center Campus may be seen as movement toward consolidation.

INTERNET RESOURCES

The following websites lead to the social work page in each of the services' web pages. Located here are additional links to more detail about military social work and affiliated organizations. Information about employment and current openings are available on these sites.

U.S. Air Force

(www.airforce.com/careers/detail/clinical-social-worker/)

U.S. Army

(www.armymedicine.army.mil/prr/social_work.html)

U.S. Navy

(www.navy.com/careers/healthcare/clinical-care/social-work.html)

U.S. Public Health Service

(www.usphs.gov/profession/healthservices/requirements.aspx#Social)

U.S. Department of Veterans Affairs

(www.socialwork.va.gov/socialworkers.asp)

Discussion Questions

1. What are some differences and similarities in serving as a commissioned social work officer and as a civilian social worker?
2. What core public health social work competencies will be required as a military social worker?
3. How is life different for families of military service members from other, nonmilitary families?
   (a) What do you think are the most stressful aspects of military life?
   (b) What interventions have the potential for reducing stress among military family members?
   (c) How might concerns about family coping impact the deployed service member?
4. What issues will confront returning deployed service personnel and their families?
5. What services are included in the following categories: armed services, uniformed services, and military services?
   (a) When does someone become eligible for VA services?

REFERENCES

Association of Military Surgeons of the United States. (2011). Uniformed Services Social Workers Conference Agenda for 8 November 2011. *AMSUS Annual Conference November 2011.* Retrieved from http://amsusmeeting.org/WordPress/wp-content/uploads/2011/08/AMSUS-Preliminary_Final-Program.pdf

Council on Social Work Education. (2010). *Advanced social work practice in military social work.* Alexandria, VA: Author.

Daley, J. G. (Ed.). (1999). *Social work practice in the military.* Binghamton, NY: The Haworth Press.

Flynn, M., & Hassan, A. (2010, Spring/Summer). Unique challenges of war in Iraq and Afghanistan. *Journal of Social Work Education, 46*(2), 169–173.

Harris, J. (1999). History of army social work. *Social work practice in the military.* Binghamton, NY: The Haworth Press.

Jenkins, J. L. (1999). History of air force social work. In J. G. Daley (Eds.), *Social work practice in the military* (pp. 27–46). Binghamton, NY: The Haworth Press.

Kelly, D. C., Howe-Barksdale, S., & Gitelson, D. (Eds.). (2011). *Treating young veterans: Promoting resilience through practice and advocacy.* New York: Springer Publishing.

Knox, J., & Price, D. H. (1999). Total force and the new American military family: implications for social work practice. *Families in Society, 80*(2), 128–136.

Mahoney, C. (2009, April 4). Navy medicine commemorates social worker awareness month. *Navy Medicine, Issue 4.* Retrieved September 21, 2012 from http://www.med.navy.mil/bumed/comms/MEDNEWS/Documents/MN%20April%202010%202009.pdf.

Making the Difference. (2011). Social work jobs in federal government. *Federal Careers.* Retrieved May 11, 2011, from http://www.makingthedifference.org/federalcareers/socialwork.shtml

National Association of Social Workers. (1965). *Mental health and psychiatric services.* New York: National Association of Social Workers.

Savinsky, L., Illingworth, M., & DuLaney, M. (2009). Civilian social work: Serving the military and veteran populations. *Social Work. 54*(4), 327–339.

Simmons, C. A., & Rycraft, J. R. (2010). Ethical challenges of military social workers serving in a combat zone. *Social Work, 55*(1), 9–18.

Social Work Professional Advisory Group. (2010). Meeting Minutes for March 11, 2010. Retrieved from http://usphs-hso.org/pags/swpags

Tarpley, A. A. (1999). The future of air force social work. In: J. G. Daley (Eds.), *Social work practice in the military* (pp. 329–342). Binghamton, NY: The Haworth Press.

United States Department of Veterans Administration, Office of Academic Affairs (2010). *History of VA social work.* Washington, D.C. Retrieved September 21, 2012 from http://www.socialwork.va.gov/about.asp.

Uniformed Services Social Workers. (2011, September). *Program for the Annual Meeting.* International Journal of AMSUS: The Society of the Federal Health Agencies.

Wheeler, D. P., & Bragin, M. (2007). Bringing it all back home: Social work and the challenge of returning veterans. *Health and Social Work, 32*(4), 297–300.

Wittman, M., & Kissel, S. (1979, April 18). *History of social work in the Public Health Service.* Presentation given at the 14th annual meeting of the USPHS Professional Association, Phoenix, Arizona.

PART V

Policy and Administration

*A*s public health social workers engage in working with individuals, families, groups, and communities, they must be aware of macro-level factors that affect the well-being of all groups. Access to health care, insurance-reimbursement policies, and workforce development issues play major roles in the health of all Americans. The chapters in this section address these important points.

Chapter 18 focuses on the ongoing issue of access to health care. For many Americans, the topic of health access and health insurance, including differences among fee-for-service plans, managed care organizations, health maintenance organizations, preferred provider organizations, Medicare, Medicaid, and health care for armed services personnel, are mind-boggling. This chapter provides descriptions of each of these funding mechanisms along with additional information to help you in your learning.

Chapter 19 addresses workforce issues in the fields of public health and social work. As our nation addresses increasingly more complicated health concerns, our public health workforce will need to be up to the task of practicing with a high level of skill at the micro, mezzo, and macro levels of practice.

As you read these chapters, think about what you consider to be the most pressing health issues in the United States at this time. The issues could be eliminating minority health disparities, discovering more effective treatments for chronic health conditions, or finding cures for various communicable diseases. Write down some of the current policies that are in place to address these issues. What demands do you believe will be placed on the public health workforce to address these issues, bearing in mind the increased longevity and the lack of access to health care many Americans face?

CHAPTER 18

Health Insurance and Access in the United States

Julia F. Hastings and Robert H. Keefe

INTRODUCTION

O ne of the goals of the U.S. public health 2020 agenda is to create a society where all people live long and healthy lives (U.S. Department of Health and Human Services, 2010). The federal government supports this goal in its *Healthy People 2020* report. The four goals of *HP2020* are (1) to attain high-quality, longer lives free of preventable disease, disability, injury, and premature death; (2) to achieve health equity, eliminate dispar-ities, and improve the health of all groups; (3) to create social and physical environments that promote good health for all; and (4) to promote quality of life, healthy development, and healthy behaviors across all life stages (U.S. Department of Health and Human Services, 2010). The challenge to meet these goals for an estimated population of 313,380,060 Americans (U.S. Bureau of the Census, 2012) where the median household income is $49,445 (DeNavas-Walt, Proctor, & Smith, 2011) is met largely through a unique health care delivery system that is built on disconnected subsys-tems of health insurance options. Frequent political debates focus on whether American families can "afford" good health. These particular debates intrigue academics, politicians, and the health professionals provid-ing health services.

In contrast to other developed countries, the United States does not have one national health insurance program that entitles all its citizens to receive basic health care services. Other nations, which have a government health care program, commonly refer to their program as "universal access," which is funded by tax dollars. Although to date, the current larger health care delivery system has evolved in response to concerns about increased cost, limited access, and poor quality, all Americans are not entitled to universal access.

Major components of the fragmented American health care delivery system include managed care; the military health care system; and the public subsystem of programs for vulnerable populations, including Medicare and Medicaid. The challenge that each of these fragmented components presents is building a universal health care system when there are multiple barriers to expanding access to health care while at the same time containing overall costs and maintaining expected levels of quality.

To make learning how persons "pay for" health care in the United States easier, this chapter covers the major components of health insurance (private, military, and public). The chapter begins by providing a broad understanding of how the parts of the health care system function via its financial support. Discussion also focuses on the population of people often referred to as "the uninsured" and how they access health care. We begin by learning the distinctions between the components behind health care delivery: private insurance, the military health system, and public insurance (i.e., Medicare and Medicaid).

COMPONENTS OF THE U.S. HEALTH INSURANCE SYSTEM

Private Insurance

Nearly 55.3% of the American population have employment-based health insurance (DeNavas-Walt et al., 2011), commonly referred to as "private health insurance." Employer-sponsored health insurance emerged out of the worker's compensation laws of the early 1900s that later expanded the types of services covered throughout the 20th century (Shi & Singh, 2010). Although a number of key factors spawned the growth of private health insurance, it essentially began as a means for employers to maintain their workforce by providing income for individuals experiencing a temporary disability resulting from injury or sickness that prevented individuals from being compensated for work performed (Shi & Singh, 2010). Today, private health insurance has become a permanent feature of employment benefits provided to employees and their dependents. The benefit involves reimbursing the health care provider for the cost of services rendered (Claxton, Rae, Panchal, Lundy, & Damico, 2011). For 2011, Claxton et al. (2011) estimated that the annual premium for employer-sponsored health insurance was $5,429 for a single person and $15,073 for a family. It is important to note that significant variation in annual premiums exists as a result of the type of benefit coverage, cost sharing, and geographic variations in the cost of care. In essence, the insurer estimates the overall risk for the cost of health care services among targeted groups (e.g., factory workers, construction workers, office staff) and then charges monthly premiums to be paid by the individual or one's employer.

Military Health System

The military health care system is comprehensive and covers preventive as well as other treatment services that are provided by salaried health care personnel, many of whom are in the military or uniformed services themselves (Shi & Singh, 2010; U.S. Department of Defense [DoD], 2012b). Medical care for wounded military personnel prior to the Civil War began with the regimental surgeon and the surgeons' mates at the battle site. Care was provided locally and limited to available supplies. Military medical care eventually became more efficient. With improvements in communication during combat, transportation of the injured, and effective treatments for disease and injury, instead of medical care available only at the battle site, injured soldiers were being transported to "combat theaters" (U.S. Department of Defense [DoD], 2012a), which led to more comprehensive medical attention that helped to return soldiers to their duties with better health outcomes. Although military personnel received much-improved medical care, it was not coordinated across the service branches. Instead, the Army, Navy, and Air Force each created separate medical services (U.S. Department of Defense [DoD], 2012a).

The creation of the Department of Defense (DoD) in 1949 led to changes in how military personnel were provided medical care. Medical services were expanded to include military dependents, more federal facilities, and a unified system of health care for the armed forces. This expanded service became known as the Civilian Health and Medical Program of the Uniformed Services (CHAMPUS; U.S. Department of Defense [DoD], 2012a). Similar to the private and public insurance sections, the CHAMPUS system experienced escalating health costs. The rise in cost for military health care led to the establishment of a demonstration project that introduced "managed care" features to service provision from a corporation called Health Net (U.S. Department of Defense [DoD], 2012a). The "managed care" demonstration project covered only California and Hawaii (U.S. Department of Defense [DoD], 2012a). By 1993, the DoD initiated new plans for a nationwide managed care program. In May 1997, TRICARE (www.tricare.mil) was awarded the contract to administer a health care program for uniformed service members, veterans, and their families (U.S. Department of Defense [DoD], 2012b). TRICARE is a program that provides health care resources to over 9.5 million individuals in the uniformed services (U.S. Department of Defense [DoD], 2012b). Administratively, TRICARE divided the United States into 12 regions; each region coordinates the health care needs of all military medical treatment facilities in its region.

Public Insurance

As public health social workers, we recognize medical care as essential to a minimum standard of living. Furthermore, we believe no one should suffer or die because of a lack of financial resources to obtain medical treatment. In response to the declining health and the inability of low-income and elderly populations to pay medical bills, the federal government assumed the major responsibility of providing health care through Medicaid and Medicare. The Medicare and Medicaid programs were established in 1965 as amendments to Title XIX of the Social Security Act. Medicaid provides health care coverage to persons receiving federally supported public assistance (Hoffman & Schlobohm, 2000). It is a means-tested entitlement program that is jointly funded by federal and state funds. Each state designs and administers its own program under broad federal regulations. As such, income eligibility levels, services covered, and the method for and amount of reimbursement for services differ from state to state (House Committee on Ways and Means, 2008).

Since 1965, the Medicaid program has grown in scope and increasingly helps to provide medical services to needy persons. Its role in today's health care system includes providing health coverage to people with disabilities, financing long-term care, and assisting low-income Medicare beneficiaries with costs for treatment (Centers for Medicare & Medicaid Services, 2012b). Medicare, by contrast, is a universal program designed to help the elderly regardless of income status. The Medicare program covers most hospital and medical costs for persons 65 years of age and older as well as persons who are disabled Social Security beneficiaries (House Committee on Ways and Means, 2008). The two questions that constantly surround both public health care programs are (1) what type of health care conditions and (2) how much service benefit (e.g., prescription drugs) should be provided? Both programs are massively expensive and have been the subject of much political discourse concerning financial cuts.

In sum, the delivery of health care via the health insurance industry involves a multitude of government agencies involved in financing health care, medical and health services research, and providing regulatory oversight for the various aspects of the health care delivery systems (U.S. Bureau of the Census, 2012; National Center for Health Statistics, 2012; U.S. Bureau of Labor Statistics, 2011).

MAJOR SYSTEMS OF HEALTH CARE DELIVERY

The rapid increase in costs of providing health care signaled to employers and insurance companies alike to seek ways to contain expenditures. Managed care emerged as the solution to rising costs of the 1990s and continues to play a major role in health care service delivery (Kane et al., 1996). Although the military and the government-supported health care systems are different and separate forms of health care provision, their goals are similar—to contain costs.

Managed Care

Managed care is a system of health care delivery that is mainly defined by three aspects (Shi & Singh, 2010):

1. Achieves efficiency by integrating the basic functions of health care delivery;
2. Controls (manages) utilization of medical services;
3. Determines the price at which the services are purchased and, consequently, how much the providers get paid.

The managed care system is financed by the employer or government entity. Instead of purchasing coverage from a traditional insurance company, the employer (financier) contracts with a managed care organization (MCO). Under a managed care framework, MCOs become responsible for monitoring financing, providing health insurance, delivering health care, and paying for services (Kane et al., 1996). MCOs operate independently and remain in charge of collecting premiums for insuring groups of people (enrollees) through contracts with physicians, clinics, and hospitals. The MCO functions as an insurance company and promises to provide health care services contracted under the health plan to the members (enrollees) of the plan and their dependents (Kane et al., 1996). Further, the MCO is responsible for negotiating with providers who are typically paid either through a capitation (per head) fixed payment arrangement or a discounted fee.

Capitation means that the health care provider is paid a fixed sum each month per enrollee regardless of whether or not the enrollee utilizes the health care provider's services (Zuvekas & Cohen, 2010). The health care provider is therefore responsible for providing medically necessary health care services. According to Shi and Singh (2010), the provider can bill the MCO for each health care service performed, but the reimbursed fee is prenegotiated at a discount from the regular charge. For the providers, the trade-off for discounted services is being included in the "network" as a participating provider and basically, being guaranteed a share of the patient population while at the same time risking not being reimbursed for services in the event that the enrollee accesses medical services from the provider after the capitated amount is exhausted.

Although MCOs have enjoyed growth, other types of managed care plans such as preferred-provider organizations (PPOs) and health maintenance organization (HMOs), evolved to offer selected health plans to employees. The managed care sector includes approximately 405 licensed HMOs and 925 PPOs (Shi & Singh, 2010). On the whole, managed care insurance represents the adopted manner for delivering health care to everyone across markets—private, military, and public.

Military Health Care System

The military health care system provides comprehensive preventive services free of charge for active-duty military personnel of the U.S. Army, Navy, Air Force, Coast Guard, and certain uniformed nonmilitary services such as the U.S. Public Health Service and the National Oceanographic and Atmospheric Association (Shi & Singh, 2010; U.S. Department of Defense [DoD], 2012b). Ambulatory care services are often provided close to the military personnel's place of employment, and hospital services are provided at military base hospitals, sick bays aboard ship, or at dispensaries (Shi & Singh, 2010; U.S. Department of Defense [DoD], 2012b). Regional military hospitals provide more comprehensive services, while long-term care is provided through U.S. Department of Veterans Affairs (VA) facilities to certain retired military personnel. Family members of active-duty or retired career military personnel are either treated at the hospitals or dispensaries or are covered by TRICARE (www.tricare.mil/).

The VA (www.va.gov/) health care system is available to retired veterans of previous military service, with priority given to veterans who have disabilities with a primary focus on hospital, mental health services, and long-term care (Department of Veterans Affairs, 2012). The VA is one of the largest and oldest (1946) integrated health care systems in the world, consisting of 152 medical centers, nearly 800 community-based outpatient clinics, 135 community living centers, 278 vet centers, and 48 domiciliaries (Department of Veterans Affairs, 2012). The VA's mission is to provide medical care, education and training, research, contingency support, and emergency management for all veterans, their dependents, surviving spouses, children, or parental figures of deceased veterans, uniformed service members, and present or former reservists or National Guard members as defined by the Department of Defense (Department of Veterans Affairs, 2012). The entire VA system is organized into 23 geographically distributed Veterans Integrated Service Networks (VISNs; Department of Veterans Affairs, 2012). Each VISN coordinates the activities of the hospitals, outpatient clinics, nursing homes, and other facilities located within its jurisdiction. Further, each facility is responsible for improving efficiency by reducing unnecessary service duplication, and costs, and emphasizing preventive services.

HEALTH INSURANCE PAYMENT

Individuals with private or government (public) insurance are limited to accessing health services at medical facilities that accept the particular type of medical insurance they carry. Visits to facilities outside the insurance program's network are usually either not covered or require patients to bear more of the cost than they would have to bear had they received services at facilities inside the insurance program's network.

Hospitals negotiate with insurance programs to set reimbursement rates. Rates for some government insurance programs are determined by federal laws. The fees for services paid provided by a doctor for health care procedures is generally less than the out-of-pocket fee paid by an uninsured person (Kane et al., 1996). In return for this discount, the insurance company includes the doctor as part of its network, which means more patients are eligible for lowest-cost treatment. The negotiated rate may not cover the cost of the service, but providers (hospitals and doctors) can refuse to accept a given type of insurance, including Medicare and Medicaid. Low reimbursement rates have generated complaints from providers and some patients who have difficulty finding local providers who treat certain types of medical services and who accept Medicaid and Medicare (Holahan & Yemane, 2009; Kane et al., 1996; Miranda et al., 2003).

Private Insurance

Most Americans under 65 years of age receive their health insurance coverage through their employer under a group coverage plan. Service providers contract with MCOs so as to be part of network provider panels. Provider networks are used to reduce costs by negotiating favorable fees from providers, selecting cost-effective providers, and creating financial incentives for providers to practice more efficiently.

PPOs and HMOs

The name *health maintenance organization* stemmed from the idea that the HMO's purpose would be to maintain the enrollee's health, rather than merely to treat his or her illness. Thus, HMOs typically cover preventive health care. HMOs can develop and disseminate guidelines on cost-effective care, while the enrollee's primary care physician can act as a patient advocate and care coordinator, thus helping the patient negotiate the complex health care system. In recent years, the HMO model has evolved toward a less tightly managed model, such as the PPO model. PPOs also negotiate discounted fees with health care professionals, who more and more maintain contracts with several health plans, each plan consisting of different referral networks, diagnostic facilities, and varying practice guidelines. The enrollee's primary care physician can facilitate patient care by referring the enrollee to other medical professionals. In most cases, the physician's referral is not necessary as long as the enrollee remains within the network of contracted providers.

Public Insurance

Government-supported programs cover about one-third of the U.S. population, including the elderly, the disabled, children, veterans, and some adults with very low incomes (Shi & Singh, 2010). Federal law mandates public access to emergency services regardless of one's ability to pay (Zibulewsky, 2001). Government-funded programs include Medicare, a government-financed system of health insurance for Social Security beneficiaries. Medicare reimburses medical care to persons who are 65 years of age and older, are disabled, or have end-stage renal failure (Centers for Medicare & Medicaid Services, 2012c). This program is financed by employer and employee contributions based on earnings and other federal tax revenues. Medicare comprises four main parts—Part A, Part B, Part C, and Part D (Centers for Medicare & Medicaid Services, 2012c).

Part A (hospital insurance) pays for four basic types of services: (a) services provided in and by hospitals; (b) limited stays in skilled nursing facilities; (c) some services, including nursing care and speech, physical, and occupational therapy for people under a physician's care who are confined to their homes; and (d) hospice care, which involves health, homemaker, and other social services provided either at home or in a supportive, homelike facility for people suffering from a terminal illness.

Part B (supplementary medical insurance) supplements benefits provided by Part A in that it covers physicians' fees, diagnostic x-rays or laboratory tests, surgical dressing and devices, purchases for rental of durable medical equipment (e.g., wheelchairs, hospital beds), ambulance services, and prosthetic devices. Part B does *not* cover dental or vision care, routine physical examinations, and long-term nursing care.

Part C (Medicare Advantage—Medicare Modernization Act, 2003) plans are private health plans that provide health care coverage in addition to benefits and services not covered by Medicare alone.

Part D (prescription drug coverage—Medicare Modernization Act, 2003) provides Medicare beneficiaries with assistance paying for prescription drugs. Coverage is not provided within the traditional Medicare program. Instead, persons must enroll in one of many hundreds of Part D plans offered by private companies. Each plan has different costs and benefits that vary from year to year.

Medicaid provides health care coverage to nearly 60 million low-income Americans (including children, pregnant women, parents, seniors, and individuals with disabilities) in all states except Arizona (Centers for Medicare & Medicaid Services, 2012b). For many people with limited incomes who cannot afford medical care, the Medicaid program helps pay for some or all of their medical bills. Eligible persons must be U.S. citizens or lawfully admitted immigrants and must meet certain requirements in order to be eligible (Centers for Medicare & Medicaid Services, 2012b). Immigrant access to Medicaid and its associated services remains a highly debated topic for states (Nam, 2011; Snowden, Masland, Peng, Lou, & Wallace, 2011; Sommers, 2010). While states set individual eligibility criteria based on federal minimum standards, certain populations must be covered. Some examples of the mandatory Medicaid-eligible groups can include the following:

- Limited-income families with children, as described in Section 1931 of the Social Security Act, who meet certain eligibility requirements in the state's Aid to Families with Dependent Children (AFDC) plan, which went into effect on July 16, 1996;
- Supplemental Security Income (SSI) recipients (or in states using more restrictive criteria—aged, blind, and disabled individuals who meet criteria that are more restrictive than those of the SSI program and that were in place in the state's approved Medicaid plan as of January 1, 1972);
- Infants born to Medicaid-eligible pregnant women. Medicaid eligibility must continue throughout the first year of life so long as the infant remains in the mother's household and the mother remains income eligible, or would be income eligible if she were still pregnant;
- Children under age 6 and pregnant women whose family income is at or below 133% of the federal poverty level. (The minimum mandatory income level for pregnant women and infants in certain states may be higher than 133% if, as of certain dates, the state had established a higher percentage for covering those groups.) States are required to extend Medicaid eligibility to all children born after September 30, 1983, until age 19 (or such earlier date as the state may choose) in families with incomes at or below the federal poverty level. Once eligibility is established, pregnant women remain eligible for Medicaid through the end of the calendar month in which the 60th day after the end of the pregnancy falls, regardless of any change in family income. States are not required to have a resource test for these poverty-level-related groups. However, any resource test imposed can be no more restrictive than that of the AFDC program for infants and children and the SSI program for pregnant women;
- Recipients of adoption assistance and foster care under Title IV-E of the Social Security Act;

- The medically needy, such as certain groups of women who are in need of treatment for breast and cervical cancer and persons diagnosed with tuberculosis;
- Special protected groups who may remain Medicaid eligible for a period of time. Some examples include people who lose SSI payments due to earnings from work or increased Social Security benefits, and families who are provided 6 to 12 months of Medicaid coverage following loss of eligibility under Section 1931 due to earnings, or 4 months of Medicaid coverage following loss of eligibility under Section 1931 due to an increase in child or spousal support.

States have some discretion in determining which groups their Medicaid programs will cover and the financial criteria for eligibility. To be eligible for federal funds, states are required to provide Medicaid coverage for most people who receive federally assisted income maintenance payments, as well as for related groups who do not receive cash payments.

The Medicaid program represents a partnership between the federal government and each participating state to pay for the health care of low-income people. States are free to create and administer their own Medicaid programs. Medicaid does not pay money to the enrollee; instead, it sends payments directly to the health care provider. As a result, Medicaid is not an insurance program, but it operates like one. As such, each state determines the type, amount, duration, and scope of services within broad federal guidelines. Examples of "mandatory benefits" include inpatient hospital services, physician series, rural health clinic service, transportation to medical care, and laboratory and x-ray services.

This list is not exhaustive. Other mandatory services can be found by searching the Medicaid website (Medicaid.gov). States can offer other "optional" health benefits through the Medicaid program, such as prescription drugs, hospice, case management, dentures, dental services, optometry services, and podiatry services (Centers for Medicare & Medicaid Services, 2012b). Although many of the optional benefits are acknowledged by service providers and consumers alike to be essential to maintaining good health (Hastings & Hawkins, 2009; Snowden & Pingitore, 2002), the trend has been for states to abandon these options due to cost-containment measures (Holahan & Yemane, 2009; Kibicho & Pinkerton, 2012).

Children's Health Insurance Program (CHIP). Title XXI amendment of the Social Security Act in 1997 (and reauthorized in February 2009) represents the most recent addition to the American public health safety net. Its implementation has meant that increased numbers of children in the United States have a regular source of health care, including preventive services. Like Medicaid, CHIP is jointly funded by states and the federal government (Centers for Medicare & Medicaid Services, 2012a). CHIP's purpose is to enable states to initiate and expand child health assistance to uninsured, low-income children through: (1) a new program that meets special requirements, (2) expanding eligibility for children under the state's Medicaid program, and (3) a combination of both.

CHIP is available to families with incomes up to 200% of the federal poverty level (Centers for Medicare & Medicaid Services, 2012a). CHIP provides comprehensive benefits that include early and periodic screening, and diagnostic and treatment services, which include mental health and dental services (Centers for Medicare & Medicaid Services, 2012a).

Vulnerable Populations' System of Care

Due to the severe economic downturn felt in the early 2000s, the term "most vulnerable" can be defined much more broadly than when the "poor" were originally defined in the Social Security Act of 1935—single mothers, children, the unemployed, disabled adults, and the elderly. The nation's new vulnerable now include a large population of low-income persons who were once considered part of the middle class, who had access to private health insurance, and now find themselves unemployed and unable to qualify for public insurance assistance.

The American health care "safety net" was established after 1965 to ensure that regardless of social or economic condition, no American citizen would lack access to essential health care services. Today's health care safety net is a complex array of entitlement programs, specialty services (such as dialysis and care for persons with HIV/AIDS), hospital-based programs, and emergency services designed to facilitate access to vital health care for many medically underserved, uninsured, or underinsured persons. The modern health care "safety net" includes community health centers, physicians' offices, hospital outpatient and emergency departments, and mental health facilities designed to serve vulnerable populations. These service providers often offer comprehensive medical services that include language translation, transportation, outreach, nutrition, health education, social support, case management, and child care services. Each provides "wrap-around" services to reduce access barriers to health care services.

The Uninsured

Some Americans do not qualify for government-provided health insurance, are not provided health insurance by an employer, are unable to afford insurance, or choose not to purchase private health insurance. This population is referred to as "the uninsured" and in recent years has become a source of considerable political national controversy. It is widely argued that not having health insurance will have adverse consequences for the health of the uninsured individual. However, others argue that some of the uninsured have access to needed health care services at hospital emergency rooms, community health centers, or other safety net facilities offering charity care and therefore, enrolling in health care insurance to maintain one's health is largely unnecessary. The costs of treating the uninsured must often be absorbed by providers as charity care, passed on to the insured via cost shifting and higher health insurance premiums, or paid by taxpayers through higher taxes. However, hospitals and other providers are reimbursed for the cost of providing uncompensated care via a federal-matching fund program.

CURRENT ISSUES IN HEALTH POLICY

In 2010, the Patient Protection and Affordable Care Act (PPACA) was passed. The act includes various new regulations, with one of the most notable being a health insurance mandate that requires all Americans and legal residents to purchase health insurance. Those without coverage will pay a tax penalty of $695 per year up to a maximum of three times that amount ($2,085) per family. Exemptions will be granted for financial hardship, religious objections, American Indians, those without coverage for less than three months, undocumented immigrants, incarcerated persons, those for whom the lowest cost plan option would exceed 8% of an individual's income, and those with incomes below the tax-filing threshold. Other provisions include covering preventive benefits without cost sharing, extending health benefits to children of covered workers until the child reaches 26 years of age, and expanding Medicaid and CHIP. Additional information about the PPACA can be found at www.healthcare.gov/law/full or http://healthreform.kff.org (Henry J. Kaiser Family Foundation, 2012).

Underserved Populations

Certain populations in the United States face greater challenges than the general population in accessing timely and needed health care services. These populations are at greater risk of poor physical, psychological, and/or social health (Alegría et al., 2006; Kumanyika & Morssink, 2006; Ponce et al., 2009; Williams et al., 2007). The causes of their vulnerability are largely attributable to unequal social, economic, health, and geographic conditions. These population groups consist of racial and ethnic minorities, gay/lesbian/bisexual/transgendered persons, uninsured children, women, individuals living in rural areas, the homeless, the mentally ill, the chronically medically ill and disabled, and people living with HIV/AIDS.

People designated as members of one or more of the above groups means that they are more vulnerable than the general population and experience greater barriers in accessing care, obtaining finances for their care, and racial or cultural acceptance. To address this problem, the National Institutes of Health has devoted funding to researchers to uncover why significant differences in health exist across the various racial/ethnic groups. The federal initiatives that have served primarily to generate national attention on racial disparities in health care can be found in Table 18.1.

TABLE 18.1   Federal Programs to Eliminate Racial and Ethnic Disparities

FEDERAL PROGRAM	DESCRIPTION	YEAR
Indian Health Service	An agency within the U.S. Department of Health and Human Services with the mission to be the principal advocate and provider of health services to American Indians and Alaska Natives.	1955
Migrant Health Center Program	Established by the Migrant Health Act to provide medical and support services to migrant farm workers and their families.	1962
U.S. Office of Minority Health (OMH)	Created from the *Secretary's Task Force Report on Black and Minority Health*. The office is dedicated to improving the health of racial and ethnic minority populations through the development of health policies and programs that will help eliminate health disparities. OMH was reauthorized by the Patient Protection and Affordable Care Act of 2010 (P.L. 111-148). http://minorityhealth.hhs.gov/templates/browse.aspx?lvl=1&lvlID=7	1986
The Office of Research on Minority Health (ORMH)	Established, with the encouragement of Congress, by the Director of the National Institutes of Health (NIH) to research minority health disparities.	1990
Minority Health Initiative (MHI)	The centerpiece of the ORMH agenda, the MHI was launched and initially funded at $45 million. This multiyear biomedical and behavioral research and research-training program co-funds through its partnerships (1) interventions to improve prenatal health and reduce infant mortality; (2) studies of childhood and adolescent lead poisoning, HIV infection and AIDS, and alcohol and drug use; (3) research in adult populations focused on cancer, diabetes, obesity, hypertension, cardiovascular diseases, mental disorders, asthma, visual impairments, and alcohol abuse; and (4) training for faculty and for students at all stages of the	1992

(Continued)

TABLE 18.1 Federal Programs to Eliminate Racial and Ethnic Disparities *(Continued)*

FEDERAL PROGRAM	DESCRIPTION	YEAR
	educational pipeline—from precollege and undergraduate through graduate and postdoctoral levels.	
National Center on Minority Health and Health Disparities	The center was established by the passage of the Minority Health and Health Disparities Research and Education Act of 2000, Public Law 106-525, which was signed by the President of the United States on November 22, 2000. The purpose of the NCMHD was to expand the infrastructure of institutions committed to health disparities research and to encourage the recruitment and retention of highly qualified minority and other scientists in the fields of biomedical, clinical, behavioral, and health services research: (1) the Endowment Program, (2) the Loan Repayment Program for Health Disparities Research, and (3) the Extramural Clinical Research Loan Repayment Program for Individuals from Disadvantaged Backgrounds.	2000
National Institute on Minority Health and Health Disparities	On March 23, 2010, the Patient Protection and Affordable Care Act (P.L. 111-148) was passed and redesignated the NCMHD as an Institute, renamed the National Institute on Minority Health and Health Disparities (NIMHD). The law gave the NIMHD authority to plan, review, coordinate, and evaluate the minority health and health disparities research and activities conducted and supported by the NIH institutes and centers. In addition, it transferred all of the responsibilities of the NCMHD to the NIMHD and expanded the eligibility criteria for the Research Endowment program to include institutions with an active NIMHD Center of Excellence grant.	2011

CONCLUSIONS

Given the advances in medical technology, economic changes, cultural beliefs about health, and social mores determining who is deserving of receiving health care, the future of health care delivery is unknown. Trends for adapting to the future insurance landscape appear to be quite creative. For example, more hospitals are merging with one another in order to create new physician networks. A possible extension of the newly formed hospitals is the possibility that hospitals will contract directly with employers for health care services, which cuts out insurance and MCO measures. Another response to PPACA, the new federal legislation requiring health care insurance, might be an increase in the public's demand for more health care services because of greater costs in insurance coverage.

An unintended consequence of reforming the health care system is that the employed might receive fewer raises because their employers might use the undistributed monies to pay higher insurance premiums for workers. If raises are done away with, the employee would most likely pay higher out-of-pocket costs for one's health care. These possibilities represent only a few outcomes that might gain more traction in political health care debates. To navigate the health care system, whether it be through private, military, or public insurance, public health social workers will need to be prepared to help individuals decide about how to live healthier lives. The upside to the patchwork of health care service subsystems is that more changes, hopefully for the better, are expected. However, the downside to the vast fragmented health care system is that access to health care will continue to be not enjoyed by all Americans. No country in the world supports a perfect health care system. In total, we all just try to protect ourselves from life's health uncertainties.

CLASSROOM EXERCISES

Exercise 1

Esperanza Hernandez is a 30-year-old, widowed, Hispanic female who has recently become a U.S. citizen. She and her three children—Martin 8, Selena 6, and Jose 5—immigrated to the United States from Mexico. Martin and Selena were born in Mexico; Jose was born in the United States. Esperanza recently lost her job at a small factory in southern California. The county department of social services became involved when a school social worker began to suspect that Esperanza's three children were not being properly cared for at home. The school social worker noted the children had missed several days of school, frequently fell asleep during class, and went without lunch.

The county child protective services worker investigating the case interviewed the three children at school and concluded that the children were not being physically abused. However, the worker noted that the children claimed that they rarely had enough food at home, their mother was away much of the time looking for work, and there was no one available to supervise them until their Aunt Corazon recently arrived in the United States illegally to help care for them in their mother's absence. The worker interviewed Esperanza, who corroborated her children's accounts of life at home and stated that she had sent for Corazon to come help the family because she was unable to look for a new job and care for her children. Esperanza stated that when she lost her job, she was unable to afford the COBRA payments to continue her insurance coverage and so the family was unable to access health care. She expressed much shame about the state her family is in but did not know what to do.

Discussion Questions

1. Where would you begin in your work to help the Hernandez family?
2. What would you do to help the family begin receiving Medicaid?
3. Given that many communities around the country have few doctors willing to accept new Medicaid clients, what would you do to assure the family receives prompt medical care?
4. If the Hernandez family were to relocate to your state, what policies are in place that would help them to attain the necessary health services?

Exercise 2

Many elderly individuals across the country have found Medicare benefits to be confusing. Social workers and other professionals who provide services to the elderly have also found Medicare benefits to be confusing. To address this problem, each year the federal government publishes a pamphlet titled "Medicare and You." Some elderly people state that they still find the policies confusing and frequently turn to social workers for help in understanding their benefits.

Assignment Details

For this assignment, go to the Medicare website (www.medicare.gov). Review each part (Medicare Parts A, B, C, and D) and develop an information guide or brochure that you would use to help elderly individuals in one of the following health care settings that mostly closely matches your professional interests as an aspiring public health social worker:

1. Inpatient hospital
2. Skilled nursing facility
3. Outpatient physician's office
4. Allied health professional's office (i.e., speech therapist, physical therapist, occupational therapist)
5. In-home hospice services

Exercise 3

Asenath Daniels is a 22-year-old African American female soldier enlisted in the U.S. Army and deployed to Iraq. While in Iraq, some of her fellow soldiers note that she seems to be having difficulty with sleep, gets "excited" very easily, is tearful, and obsessed with checking locks on the doors and windows of the rooms she enters. After meeting with Asenath, you diagnose her condition as posttraumatic stress disorder (PTSD).

Although PTSD responds well to cognitive-behavioral treatment, Asenath is uncertain if she is ready to delve into all of the issues surrounding the trauma and is also worried that the military might find out she is seeking behavioral health care. She is concerned that if the military were to find out that she has PTSD, they might not call her back for duty in the future.

Assignment Details

For this assignment, go to www.tricare.mil and look into the benefits for "Mental Health and Behavior" care and find out:

1. What types of therapy are covered (e.g., individual therapy)
2. What are the policies concerning privacy of patient information
3. What other local community services that are not affiliated with the military might be appropriate for you to refer Asenath to

INTERNET RESOURCES

National Library of Medicine (NLM): American Indian Health

(http://americanindianhealth.nlm.nih.gov/index.html)

This site brings together health resources relevant to American Indians. The content includes consumer health information, research, policies, and various resources and databases for researchers and students.

The National Alliance for Hispanic Health

(www.hispanichealth.org/)

The National Alliance for Hispanic Health is a nonprofit organization begun in 1973. It focuses on improving the health of Hispanics and reaches more than 15 million Hispanic consumers nationwide.

The Kaiser Family Foundation

(www.kff.org/minorityhealth/index.cfm)

This website, sponsored by the Kaiser Family Foundation, focuses on a wide range of topics, including specific illnesses, third-party payers, and policies affecting the health of racial and ethnic minorities.

The United States Census Bureau

(www.census.gov/hhes/www/hlthins/)

This website is sponsored by the U.S. Bureau of the Census and provides data on health insurance as collected by three national surveys from 50 states, the District of Columbia, and Puerto Rico. Additional links provide downloads of research briefs, reports on health insurance by poverty and other sociodemographic characteristics, and related sites on health care demographics.

The Official U.S. Government Site for Medicare

(www.medicare.gov/default.aspx)

This website provides valuable information on Medicare, including health management for the elderly, details on each part of Medicare, policy updates, and help and support for Medicare beneficiaries.

The Center for Medicaid and CHIP Services (CMCS)

(http://medicaid.gov/)

This link provides much information, including Medicaid enrollments by state; federal versus state costs per state; federal policies, including the Affordable Care Act and Medicaid 1115 waivers; and links to other government and health care websites.

The Gay and Lesbian Medical Association (GLMA)

(http://glma.org)

The Gay and Lesbian Medical Association provides information on health care and referrals to GLBT physicians for GLBT individuals around the country. The GLMA is a multidisciplinary organization open to all GLBT health professionals.

United States Department of Veterans Affairs

(www.va.gov/health/default.asp)

The Veterans Health Administration website provides valuable information on the health care resources available to veterans.

REFERENCES

Alegría, M., Cao, Z., McGuire, T. G., Ojeda, V. D., Sribney, B., Woo, M., et al. (2006). Health insurance coverage for vulnerable populations: Contrasting Asian Americans and Latinos in United States. *Inquiry—Excellus Health Plan, 43*(3), 231–254.

Centers for Medicare & Medicaid Services. (2012a). *Children's Health Insurance Program.* Retrieved April 12, 2012, from http://www.medicaid.gov/Medicaid-CHIP-Program-Information/By-Topics/Childrens-Health-Insurance-Program-CHIP/Childrens-Health-Insurance-Program-CHIP.html

Centers for Medicare & Medicaid Services. (2012b). *Medicaid.gov: Keeping America healthy.* Retrieved April 12, 2012, from http://www.medicaid.gov/

Centers for Medicare & Medicaid Services. (2012c). *Medicare.* Retrieved April 12, 2012, from http://www.cms.gov/Medicare/Medicare.html

Claxton, G., Rae, M., Panchal, N., Lundy, J., & Damico, A. (2011). *Employer health benefits: 2011 annual survey.* Washington, DC: Henry J. Kaiser Family Foundation and Health Research & Educational Trust.

DeNavas-Walt, C., Proctor, B. D., & Smith, J. C. (2011). *Income, poverty, and health insurance coverage in the United States: 2010.* Washington, DC: U.S. Government Printing Office.

Department of Veterans Affairs. (2012). *Health care.* Retrieved April 11, 2012, from http://www.va.gov/health/default.asp

Emergency Medical Treatment and Active Labor Act § 1395 (1986).

Hastings, J. F., & Hawkins, J. M. (2009). Health insurance and diabetes among multiracial men: The mediation effects of usual source of care. *American Journal of Men's Health, 4*(3), 207–217.

Henry, J. Kaiser Family Foundation. (2012). *Health reform source.* Retrieved April 13, 2012, from http://healthreform.kff.org/timeline.aspx

Hoffman, C., & Schlobohm, A. (2000). *The Kaiser Commission on Medicaid and the Uninsured: Chart book* (2nd ed.). Washington DC: Henry J. Kaiser Foundation.

Holahan, J., & Yemane, A. (2009). Enrollment is driving medicaid costs—But two targets can yield savings. *Health Affairs, 28*(5), 1453–1465.

House Committee on Ways and Means. (2008). *Green book.* from http://www.gpoaccess.gov/wmprints/green/index.html

Kane, R., Kane, R., Kaye, N., Mollica, R., Riley, T., Saucier, P., et al. (1996). The basics of managed care. In R. Kane, & L. Starr (Eds.), *Managed care: Handbook for the aging network.* Minneapolis, MN: National LTC Resource Center.

Kibicho, J., & Pinkerton, S. D. (2012). Multiple drug cost containment policies in Michigan's Medicaid program saved money overall, although some increased costs. *Health Affairs, 31,* 4816–4826.

Kumanyika, S. K., & Morssink, C. B. (2006). Bridging domains in efforts to reduce disparities in health and health care. *Health Education & Behavior, 33*(4), 440–458.

Miranda, J., Duan, N., Sherbourne, C., Schoenbaum, M., Lagomasino, I., Jackson-Triche, M., et al. (2003). Improving care for minorities: Can quality improvement interventions improve care and outcomes for depressed minorities? Results of a randomized, controlled trial. *Health Services Research, 38,* 613–630.

Nam, Y. (2011). Welfare reform and elderly immigrants' health insurance coverage: The roles of federal and state medicaid eligibility rules. *Journal of Gerontological Social Work, 54*(8), 819–836.

National Center for Health Statistics. (2012). *Health, United States, 2010*. Retrieved April 14, 2012, from http://www.cdc.gov/nchs/hus/healthinsurance.htm

Ponce, N., Tseng, W., Ong, P., Shek, Y. L., Ortiz, S., & Gatchell, M. (2009). *The state of Asian American, Native Hawaiian and Pacific Islander health in California report*. Los Angeles: University of California, Los Angeles.

Shi, L., & Singh, D. A. (2010). *Essentials of the U.S. health care system*. Sudbury, MA: Jones and Bartlett.

Snowden, L. R., Masland, M. C., Peng, C. J., Lou, C. W.-M., & Wallace, N. T. (2011). Limited English proficient Asian Americans: Threshold language policy and access to mental health treatment. *Social Science & Medicine, 72*(2), 230–237.

Snowden, L. R., & Pingitore, D. (2002). Frequency and scope of mental health service delivery to African Americans in primary care. *Mental Health Services Research, 4*, 123–130.

Sommers, B. D. (2010). Targeting Medicaid: The costs and enrollment effects of Medicaid's citizenship documentation requirement. *Journal of Public Economics, 94*(1–2), 174–182.

U.S. Bureau of Labor Statistics. (2011). *Unemployment rate: Civilian labor force*. Retrieved April 1, 2012, 2012, from http://www.bls.gov/data/home.htm

U.S. Bureau of the Census. (2012). *Current population*. Retrieved April 12, 2012, from http://www.census.gov

U.S. Department of Defense. (2012a). *Military health system: History*. Retrieved April 14, 2012, from http://www.health.mil/About_MHS/History.aspx

U.S. Department of Defense. (2012b). *TRICARE*. Retrieved April 14, 2012, from http://www.tricare.mil

U.S. Department of Health and Human Services. (2010). *Healthy People 2020*. Retrieved April 10, 2012, 2012, from http://www.healthypeople.gov/2020/default.aspx

Williams, D. R., Haile, R., Gonzales, H. M., Neighbors, H. W., Baser, R., & Jackson, J. A. (2007). Disentangling mental health disparities: The mental health of Black Caribbean immigrants: Results from the National Survey of American Life. *American Journal of Public Health, 97*, 52–59.

Zibulewsky, J. (2001). The Emergency Medical Treatment Act and Active Labor Act (EMTALA): What it is and what it means for physicians. *Proceedings* (Baylor University Medical Center), *14*(4), 339–346.

Zuvekas, S. H., & Cohen, J. W. (2010). Paying physicians by capitation: Is the past now prologue? *Health Affairs, 29*(9), 1661–1666.

CHAPTER 19

Workforce Issues

Bari Cornet

INTRODUCTION

S ocial work and public health have long been recognized as highly compatible fields that have at times overlapped (Carlton, 1988). Among the earliest programs was the Maternal and Child Health program (MCH), which emerged from the settlement house movement and the U.S. Children's Bureau (Evans, 1985). Since the 1920s, social workers have been placed within the U.S. Public Health Service doing direct clinical work, program planning, and consultation (Leukefeld, 1989) with individuals, families, and groups, dealing with a broad array of issues and public health agencies. To be effective, public health social workers and public health professionals must work together to address the myriad health problems that need our attention throughout the United States. As noted by Watkins (1985), "the major health problems to be solved today are those which require social work intervention" (p. 17).

The interest in integrated education between social work and public health was first noted with the formation of the Social Work Committee of the U.S. Public Health Service (National Association of Social Workers [NASW], 2006). The public health social work profession has recognized the need for enhanced communication and linkages (Wilkinson, Copeland, & Rounds, 2000), the impact of the combined professional training on careers (Ruth, Geron, & Chiasson, 2002), and the integration of individual programs (Coulter & Hancock, 1989, Terrell, 1984).

A logical question to ask is, what makes a public health social worker? A public health social worker uses skills in social epidemiology to assess, plan, intervene, and evaluate the quality of services. A medical social worker does not necessarily integrate both public health knowledge and skills but retains the separate and unique perspective of social work, while the public health social worker integrates the public health and social work perspectives. Although the exact number of public health social work practitioners is hard to estimate, it is clear that there are many social workers practicing in health settings who, although not formally trained in public health, integrate the two fields (Ruth & Sisco, 2008). Schools of social work, however, rarely prepare practitioners for an integrated approach. Books and articles in the field of social work in health may recognize public health issues (e.g., policy, population, prevention); however, public health issues are often not included in discussions of mainstream social work interventions (Gehlert & Browne, 2006, Kerson, 1989).

WHAT IS PUBLIC HEALTH SOCIAL WORK?

While the core functions of public health (assessment, policy development, and assurance) fit well with all branches of social work regardless of practice setting (Ruth & Sisco, 2008), public health social work differs from other branches of social work practice in that it integrates the two fields of public health and social work. Whether the relationship is interdisciplinary, multidisciplinary, or transdisciplinary, public health social work requires much collaboration.

Collaborative efforts among public health social workers and other professionals occur most often in the multidisciplinary practice settings in which practitioners from different fields work side by side, each bringing their unique and discipline-specific perspective to address issues. A common example is the multidisciplinary team meetings that occur in many medical settings. A multidisciplinary team may include the primary care physician (who focuses on the patient's overall medical condition), a physician special- ist (who focuses on the intricacies of the management of the patient's specific disorder), the nurse (who focuses on the day-to-day management of the patient's illness), a social worker (who focuses on the patient's family dynamics that will facilitate or hinder successful discharge), a case manager (who focuses on the community resources the patient needs upon discharge), and perhaps a representative of a community facility to which the patient may be discharged. Each of these individuals focuses on the best interests of the patient, but through their own unique professional lens. The challenge for each profession is that it must overcome the limits of its discipline-specific lens and develop collaborative practice methods that will help each patient (Aronoff, 2008; Moxley, 2008).

Historically, public health and social work developed along parallel tracks (Turnock, 2004). While social work focused on the protection of individual children and their families and the deserving poor, public health focused on population-level issues of devastating and recurrent diseases. Social work conducted individualized, micro-level assessments that considered a person's individual relationships to one's community, society, and the environment. Public health used community, macro-level assessments, such as epidemiology, that considered the larger communities in which people lived.

As mortality (i.e., death) from many persistent diseases began to decrease, public health began to focus more on morbidity (i.e., poor health) that affected quality of life. An example of this change in focus is the decline in rates of infant mortality. Although medical interventions such as good prenatal care, nutrition, and exercise significantly reduced mortality, they could not fully eliminate morbidity due to, for example, low birth weight, which results in respiratory and feeding problems as well as anemia.

Epidemiological investigators began to realize the importance of social, behavioral, and environmental factors, which had, up to that point, been the domain of social work. Together, the two professions looked at the social determinants of health, including childhood lead poisoning, teen pregnancy, cancer, HIV/AIDS, and obesity. Remediation of these disorders required the skills of professionals from both fields working together.

Public health social workers focused on the population level by integrating skills to affect the individual in one's environment. The goals were to advocate for changing societal conditions while at the same time advocating on behalf of the needs of specific individuals. Each goal focuses on functioning for the optimal health and well-being of their clients/communities.

DIFFERENT LEVELS OF THE PROFESSION/PERSPECTIVE AND THEIR IMPORTANCE

Some estimates conclude that there are as many as 425,000 public health practitioners, among whom public health social workers constitute a very small portion (Turnock, 2006). A controversy in the public health field is whether a practitioner must have an advanced degree in a health field (e.g., MPH, DrPH, PhD) to rightfully be considered a public health professional. Another consideration is whether the individual has a professional certification (e.g., CHES or RD). As public health social workers, we prefer not to make a distinction between professional and nonprofessional, because doing so implies that only those with advanced degrees can function with the integrated perspective, which is not only false but also widens the gap between the practitioners and the community. For example, the term "community health worker" has grown over the past decade as distinct from someone who is professionally trained.

Turnock (2006) reported that only 20% of public health professionals in the United States have formal training in public health; the other 80%

acquired their skills on the job. The training can range from specific skills, such as community needs assessment, to grounding in the public health-essential services and core values. Much of the funding for training for public health (whether academic or in the community) comes from the Health Resources and Services Administration (HRSA) and from the Centers for Disease Control and Prevention. Each of these funding sources encourages a unified body of public health professionals to provide an inter-disciplinary approach to assessing community problems and developing practical solutions to those problems, which is the hallmark of public health practice (Turnock, 2006).

WHERE DO PUBLIC HEALTH SOCIAL WORKERS WORK?

The range of opportunities available for social workers who combine the public health and social work perspectives is as wide as the public health field itself: Among the 10 essential public health services, nearly all public health occupations and titles are actively involved in evaluating the effective-ness, accessibility, and quality of personal and population-based health ser-vices (Turnock, 2006).

In 1979, the Surgeon General of the U.S. Department of Health and Human Services (DHHS) published *Healthy People: The Surgeon General's Report on Health Promotion and Disease Prevention*. This report led to *Healthy People 1990: Promoting Health/Preventing Disease—Objectives for the Nation*. This planning document is revised every decade, with the most recent (*Healthy People 2020*) released in December 2010. *Healthy People 2020* has several additions that argue for the inclusion of a social work perspective within public health. Several new topic areas were added, including Social Determinants of Health, Health-Related Quality of Life and Well-Being, and Older Adults. The section on Social Determinants of Health includes the statement that individuals' choices are influenced in part by the nature of their social relationships:

> The conditions in which people live determine, in part, why some Americans are healthier than others and why Americans are generally not as healthy as they could be. Lack of options for healthy, affordable food and safe places to play in some neighborhoods makes it nearly impossible for residents to make healthy choices. In contrast, people living in neighborhoods with safe parks, good schools, and high employment rates are provided with some of the key requirements to better health. (DHHS, 2010)

The section on Health-Related Quality of Life and Well-Being states that this is a multidimensional concept that includes domains related to physical, mental, emotional and social functioning. It goes beyond direct measures of population health, life expectancy and causes of death, and focuses on the impact health status has on quality of life. A related concept of Health-Related Quality of Life is well-being, which assesses the positive aspects of a person's life, such as positive emotions and life satisfaction (DHHS, 2010).

A specific population area that was added to *Healthy People 2020* is Older Adults. This topic and its objective areas include both Health Services and Quality of Life. Two of the three descriptive objectives are within the realm of social work: Individual Behavioral Determinants of Health in Older Adults and Social Environment Determinants of Health in Older Adults (DHHS, 2010).

AN INTEGRATED PUBLIC HEALTH SOCIAL WORK PERSPECTIVE

In an effort to provide some consistency and cohesion, Public Health Social Work Standards and Competencies (Rounds, 2005) were promulgated by a leadership group from the Social Work section of the American Public Health Association (APHA):

> The major characteristic of public health social work is an epidemiological approach to identifying social problems affecting the health status and social functioning of all population groups, with an emphasis on intervention at the primary prevention level. Public health social workers focus on the promotion of positive health behaviors in the development of lifestyles by individuals, families and groups; enhancement by the environment; and avoidance of risks. They assess the health needs of the target population and determine the association between social factors and the incidence of health problems. They plan and implement intervention strategies based on the five levels of prevention. They emphasize reducing the social stress associated with health problems and determining the social supports that promote well-being and provide protection against ill health and minimize disability and institutionalization.

> The practice of public health social work is usually conducted within the context of a multi-disciplinary setting where social workers participate with other health and human service professionals in assuring all persons in the target population have access to health care and social services. Public health social work is a blending of roles: provider of direct services, researcher, consultant, administrator, program planner, evaluator and policymaker. Each function is dependent upon the other in assuring the health and social needs of the total population. (Rounds, 2005)

WHAT ARE THE NEEDED SKILLS?

The challenge of developing a unified vision of public health practice encompasses the notion of multiple professions, each governed by its own core functions, standards, and codes of ethics. Public health social work is no different. Not only is public health social work shaped by public health core functions but also by the code of ethics and practice standards set forth by NASW and the standards of the Council on Social Work Education—the accrediting body for all schools and departments of social work in the United States and Canada. We will first discuss the efforts of the two disciplines separately, and then the integrated public health social work document.

A variety of attempts have been made to characterize public health practice, starting with a survey of various state programs in 1914, which was followed in the 1920s by APHA reviews of both urban and rural practice. The Emerson Report in 1945 made recommendations about the level of public health practice, including six basic functions (vital statistics, sanitation, communicable disease control, maternal and child health, health education, and laboratory services; Turnock, 2004). APHA continued to reexamine and redefine this outline of services for a number of years. In 1988, the Institute of Medicine Committee on the Future of Public Health issued a report that identified three core functions (assessment, policy development, and assurance), which comprise 10 essential services.

Assessment (core function)
1. Monitor health status to identify and solve community health problems
2. Diagnose and investigate health problems and health hazards in the community

Policy Development (core function)
3. Inform, educate, and empower people about health issues
4. Mobilize community partnerships and action to identify and solve health problems
5. Develop policies and plans that support individual and community health efforts

Assurance (core function)
6. Enforce laws and regulations that protect health and ensure safety
7. Link people to needed personal health services and ensure the provision of health care when otherwise unavailable
8. Ensure the provision of a competent public and personal health care workforce
9. Evaluate effectiveness, accessibility, and quality of person- and population-based health services
10. Conduct research to seek out new insights and innovative solutions to health problems

Healthy People 2020 sets out a methodology for the implementation of its objectives, which is referred to as MAP-IT (Mobilize . . . Assess . . . Plan . . . Implement . . . Track). Both of these frameworks provide a direction for the skills needed for public health practitioners, including public health social workers.

Academic programs must include curriculum content in five areas: (1) epidemiology, (2) biostatistics, (3) health and social behavior, (4) environmental health, and (5) policy. The perspective that this creates is laid over the discipline-specific training and ethical standards of social work. Social work education programs must include study in five areas (policy, research, human behavior in the social environment, practice methodology, and human diversity). The focus of social work education is on underserved and vulnerable populations in society. The Preamble to the professional code of ethics states:

> The primary mission of the social work profession is to enhance human wellbeing and help meet the basic human needs of all people, with particular attention to the needs and empowerment of people who are vulnerable, oppressed, and living in poverty. A historic and defining feature of social work is the profession's focus on individual wellbeing in a social context and the wellbeing of society. (NASW, 2008)

While these two perspectives are highly compatible, they view the issues through different lenses. A group of public health social work leaders gathered in 1998 to attempt to identify exactly what public health social workers do in order to create a vision of the future of the profession. Out of this meeting the Public Health Social Work Standards and Competencies was developed (Rounds, 2005). The document includes 14 professional standards and 5 core competencies.

Note the degree to which public health core functions and social work standards are combined. For example, public health social work Professional Standard #1 ("Public Health Social Work uses social epidemiology principles to assess and monitor social problems affecting the health status and social functioning of at-risk populations within the context of family, community and culture") combines the public health core function and skill (social epidemiology. . .to assess and monitor) with the social work focus on "at-risk. . .in the context of family, community and culture."

While the two disciplines meld seamlessly, there are occasional tensions and conflicts that are often between the individual versus the population perspectives. An example is the debate over a policy that would require all health care workers (including volunteers) to be fully immunized. The public health argument is that health care workers are in the position of potentially spreading disease because of their proximity to disease and their widespread circulation within the community. Immunization is needed to protect the general population. In contrast, the social work view is to protect the rights of individual choice and self-determination.

SPECIFIC CONTENT AREAS

Public health social workers practice in a wide range of areas and domains; the most common are the traditional areas of infectious disease, maternal and child health, chronic disease and disability, and sociobehavioral issues.

Historically, infectious disease and related environmental vectors included diseases such as cholera and smallpox. With better control and eradication of these diseases the focus shifted to emerging and reemerging diseases such as HIV/AIDS, tuberculosis, and measles. To eradicate these diseases and their social impact, public health social workers practice all three core public health functions in these areas.

POLICY CONSIDERATIONS

> In order to better serve vulnerable populations, social work must continue to study and analyze workforce trends and emerging service delivery systems. Understanding and advocating for the value of social work services is central to the vitality and relevance of the profession in improving social conditions for all persons. (Weismiller & Whitaker, 2008)

There are several policy initiatives that can further the development of a public health social work workforce. The first group of these has to do with furthering the development of public health and social work training programs. There are several federal and state initiatives that can be pursued. Federal training grants exist in Maternal and Child Health and in Mental Health (the U.S. Department of Health and Human Services, 2011).

Another federal initiative is loan forgiveness programs, part of HRSA's Bureau of Health Professions. Either directly, or through matching grants to the states, primary health professionals who provide full-time clinical services in a public or nonprofit setting located in a federally designated Health Professional Shortage Area are eligible (the U.S. Health Resources and Services Administration, 2011).

The National Health Service Corps Loan Repayment Program is available to public health social workers who join the Corps. The amount available ranges from $60,000 (for two years of service in the Corps) to full debt repayment (for 6 or more years of service). To be eligible, one must be a licensed practitioner (e.g., a licensed clinical social worker) in the state in which one is working. While legislation establishing a number of programs on both the state and federal levels has been adopted, funding allocations can vary. More information is available from http://nhsc.hrsa.gov/loanrepayment/.

A second area of policy development that addresses the use of public health social work professionals is related to professional organizations. At the 2005 Social Work Congress, NASW established several initiatives that are relevant to understanding the public health and social work connection (NASW, 2005). Three of these are (1) participate in politics and policy where by major decisions are being made about behavioral health, (2) take the lead in advocating for quality universal health care, and (3) elevate the public's awareness of the efficacy and cost-effectiveness of social work practice in health care (NASW, 2005). The Social Welfare Reinvestment Initiative (NASW, 2007) is designed to strengthen the process in four arenas: (1) legislative and political advocacy, (2) public education, (3) workforce development, and (4) stakeholder engagement.

Additionally, professional organizations, as well as state and local agencies, can either facilitate or impede collaboration. There are often funding or structural limitations and requirements can impede collaboration. Two examples are (1) categorical funding and (2) workplace structural issues that do not recognize an integrated job classification. The challenge to the profession is to address these issues and advocate removing these barriers.

TRAINING FOR PUBLIC HEALTH SOCIAL WORK

Public health and social work grew from similar roots. Both were interested in social reform. Both came from the Charity Organizations Society of 1887 to deal with poverty in urban slums, both were involved in the control of communicable diseases (especially in congested areas), and both were concerned with immigrant populations in urban centers. Moreover, they have shared historic core missions that include the belief in the worth and dignity of the individual, the commitment to improved quality of life for all individuals, and the desire to promote social justice that protects and enhances community well-being and that ameliorates complex social health problems.

Many of the major health problems to be solved today require social work interventions. Advances in medical technology have virtually eliminated handicapping conditions resulting from infectious diseases such as tuberculosis. However, those same advances have enabled persons to survive with handicapping conditions and lifelong chronic illnesses, which require social workers to intervene to enable individuals to obtain services that allow them to continue living independently in the community.

The two fields rely on each other's expertise. Epidemiology comes from public health and psychosocial determinants of health come from social work. Community organizing comes from both, at different times. Analysis of the social environment comes from social work. The prevention perspective of public health takes its methodology from both disciplines. Primary prevention (to prevent conditions that might lead to illness or disability) comes from public health. Secondary prevention (to intervene after a disease process has begun) often comes from social work. Tertiary prevention (to restore functioning or rehabilitation for improved functioning) also comes from social work. Discussion of the relationship between the two disciplines is not new. The creation of the Children's Bureau in 1912 recognized the importance of viewing the "whole child" and the interrelated problems of child health, dependency, delinquency and child labor ... using specialists from many fields (Hutchins, 1994).

Two of the early proponents of the interrelationship between social work and public health were Virginia Insley and Juanita Evans. Both were social workers who were influential within the U.S. Public Health Service.

> Social workers were brought into maternal and child health programs to apply their special knowledge and skills to the total planning, organization and delivery of health services for mothers and children. Their knowledge and skill in identifying and dealing with social needs of mothers and children, understanding of the dynamics of human relationships, knowledge of available community services, and ability to organize social services were major contributions of social work from the outset. (Insley, 1977)

> Social factors related to prevention and treatment are a major responsibility of social work. Therefore, it is particularly important that initial planning and continued attention be given to the social component in the overall design for delivery of health services to families. (Evans, 1985, p. 13)

While public health social work training institutes have focused on MCH, the academic joint degree programs have been much broader. The joint degrees began in the early 1980s and now number approximately 23 (Cornet, 2002; McClelland, 1985; Terrell, 1984). Various names (*joint, concurrent, dual, combined*) have been given to the programs, but there is no consistency in meaning. The length of time for students to complete the programs ranges from $2\frac{1}{2}$ to $3\frac{1}{2}$ years. Some have simultaneous admissions, while others have sequential admissions. Some are separate and coordinated; others are fully integrated.

In recognition of the need for social workers to be able to function effectively in both the health and social work arenas, many schools and departments of social work have added specializations or concentrations in health. As early as 1982, 44 (51%) of the 87 master of social work programs in the country had health specializations (Coulter & Hancock, 1989). At about this time, the first joint master of social work/master of public health degree programs began. Most of the programs were (and still are) closely associated with MCH (Cornet, 2002), in spite of the fact that there was broad acceptance that public health social workers functioned in a wide range of fields, such as family violence, adolescent problems, divorced women, young children in day care, geriatrics, homelessness, malnourishment, farm families, communicable disease control, and environmental concerns.

FUTURE/KEY ISSUES

Public health social workers face a number of issues and challenges. These can roughly be divided into issues of need in the community and issues of professional development.

Community Need

Health care issues, including health reform, have become current political concerns. One of the challenges for all public health practitioners is to shape the public health debate to recognize both the importance of public health and its focus on wellness, rather than on pathology. In the United States, we as public health social workers must do a better job of presenting a strong case for preventative care on local, state, and federal levels.

Another area for intervention is the education of other public health disciplines (e.g., public health nursing and health education) as to the significant and unique contributions that public health social workers can make to everyone's understanding of social and behavioral health issues that affect and motivate the individual client, family, or community to grow and change. Another related intervention is the education of our own discipline (i.e., social work) about the impact that public health core functions can have in adequately serving those clients who are part of our traditional mandate (Ruth & Sisco, 2008). Embracing public health social work principles may be the way of returning social work to a prominent position in the discussions on health and community development (Stoesz, 2002).

Professional Development

All professional social workers have an obligation to remain current in their knowledge and practice. As a consequence, public health social workers must continue to engage in professional development. Their participation can be as a learner or a presenter. As public health social workers, we possess many skills and talents that help to alleviate the pain and suffering the many individuals we work with endure.

In our work, we should informally refer to ourselves as "public health social workers." The challenge is that the meaning of "public health social worker" is somewhat oblique. A practitioner is more likely to be identified as a "community planner" or "program manager" or by whatever one's job function is. This is particularly challenging in light of the ideal of transdisciplinary practice described earlier.

Another aspect of professional identification is organizational. Although there are certain affiliations specifically for public health social workers (Social Work section of the APHA, Association of State and Territorial Public Health Social Workers), most social workers tend to identify with the professional organization that reflects their work focus. For example, social workers in APHA who work in the area of MCH are more likely to affiliate with the MCH section. Within the formal social work associations (e.g., NASW and the Council on Social Work Education), the focus of social workers interested in health is social work in health—not public health. This invisibility of public health social work in professional organizations is a major issue that we need to address (Bracht, 2000). A stronger identification with public health social work organizations is paramount if we are to have a stronger influence at the policy and program levels. However, it is not clear which comes first: more visibility or more influence.

A somewhat different, although related issue for both social work and public health social work is recruiting and retaining practitioners (Blosser, Cadet, & Downs, 2010). This issue has several different aspects. The social work perspective values the full participation and inclusion of the range of communities being served. The profession needs to reflect the increasing diversity of the population and communities. Thus, current practitioners must work with the academic institutions to identify and value the unique understanding and perspectives that these (often underserved) communities bring to the assurance of the public's health. This will also aid in the development of new and emerging professionals to fill the void left by many retiring practitioners and for a succession of planning for agency executives.

CLASSROOM EXERCISES

For this assignment, you are to assume the role of student representative to your social work program. The social work program director has been informed by the community's public health agencies that there is a shortage of public health social workers. To address this problem, you and three faculty members are charged with reviewing the courses currently offered in your social work program and to make recommendations on how to include content in the five key areas (epidemiology, biostatistics, health and social behavior, environmental health, and policy).

To complete this project, you must first review the course syllabi in the four curriculum areas (human behavior and social environment, policy, social work practice, and research) in your social work program. Second, do a literature search on one the five content areas (e.g., epidemiology) for one course in each curriculum area. Third, come up with two peer-reviewed journal articles in each curriculum area. Fourth, write an annotated bibliography for each of the articles to present to the program director.

INTERNET RESOURCES

1. Public Health Social Work

(http://publichealthsocialwork.org/)

2. *US News and World Report*: Best Careers 2011: Medical and Public Health Social Worker

(http://money.usnews.com/money/careers/articles/2010/12/06/best-careers-2011-medical-and-public-health-social-worker)

3. How to Become a Social Worker: Public Health Social Worker Requirements

(www.howtobecomeasocialworker.net/Public-Health-Social-Worker-Requirements.html)

4. U.S. Bureau of Labor Statistics: Occupational Employment and Wages, May 2010, Health Care Social Workers

(www.bls.gov/oes/current/oes211022.htm)

REFERENCES

Aronoff, N. (2008). Interprofessional & partnered practice. In *Encyclopedia of social work* (Vol. 2, pp. 533–536). Washington, DC: National Association of Social Workers.

Blosser, J., Cadet, D., & Downs, L. (2010). Factors that influence retention and professional development of social workers. *Administration in Social Work*, *34*(2), 168–177.

Bracht, N. F. (2000). Prevention: Additional thoughts. *Social Work in Health Care*, *30*(4), 1–6.

Carlton, T. (1988). The public's health. *Health and Social Work*, *13*, 242–244.

Cornet, B. (2002). *Public health social work programs.* Unpublished report, University of California at Berkeley.

Coulter, M. L., & Hancock, T. (1989). Integrating social work and public health education: A clinical model. *Health and Social Work*, *14*(3), 157–164.

Evans, J. (1985). Mission. In A. Gitterman, R. B. Black, & F. Stein (Eds.), *Public health social work in maternal and child health: A forward plan* (pp. 13–16). Washington, DC: Division of Maternal and Child Health.

Gehlert, S., & Browne, T. A. (2006). *Handbook of health social work*. Hoboken, NJ: John Wiley & Sons, Inc.

Hutchins, V. L. (1994). Maternal and child health bureau. *Pediatrics*, *94*, 695–699.

Insley, V. (1977). Health services: Maternal and child health. In *Encyclopedia of social work* (Vol. 1, pp. 552–560). Washington, DC: National Association of Social Work.

Kerson, T. S. (1989). *Social work in health settings: Practice in context*. Binghamton, NY: Haworth Press.

Leukefeld, C. G. (1989). Social workers celebrate the centennial of the U.S. Public Health Service. *Health and Social Work*, *14*(3), 153.

McClelland, R. (1985). Joint degrees: Do they strengthen or weaken the profession? *REFJ of Social Work Education*, *21*(1), 20–26.

Moxley, D. (2008). Interdisciplinarity. In *Encyclopedia of Social Work* (Vol. 2, pp. 468–472). Washington, DC: National Association of Social Workers.

National Association of Social Workers. (2005). *Social work imperatives for the next decade*. Retrieved February 28, 2011, from www.nasw.org

National Association of Social Workers (2006). Center for Workforce Studies. Retrieved February 28, 2011 from www.nasw.org.

National Association of Social Workers (2007). NASW News 52:2, February 2007. Retrieved February 28, 2011.

National Association of Social Workers. (2008). *Code of ethics—Revised 2008*. Retrieved February 28, 2011, from www.nasw.org

Rounds, K. (Ed.). (2005). *Public health social work standards and competencies*. School of Social Work, University of North Carolina.

Ruth, B., Geron, S. M., & Chiasson, E. (2002). *Dual degree programs in public health and social work: comparing graduates*, Paper presented at the 130th Annual Meeting of the American Public Health Association.

Ruth, B., & Sisco, S. (2008). Public health. In *Encyclopedia of Social Work*, (Vol. 3, pp. 476–483). Washington, DC: National Association of Social Work.

Stoesz, D. (2002). From social work to human services. *Journal of Sociology and Social Welfare*, *29*(4), 19–37.

Terrell, P. (1984). The MSW/MPH Dual Degree Program. Unpublished report, MSW/MPH Dual Degree Program, University of California, Berkeley.

Turnock, B. J. (2004). *Public health: What it is and how it works*. Sudbury, MA: Jones & Bartlett Publishers.

Turnock, B. J. (2006). *Public health: Career choices that make a difference*. Sudbury, MA: Jones & Bartlett Publishers.

U.S. Department of Health and Human Services. (2010). *Healthy People 2020*. Retrieved February 28, 2001, from www.HealthyPeople.gov

U.S. Department of Health and Human Services. (2011). *Loan forgiveness programs for social workers*. Retrieved February 28, 2011 from www.hhs.gov

U.S. Health Resources and Services Administration. (2011). *Loan repayment*. Retrieved from http://nhsc.hrsa.gov/loanreparyment/

Watkins, E. L. (1985). The conceptual base for public health social work. In A. Gitterman, R. B. Black, & F. Stein (Eds.), *Public health social work in maternal and child health: A forward plan.* (pp. 17–34). Washington, DC: Division of Maternal and Child Health.

Weismiller, T., & Whitaker, T. (2008). Social work profession: Workforce. In *Encyclopedia of Social Work* (Vol. 4, pp. 164–168). Washington, DC: National Association of Social Workers.

Wilkinson, D. S., Copeland, V. C., & Rounds, K. A. (2000). *Dual or joint MSW/MPH programs—Collaborating to improve our offerings.* Paper presented at 128th Annual Meeting, American Public Health Association, Boston, MA.

CHAPTER 20

Emerging Issues and Conclusion

Abigail M. Ross, Betty J. Ruth, Robert H. Keefe, and Derek R. Smith

INTRODUCTION

This book has focused on many key issues in the field of public health social work. Several of these issues have been of concern for years (e.g., negative maternal and child health outcomes, substance abuse, and mental illness), and others have emerged more recently (e.g., the increasing rates of HIV infections in communities of color and the ethical issues surrounding genetic testing), while still others, although long standing, have become more pressing due to recent media and public attention (e.g., the spread of disease due to increased globalization and the increase in natural or human-made disasters). Newer issues that require our attention include the intersection of aging, disability, and chronic disease; the ever-burgeoning uninsured and underinsured population in the United States; and the health needs of recent immigrants, refugees, and their families.

The purpose of this book was to provide an overview of the various public health issues that public health social workers must attend to. Consequently, other important issues, such as the alarming rates of childhood obesity, tobacco use, and ongoing environmental degradation, were not included. Given the protracted nature of the "great recession," the legal challenges to the Patient Protection and Affordable Care Act (PPACA), and the explosive political climate as it relates to health care, it is likely that by the time this book appears in print other health concerns will have surfaced.

THE EMERGING CONTEXT OF THE NATION'S PUBLIC HEALTH

The health status of Americans continues to be an issue for health care professionals nationwide. Despite the fact that the United States is spending more than any other country on health care services, Americans do not appear to be living healthier lives. Recent financial projections indicate that by the year 2020 the United States will commit one-fifth of its gross domestic product to health care (Truffer et al., 2010). It is highly unlikely, however, that this spending will result in positive health outcomes for many Americans.

Taking into account some specific health indicators, data show that the United States now ranks 50th in life expectancy and 49th in infant mortality among 193 nations (CIA World Factbook, 2012 a,b). Other *social determinants of health* (SDOH), a term that refers to the broad environments in which people grow, live, and work (including race, class, gender, immigration status, sexual orientation, and disability), continue to influence health outcomes (Satcher & Higginbotham, 2008; Voelker, 2008).

Among the most serious systemic factors influencing health outcomes is the lack of health insurance and under insurance of many Americans, a problem fueled by a lackluster economy and the slow, fragile trajectory of health insurance reform. Evidence linking inadequate health insurance coverage with poorer health outcomes, including increased risk of mortality (Hadley, 2006; Institute of Medicine, 2009), particularly for people of color who are likewise much less likely to have access to ongoing health care from service providers than their White counterparts (Keefe, 2010), continues to mount.

PUBLIC HEALTH SOCIAL WORK PREPARATION

The U.S. health care system employs the majority of the nation's 500,000 social workers (Marshall, Ruth, Sisco, Cohen, & Bachman, 2011). Public health social workers must be able to negotiate the challenging terrain of physical health, mental health, and substance abuse services housed within a fragmented system that seeks to provide disease treatment over prevention, fails to contain escalating costs, and is unable to meet the needs of a significant segment of the population (Schroeder, 2007).

Given its focus on prevention, public health social workers may be the professionals most well suited to respond to ongoing health crises (Ruth & Sisco, 2008). Various studies have reported growing support for the integration of public health practice skills and competencies into the social work profession (Ruth, Ross, Marshall, & Hill, 2011; Vourlekis, Ell, & Padgett, 2001). Within the past 15 years, a working definition, as well as standards and competencies for public health social work, has been developed. In its practice standards, the National Association of Social Workers has identified prevention, health promotion, and health education as core competencies for social work practitioners in health care settings (Association of State and Territorial Public Health Social Workers, 2005; National Association of Social Workers, 2005). Likewise, the 2008 Education Program Accreditation

Standards of the Council on Social Work Education now requires that schools of social work educate master of social work (MSW) students on prevention principles, knowledge, and skills (McCave & Richel, 2011). A content analysis of nine professional social work journals revealed a doubling in the number of prevention-focused articles published between 2000 and 2008, reflecting an increased interest in research on health care (Ruth & Hill, 2010). Moreover, the proliferation of joint MSW/master of public health (MPH) programs signals interest from the next generation in transdisciplinary education in public health social work as an important pathway to an integrated skill set focused on both prevention and intervention (Ruth, Wyatt, Chiasson, Geron, & Bachman, 2006).

Simultaneously, a number of opportunities are emerging that can enhance public health social work's relevance in the health and social service sector now and well into the future.

Increased Use of Public Health Models and Approaches

The Obama Administration's newly created Prevention and Public Health Fund and National Prevention Council provides a national strategy and much-needed funding for prevention (Fielding, Teutsch, & Koh, 2012). The U.S. Department of Health and Human Services' document, *Healthy People 2020*, the nation's decennial blueprint for measuring health and well-being, was recently updated and released. This influential document emphasizes ecological and person-in-environment approaches, addresses health equity and SDOH, and focuses on community-based empowerment and culturally responsive approaches (www.healthcare.gov/prevention/nphpphc/index.html).

Both of these recent initiatives prioritize the integration of medical public health and social service approaches, use ecological language and frameworks familiar to social workers, and emphasize social justice (Braveman, Kuminyaka, & Fielding, 2011).

Integrated Health Models and Health Legislation

A significant body of research suggests that integrating and coordinating mental health and substance abuse treatment with primary care increases quality health care and improves patient outcomes, particularly in vulnerable populations or for persons living with comorbid conditions (Center for Integrated Health Services, www.integration.samhsa.gov/integrated-care-models 2011). The PPACA emphasizes developing more public health–oriented, transdisciplinary, and integrated health systems and has spurred movement toward organizing care into medical home models and using care management to coordinate ongoing care (Northridge, Glick, Metcalf, & Shelley, 2011).

Enhanced Opportunities in Community Practice

Moving public health services out of institutions and into communities provides public health social workers with expanded opportunities for practice, including engaging in community-based participatory research, emergency/disaster preparedness planning, community and neighborhood development, and primary-prevention endeavors. Each of these efforts intersect with various overarching public health initiatives outlined in *Healthy People 2020* (Davis, Cook, & Cohen, 2005; Gibson, Theodore, & Jellison, 2012).

Public Health Social Work Education

Schools and departments of social work can play an important role in promoting public health social work by integrating public health approaches throughout their curricula. This can be done by directing MSW curricula away from treatment and intervention and toward prevention strategies (McCave & Rishel, 2011). Schools and departments that have dual MSW/MPH degree programs can provide faculty with opportunities to infuse their courses of study with public health course content and provide students with scholarships and integrative activities, such as service-learning projects, that promote collaboration with other public health professionals. Schools and departments that do not have dual degree programs can infuse prevention, social epidemiology, and public health approaches into course readings and encourage "public health social work working groups" or postgraduate public health social work professional education opportunities (Ruth et al., 2011) as ways to infuse public health content into professional practice. Doctoral programs can include courses in social epidemiology and encourage students to undertake dissertations that focus on public health issues.

Public Health Social Work Practice in Agencies

Health care organizations, programs, and practitioners can use the public health model in their day-to-day operations. Examples include (1) agencies identifying issues they want to effect or prevent, and begin collecting data on those issues; (2) agencies familiarizing themselves with public health terminology and practice by framing their work in the language of social epidemiology, resilience, risk, health equity, prevention, disparities, and SDOH; (3) agencies updating old and developing new programs based on a public health social work approach; (4) MSW interns being provided with "public health" assignments in their agencies, where by they conduct program and practice evaluations and suggest ways to implement public health approaches; (5) agency administrators seeking out opportunities for academic/community partnerships, particularly with schools that have MSW/MPH programs; (6) agencies familiarizing themselves with the many uses of social epidemiology, and strengthening their program evaluation and outcomes-based research capacities; (7) employers recruiting and hiring MSW/MPH graduates for various positions within their organizations; and (8) practitioner groups starting working groups or journal groups to educate themselves on public health social work approaches.

Professional Organizations

Social work organizations are numerous, and their goals can sometimes appear disparate (Skwiot, 2007). With the integration of health, behavioral health, and substance abuse services within public health, most social workers will soon be employed in settings informed and shaped by public health goals. Consequently, professional organizations will need to continue addressing a coordinated presence and a deeper understanding of the roles of public health social workers within the public health infrastructure and explain the added value of public health social work. All social work organizations that address public health, especially the National Association of Social Workers, the American Public Health Association, and the Council on Social Work Education should form a coordinated national public health social work task force to identify and shape the future of social work's roles in these settings.

SUMMARY

Given this time of economic uncertainty, it is difficult to overstate the ethical, financial, and practical urgency associated with the need for changes in the current health care system. The legal challenges surrounding the adoption of the PPACA make its future unclear. Despite the uncertainty regarding this landmark health care reform legislation, the field of public health social work must continue to grow and develop and increase its visibility by attending to new opportunities that widen its impact and broaden its base. As these health systems change, public health social workers are well equipped to ensure that programs and services support the people they are designed to assist. Public health social work professionals must continue to evolve as professionals and take on the important role of a bridge between disciplines that have not traditionally worked together in a seamless fashion.

Dr. George Albee, a renowned psychologist and trailblazing scholar who argued in favor of the use of primary prevention in the helping professions, observed that humankind's greatest diseases and disorders were eliminated or brought under control not by exclusive focus on the individual, but on population-based approaches and prevention strategies as well (Albee & Gullotta, 1997). His words echo throughout these pages as the authors illustrate the many facets and applications of public health social work. With its timely emphasis on prevention and intervention, the future of public health social work is a bright one. We hope that this book will be part of an inspired conversation about the future of this important discipline.

REFERENCES

Albee, G., & Gullotta, T. (1997). *Primary prevention works*. Thousand Oaks, CA: Sage Publications, Inc.

Association of State and Territorial Public Health Social Workers. (2005). *Public health social work standard and competencies*. Retrieved from http://oce.sph.unc.edu/cetac/phswcompetencies_may05.pdf

Braveman, P. A., Kumanyika, S., Fielding, J., LaVeist, T., Borrell, L. N., Manderscheid, R., & Troutman, A. (2011). Health disparities and health equity: The issue is justice. *American Journal of Public Health*, *101*(Suppl 1), S149-155.

CIA—The World Factbook. (n.d.-a). *Country comparison: Infant mortality rate*. Retrieved June 1, 2012, from, https://www.cia.gov/library/publications/the-world-factbook/rankorder/2091rank.html

CIA—The World Factbook. (n.d.-b). *Country comparison: Life expectancy at birth*. Retrieved June 1, 2012, from, https://www.cia.gov/library/publications/the-world-factbook/rankorder/2102rank.html

Davis, R., Cook, D., & Cohen, L. (2005). A community resilience approach to reducing ethnic and racial disparities in health. *American Journal of Public Health*, *95*(12), 2168-2173. doi:10.2105/AJPH.2004.050146

Fielding, J. E., Teutsch, S., & Koh, H. (2012). Health reform and the Healthy People initiative. *American Journal of Public Health*, *102*(1), 30-33. doi:10.2105/AJPH.2011.300312

Gibson, P. J., Theodore, F., & Jellison, J. B. (2012). The common ground preparedness framework: A comprehensive description of public health emergency preparedness. *American Journal of Public Health*, *102*(4), 633-642. doi:10.2105/AJPH.2011.300546

Hadley, J. (2006). *Consequences of the lack of health insurance on health and earnings*. Urban Institute. Retrieved July 3, 2008, from http://www.urban.org/url.cfm?ID=1001001

Institute of Medicine. (2009). *America's uninsured crisis: Consequences for health and health care*. Washington, DC: National Academies Press. Retrieved June 1, 2012, from www.rwjf.org/files/research/20090224iomamericasuninsuredcrisis.pdf

Keefe, R. H. (2010). Health disparities: A primer for public health social workers. *Social Work in Public Health*, *25*(3/4), 237-257.

Marshall, J., Ruth, B. J., Sisco, S., Cohen, M., & Bachman, S. (2011). Social work interest in prevention: A content analysis of the professional literature. *Social Work, 56*(3), 201-211. doi:10.1093/sw/56.3.201

McCave, E. L., & Rishel, C. W. (2011). Prevention as an explicit part of the social work profession: A systematic investigation. *Advances in Social Work, 12*(2), 226-240. Retrieved from http://journals.iupui.edu/index.php/advancesinsocialwork/article/view/1444/1874

National Association of Social Workers. (2005). *NASW standards for social work practice in health care settings.* Retrieved January 11, 2007, from http://www.socialworkers.org/research/naswResearch/PublicHealth/default.asp

Northridge, M. E., Glick, M., Metcalf, S. S., & Shelley, D. (2011). Public health support for the health home model. *American Journal of Public Health, 101*(10), 1818-1820.

Ruth, B. J., & Hill, E. (2010). Social Work Interest in Prevention: Findings from an Ongoing Content Analysis. Paper presented at the 56th Annual Program Meeting of the Council on Social Work Education. Portland, OR.

Ruth, B. J., Ross, A., Marshall, J. W., & Hill, E. (2011). *Public health social work in the 21st century: Overview and examples from the field.* Society for Social Work Leadership in Health Care annual meeting, San Francisco, CA. Retrieved from http://www.ncbi.nlm.nih.gov/pmc/articles/PMC2431100/

Ruth, B. J., & Sisco, S. (2008). Public health social work. In T. Mizrahi & L. Davis (Eds.), *Encyclopedia of social work* (20th ed.). Washington, DC: National Association of Social Workers.

Ruth, B. J., Wyatt, J., Chiasson, E., Geron, S., & Bachman, S. (2006). Social work and public health: Comparing graduates from a dual-degree program. *Journal of Social Work Education, 42*(2), 429-439.

Satcher, D., & Higginbotham, E. J. (2008). The public health approach to eliminating disparities in health. *American Journal of Public Health, 98*(3), 400-403. doi:10.2105/AJPH.2007.123919

Schroeder, S. A. (2007). We can do better—Improving the health of the American people. *The New England Journal of Medicine, 357*(12), 1221-1228. Retrieved from http://www.nejm.org.ezproxy.bu.edu/doi/full/10.1056/NEJMsa073350

Skwiot, R. (2007). Scattered images: Perspectives on social work's identity challenge. *Social Impact Magazine,* 15-21. Retrieved from http://gwbweb.wustl.edu/Pages/SocialImpactFall2007.aspx

Substance Abuse and Mental Health Services Administration—Health Resources and Services Administration. (n.d.). Integrated care models. Retrieved June 1, 2012, from, http://www.integration.samhsa.gov/integrated-care-models

Truffer, C. J., Keehan, S., Smith, S., Cylus, J., Sisko, A., Poisal, J. A., et al. (2010). Health spending projections through 2019: The recession's impact continues. *Health Affairs, 29*(3), 522-529. doi:10.1377/hlthaff.2009.1074

Voelker, R. (2008). Decades of work to reduce disparities in health care produce limited success. *Journal of the American Medical Association, 299*(12), 1411-1413. doi:10.1001/jama.299.12.1411

Vourlekis, B. S., Ell, K., & Padgett, D. (2001). Educating social workers for health care's brave new world. *Journal of Social Work Education, 37*(1), 177-191. Retrieved from http://www.mendeley.com/research/educating-social-workers-health-care-s-brave-new-world/

Public Health Social Workers: Core Competencies

A. **Theoretical Base:**

Public health social workers will demonstrate knowledge and adhere to:

1. The principles of social epidemiology.
2. The principles and theories of population-based health promotion and empowerment.
3. The normal patterns of individual and family growth and development from an intergenerational and life span perspective.
4. The impact of economic, environmental, and social issues for at-risk populations.
5. The impact of protective or risk factors, for example, gender, racism, ageism, classism, sexual orientation, sexual identity, disability or religious belief, on the health and well-being of individuals, families, and communities.
6. The theories and principles of community organization, planned changed, and development.
7. The characteristics of health systems, including the dimensions of, use of, and access to health care.
8. Macro-level public health social work practice methods in the promotion and enforcement of regulations (policies and legislation) formulated to protect the health and safety of at-risk populations.

Public health social workers should demonstrate the following skills:

9. Application of macro-level public health social work methods, for example, social planning, community organization/development, and social marketing.
10. Use of demographic data.

Source: Public health social work practice project at the UNC School of Social Work. (2005). *Public health social work standards and competencies*. Columbus, OH: Ohio Department of Health. Available at http://oce.sph.unc.edu/cetac/phswcompetencies_ May05.pdf. Retrieved March 5, 2012.

11. Critical analyses of inequities in health status based on race/ethnicity, socioeconomic position, and gender.
12. Recognition of various strengths, needs, values, and practices of diverse cultural, racial, ethnic, and socioeconomic groups to determine how these factors affect health status, health behaviors, and program design.
13. Application of primary, secondary, and tertiary strategies to address the health, social, and economic issues of individuals, families, and communities.
14. Use of practice and epidemiologic theories to substantiate interventions and programming designed to promote health and behavioral change.

B. **Methodological and Analytical Process**
   Public health social workers will demonstrate knowledge and understanding of:
   1. Research design, sampling, basic descriptive and inferential statistics, and validity/reliability assessment of measures.
   2. Epidemiological/socioepidemiological concepts.
   3. The use of data to illuminate ethical, political, scientific, economic, social, and overall public health issues.
   4. Principles and key features of community needs assessment, program design, implementation, and evaluation.
   Public health social workers should demonstrate the following skills:
   5. Collection and interpretation of data from vital statistics, censuses, surveys, service utilization, and other relevant reports on social and health status for all, especially vulnerable and underserved populations.
   6. Detection of meaningful inferences from data and translation of data into information for community assessment (gaps, barriers, and strengths analysis), program planning, implementation, and evaluation.
   7. Formulation of hypotheses or research questions, in collaboration with internal or external resources, for the development and implementation of an analytical strategy to influence health and social planned change.

C. **Leadership and Communication**
   Public health social workers will demonstrate knowledge and understanding of:
   1. Organizational culture and change.
   2. Leadership and communication practices for diverse internal and external groups.
   3. Networking inter-multidisciplinary team building and group processes.

4. Social work community organization and coalition building to address the issues of social and health disparities.
5. Strategies for soliciting and maintaining consumer and other constituencies involved at all levels of an organization.
6. Strategic planning, organizational development, performance outcome measures, and program evaluation activities.

Public health social workers should demonstrate the following skills:

7. Articulate a vision and motivate staff to actualize the mission, goals, and objectives of their organization (public health).
8. Commit to individuals, families, and communities and the diverse cultural values they hold.
9. Operationalize best-practice prevention and intervention strategies to eliminate social inequity and health disparities.
10. Build on the strengths and assets of individuals, families, and communities to develop and apply innovative and creative solutions to social and health issues.
11. Apply management and organizational theories and practices to the development, planning, budgeting, staffing, administration, and evaluation of public health programs including the implementation of strategies promoting integrated service systems, especially for vulnerable populations.
12. Develop mechanisms to monitor and evaluate programs and service networks for their effectiveness and quality, including the use of performance and outcome measures.
13. Develop, implement, monitor, and evaluate grant-funded programs.
14. Develop written and oral communications skills, including accurate and effective preparation and presentation of reports to stakeholders, for example, agency boards, administrative organizations, policymakers, consumers, and/or the media using demographic, statistical, programmatic, and scientific information.
15. Communicate effectively with diverse and multicultural organizations community/consumer boards and coalitions.
16. Develop strategies to assure integrated service systems for populations at risk for health and social issues.

D. **Policy and Advocacy**

Public health social workers will demonstrate knowledge and understanding of:

1. Federal and state mandates that guide the funding and implementation of health and social services programs.
2. Synthesizing of contemporary and alternative health and social policies.

3. Legislative, administrative, and judicial processes at the national, state, and local levels.
4. The historical development and scientific basis of public health and social policies and practices for federal, state, and local agencies.

Public health social workers should demonstrate the following skills:

5. Applying critical thinking to every stage of policy development and practice.
6. Identifying essential gaps in the delivery system of health and social services.
7. Identifying public health laws, regulations, and policies related to specific programs.
8. Collecting and summarizing data relevant to a particular policy/problem.
9. Coalition building and agenda setting to address the gaps in the system of social welfare and health care.
10. Stating the feasibility and expected outcomes of and barriers to achieving each policy option and deciding on the appropriate course of action.
11. Clearly writing concise policy statements, position papers, and/or testimonies appropriate for a specific audience.
12. Implementing a program plan, including goals, outcomes, and process objectives.

E. **Values and Ethics**

Public health social workers will demonstrate knowledge and understanding of:

1. Philosophy, values, and social justice concepts associated with public health and social work practices.
2. The National Association of Social Work's Code of Ethics and the American Public Health Association Creed.
3. The philosophical concepts and rationale underlying the delivery of family-centered, comprehensive, integrated, community-based, and culturally competent public health and social services and programs, including the recognition of family and community assets.
4. Principles and issues involved in the ethical and sensitive conduct of practice and research for all, especially with vulnerable and underserved populations.
5. Ethical issues in the organization and delivery of public health services within communities and governmental agencies including the collection of data and their management analysis and dissemination.
6. State licensure and/or regulations.

Public health social workers should demonstrate the following skills:

7. Integration of professional values and principles of ethics within community and organizational practice settings.
8. Ethical conduct in program management, research, and data collection and storage.
9. Cultural competence within public health settings.
10. Partnerships with public health and social services communities and constituencies to foster community empowerment, reciprocal learning and involvement in design, implementation, and research aspects of public health and social systems.
11. Utilization of social work standards and principles in the resolution of ethical dilemmas.

The Three Core Public Health Functions and the Essential Public Health Services

Assessment

- ☐ Monitor health status to identify community health problems
- ☐ Diagnose and investigate health problems and health hazards in the community
- ☐ Evaluate effectiveness, accessibility, and quality of personal and population-based health services

Policy Development

- ☐ Develop policies and plans that support individual and community health efforts
- ☐ Enforce laws and regulations that protect health and ensure safety
- ☐ Conduct research to discover new insights and innovative solutions to health problems

Assurance

- ☐ Link people to needed personal health services and assure the provision of health care when otherwise unavailable
- ☐ Assure a competent public health and personal health care workforce
- ☐ Inform, educate, and empower people about health issues
- ☐ Mobilize community partnerships to identify and solve health problems

Essential Service: Monitor health status to identify and solve community health problems

Activities by state and/or local public health agencies

- ☐ Determine and monitor water quality
- ☐ Monitor water wells

Source: Institute of Medicine. (1988). *The Future of Public Health*. Washington, DC: National Academies Press..

- ☐ Monitor wastewater treatment and disposal
- ☐ Identification of water-quality problems
- ☐ Mosquito surveillance
- ☐ Immunizations
- ☐ Sexually transmitted disease/HIV testing and counseling
- ☐ Food-borne illness investigations
- ☐ Bio emergency preparation and coordination
- ☐ Tracking numbers of wells, including abandoned wells
- ☐ Screening for diabetes
- ☐ Conducting needs assessment
- ☐ Collection of child oral health data
- ☐ Child lead-poisoning surveillance

Essential service: Diagnose and investigate health problems and health hazards in the community

Core activities undertaken by state and/or local public health agencies

- ☐ Medical examiners
- ☐ Epidemiology
- ☐ Tuberculosis
- ☐ HIV/AIDS
- ☐ Investigation and evaluation of nuisance complaints
- ☐ Wellhead assessments and site evaluations

Essential Service: Inform, educate and empower people about health issues

Activities by state and/or local public health agencies

- ☐ Community health education and health promotion
- ☐ Public health education through the media, presentations, the Internet, displays, etc.
- ☐ HIV/AIDS risk reduction curriculum
- ☐ Child abuse education
- ☐ Domestic violence education
- ☐ WIC educational programs
- ☐ Informing and educating parties involved in nuisance investigations
- ☐ Public education about well construction

Essential Service: Mobilize community partnerships and action to identify and solve health problems

Activities by state and/or local public health agencies

☐ Forming tobacco-free coalitions
☐ Bio emergency regional collaboration
☐ Collaborative efforts with private industry to combat domestic violence
☐ Community partnerships with law enforcement, county attorneys, community betterment groups, housing authorities
☐ Referrals and collaboration with health-care providers
☐ Collaboration with WIC, public health nursing, and special-population advocates to meet the needs of special populations

Essential service: Develop policies and plans that support individual and community health efforts

Activities by state and/or local public health agencies

☐ State board of health oversight and regulatory functions
☐ Local board of health oversight and regulatory functions
☐ Public hearings
☐ Administration of state and local public health departments
☐ Monitoring of contractors/providers
☐ Community health planning
☐ Strategic and performance planning
☐ Development of a plan to address housing needs
☐ Updating of health and nuisance ordinances
☐ Development of policies on investigations, police assistance, and trespass and safety issues
☐ Board of health adoption of rules that require better management of water systems in small, rural subdivisions
☐ Determination of need for community water supplies
☐ Development of variance procedures
☐ Establishment of procedures for water well permits
☐ Establishment of civil citation authority
☐ Establishment of procedures to deal with contaminated or high risk sites
☐ Establishment of financial assistance for well sampling, plugging, or rehabilitation

Essential service: Enforce laws and regulations that protect health and ensure safety

Activities by state and/or local public health agencies

☐ Hazardous materials and sites inspections and certifications
☐ Milk inspections
☐ Professional licensure and regulation
☐ Food inspections
☐ Tanning and tattoo parlor inspections
☐ Enforcement of state/county/local health-related rules and ordinances

Essential service: Link people to needed personal health services and assure the provision of health care when otherwise unavailable

Core activities undertaken by state and/or local public health agencies

☐ Establish tuberculosis programs
☐ Public health nursing services
☐ Breast and cervical cancer early detection program
☐ Maternal and child health
☐ WIC
☐ Critical access hospitals
☐ Linkages to regional landfills for disposal options
☐ Informing the public on useful nuisance-abatement web sites

Essential Service: Assure a competent public and personal health-care work force

Core activities undertaken by state and/or local public health agencies

☐ Food service worker safety certification course
☐ Public health certification
☐ Learning management system
☐ Regional bio emergency meetings
☐ Public health practitioner performance evaluations
☐ Sanitation, water contractor training
☐ Certification of environmental health professionals

Essential service: Evaluate effectiveness, accessibility, and quality of personal and population-based health services

Activities by state and/or local public health agencies

- ☐ Data management
- ☐ Performance-plan monitoring
- ☐ Public health contract requirements
- ☐ Health needs assessments
- ☐ Tracking responses to complaints
- ☐ Permit issuance for nuisances
- ☐ Ensuring that wells are drilled by certified people
- ☐ Sealing unused, unsafe wells

Essential service: Research new insights and innovative solutions to health problems

Activities by state and/or local public health agencies

- ☐ Health needs assessments
- ☐ Bio-emergency survey participation
- ☐ Lighten Up survey participation
- ☐ Customer service evaluations
- ☐ Promotion of recycling and composting
- ☐ Study of successful public health programs in other jurisdictions
- ☐ Research on water treatment methods

Index